Vision

Vision

Pierre Buser and Michel Imbert

Translated by R. H. Kay

A Bradford Book
The MIT Press
Cambridge, Massachusetts
London, England

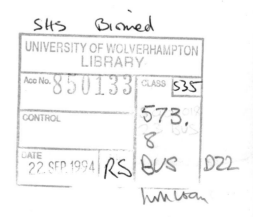

This book was set in Palatino and Univers by Achorn Graphic Services
and was printed and bound in the United States of America.

Library of Congress Cataloging-in-Publication Data

Buser, Pierre A.
  [Vision. English]
  Vision / Pierre Buser, Michel Imbert; (translated by R. H. Kay).
    p.   cm.
  Translation of: Vision.
  "A Bradford Book."
  Includes bibliographical references and index.
  ISBN 0-262-02336-9
  1. Vision. I. Imbert, Michel, 1935–   . II. Title.
  [DNLM: 1. Retina—physiology. 2. Vision—physiology.   WW 103
[B977v]
QP475.B8413   1992
599'.01823—dc20
DNLM/DLC
for Library of Congress   91-32473
                                                                   CIP

Contents

Appendix

Preface

There are five chapters in this textbook on vision. The first concerns vertebrate retinal morphology. The second reviews the principal physical characteristics of light stimuli and their classic measurement in terms of photometric and colorimetric units. The third is dedicated to discussion of some of the psychophysical laws governing visual sensations, notably absolute thresholds, retinal adaptation, visual acuity, temporal resolution, movement perception, color vision, and stereopsis. The fourth chapter examines receptor and intraretinal neuronal network functions, including retinal photochemistry, the electroretinogram, transduction mechanisms and retinal coding of the visual stimulus. The fifth and final chapter treats neural processing in the more central projection pathways and notably in the medial geniculate, the superior colliculus, and the cortical visual areas themselves.

As in the companion volume on audition, this book is written at the level of upper-level undergraduate and graduate students. It emphasizes mammalian studies, except for those areas where studies in lower vertebrates provide models that are essential for understanding some of the mammalian retinal mechanisms.

We wish to thank Dr. R. H. Kay, who is responsible for translating the French texts. We also thank the publishers and authors who have allowed the use of some of their material.

P. B., M. I.

TRANSLATOR'S NOTE

The authors and I agreed that a translation into current English language scientific usage would be better than a literal word-for-word transform. Liaison across the Channel with Dr. Buser and across the Atlantic with MIT Press editors Fiona Stevens and Katherine Arnoldi has been very friendly.

R. H. K.

Pierre Buser, Professor of the Université Pierre et Marie Curie, Paris, France, was born in 1921. His major research is concerned with sensorimotor integrative mechanisms of the central nervous system.

Michel Imbert, Professor of the Université Pierre et Marie Curie, Paris, France, was born in 1935. His major research is concerned with the neurophysiology of development in the visual nervous system.

R. H. Kay, Emeritus Fellow of Keble College, Oxford, England, was born in 1921. His major research is in sensory mechanisms, particularly of human hearing.

Vision

Structure and Organization of the Retina

The arrangement of the mammalian visual system can be summarized in the following way: Axons of the retinal ganglion cells leave the eye via the *optic nerve*. Each optic nerve decussates at the *optic chiasm*, with half its nerve fibers going ipsilaterally and the other half contralaterally. The optic tracts leaving the chiasm terminate in the corresponding thalamic relay, the *lateral geniculate body* (LGB) in its dorsal region, *pars dorsalis*. From here the optic radiations project to the corresponding *visual cortex*.

In contrast, other ganglion cell axons (or collaterals of the above population that go to the thalamus) project to two midbrain structures, the *pretectum* (PrT) and the *superior colliculus* (SC; the anterior quadrigeminal tubercle).

Certain other destinations of retinal nerve fibers have been identified; in particular, some axons reach hypothalamic, or more generally basal, structures. These axons constitute a tract called the *accessory optic tract* (AOT).

This chapter will examine in broad outline the structure of the retina as it is revealed by light microscopy and more recently by electron microscopy (EM). The general gross anatomy of the eye will not be discussed.

2 GENERAL ORGANIZATION

Roughly speaking, the *retinal receptors* (REC)—*cones* (C) and *rods* (R)—are connected via bipolar cells to the optic ganglion cells whose axons constitute the optic nerve. Examination of a radial section of the retina from the outer regions (i.e., the side near the sclera and the choroid) toward the inner regions (i.e., toward the vitreous humor and the center of the eyeball) shows the following (figure 1.1):

1. A *pigmented layer* (P)
2. A layer containing the *outer segments* (OS) and *inner segments* (IS) of the receptors C and R

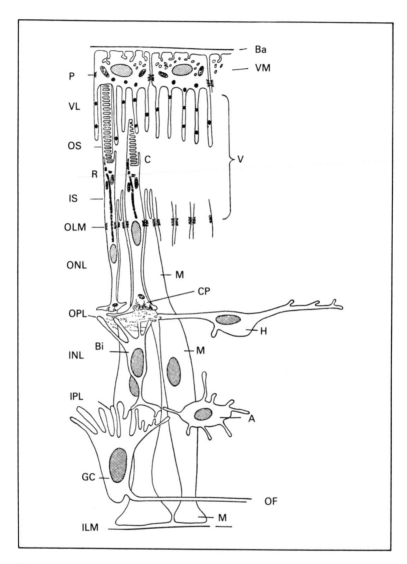

Figure 1.1
Diagram of the principal histological elements of the vertebrate retina. P, pigment
epithelium with villi (VL); Ba, basement membrane of P; VM, Verhoeff's membrane;
OLM, outer (or external) limiting membrane; R, rod; C, cone; OS, outer segment; IS,
inner segment; CP, cone pedicle; V, putative space of the primitive optic vesicle; ONL,
outer nuclear layer; OPL, outer plexiform layer; INL, inner nuclear layer; IPL, inner
plexiform layer; Bi, bipolar cell; GC, ganglion cell; OF, optic nerve fiber; ILM, inner
(or internal) limiting membrane; M, Müller cell; H, horizontal cell; A, Amacrine cell.
(From Cohen 1963)

3. The *outer nuclear layer* (ONL) formed by the nuclei of C and R
4. The *outer plexiform layer* (OPL) where the dendrites of the *bipolar cells* (Bi) and *horizontal cells* (H) meet
5. The *inner nuclear layer* (INL) containing the cell bodies of Bi and H
6. The *inner plexiform layer* (IPL), a zone where Bi cells connect with *ganglion* (GC) and *amacrine* (A) cells; this IPL zone comprises two subdivisions, an outer (a) and an inner (b) layer characterized by different connectivities
7. The layer of cell bodies of the *ganglion cells*
8. The layer of *optic nerve fibers* (OF), the axons of GC
9. The *internal (or inner) limiting membrane* (ILM)

3 RECEPTORS AND THE PIGMENT EPITHELIUM

The retina is derived initially from the *optic vesicle* (V), which in embryogenesis first comprises a cavity that is simply a prolongation of the cerebral ventricle. The interest of histologists was attracted particularly by the fate of the *neuroepithelial border* of the vesicle, which normally develops into ependymal cells. Thus it was recognized that the cells of the distal border differentiate to form the *pigment epithelium* (P) and the proximal border cells give rise to the *receptors*. Even when the ependymal cells have differentiated they remain interconnected by fine fibrils (*tonofibrils*). The latter by their clear continuity define a membrane for each side of the ventricle; the *membrane of Verhoeff* (MV) for the outer ependymal cells and the *external (or outer) limiting membrane* (OLM) at the level of the receptors.

The pigment cells are separated from more external structures by a fibrillar, more amorphous zone called *Bruch's membrane*. This comprises the basement membrane of the pigment epithelium (Ba), which is firmly in contact with the collagenous, elastic, and capillary regions of the *choroid*. The pigment epithelium, Bruch's membrane, and the choroid are thus firmly bound together. In the opposite direction, *villi* (VL) in which melanin pigment is found reach out toward the receptors. In certain nonmammalian vertebrates (fish, amphibians and birds), this pigment is redistributed according to the light intensity level. In a high luminance when the eye is light adapted, the pigment migrates within these cytoplasmic extensions toward the external limiting membrane (i.e., inward), whereas the pigment retracts toward the exterior in the dark-adapted eye (see chapter 3, section 2) at low light levels. The existence of any such migration in mammals is disputed.

One can imagine possible functional roles for the pigment epithelium. It is agreed that three are very probably correct:

• Acting as a system of "light traps" to avoid the glare of lateral scattering of light
• Underpinning the metabolism of distal elements in the retina
• Removing the disks from receptors as and when they are degraded (see below)

[In some mammalian species there is a *tapetum lucidum* situated behind the retina which is a light-reflecting layer. In mammals, this tapetum is created by modifying the structure of the choroid. Sometimes connective tissue fibers become tendinous, compact, and reflecting (ungulates, cetaceans, and elephants); sometimes, as in prosimians and carnivores, the choroid epithelial cells envelop crystalline particles, which form one or two reflecting layers (green or yellow). In general, this is an adaptation to nocturnal living. It increases the reflected light at the back of the eye and leads to a considerable lowering of the absolute intensity threshold; remember, for example, the threshold difference between cat and human.]

The receptors R and C share some common structural characteristics. They have a body, or nucleus, localized in the ONL in the vicinity of the OLM beyond which the receptor proper (R or C) extends and comprises an *inner segment* (IS) and an *outer segment* (OS) separated by an *intermediate zone* (IZ) (figures 1.1, 1.2, and 1.3).

The structure of the two REC categories varies according to species and group. For a given species, as a general rule, the diameter of R is small (in particular that of the OS), whereas that for C is greater but can vary according to the part of the retina in which it is situated.

Most of our detailed knowledge of receptor structure is derived from EM studies. The IS, whose diameter differs between C and R, contains both mitochondria and nuclei and more distal, in the IZ, two very clear centrioles with ciliary filaments; one is oriented longitudinally, the other transversely. These filaments are no doubt remnants of the cilia structures of the ependymal cells of origin.

The OS, for its part, is formed in each receptor type by a stack of disks called segments, or *saccules*. In C the saccular membrane is simply a prolongation of the general plasma membrane of the REC, so that in longitudinal section the disks (sometimes called sacs in C) show open infoldings in contact with extracellular space, while the membrane itself encloses a restricted intracellular space. This struc-

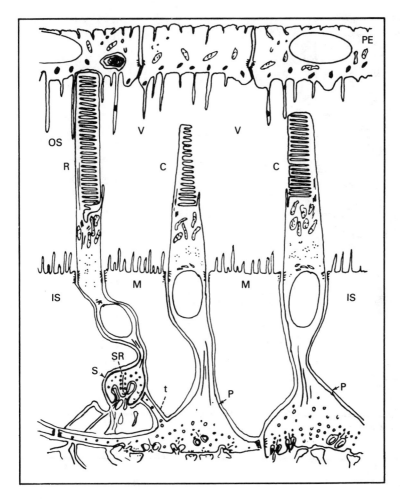

Figure 1.2
Typical vertebrate receptors and their environment. R, rods; C, cones; PE, pigment epithelium; V, ventricular space; OS, outer segment; IS, inner segment; M, Müller cell; SR, synaptic ribbon; t, lateral process (teledendrite); S, spherule; P, pedicle. (From Cohen 1972)

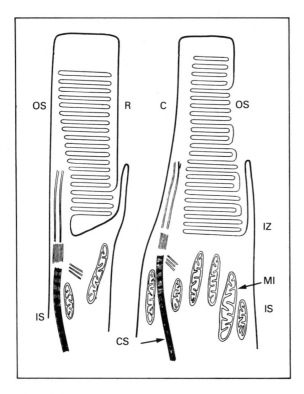

Figure 1.3
Diagram of membrane-folding in the outer segment (OS) of a rod (R) and cone (C).
IZ, intermediate zone; MI, mitochondria; IS, inner segment; CS, ciliary structure.
(From Cohen 1963)

ture is more complex in R: The continuity observed in C is only apparent in the basal part of the receptor, and elsewhere these structural elements have become closed disks that divide the OS into two regions, an intradisk space and an interdisk space (figure 1.3). In transverse sections of the REC the disks are either simple in C or lobulated or segmented in R.

Both rods and cones show a swelling at their inner end (foot) that differs with receptor type and is the level at which presynaptic contacts occur. This end of the cones forms a wide flattened *pedicle* (P) (see figure 1.2), whereas the end of the rods is a *spherule* (S).

The receptors principally make synaptic contacts with bipolar and horizontal cells (see below). These contacts can be of two types: *invaginated* when the postsynaptic prolongation is buried in a synaptic well of the pedicle or spherule, and *superficial* (or a basal flattening) when the synaptic elements make contact without invagination. Superficial synapses seem to exist only at the pedicle of cones.

The synapses of the receptors generally have accompanying mitochondria and synaptic vesicles, suggesting contacts of the familiar sort: The invaginated synapses show in addition a particular formation called the *synaptic ribbon*, approximately perpendicular to the plane of the synaptic contact and surrounded by a halo of vesicles. Direct electric synapses, *gap junctions*, are also seen at the level of these synaptic contacts (particularly at contacts made with horizontal cells).

[Remember that gap junctions, or bridged junctions, are limited zones in the surface of neuronal membranes that are very closely approximated to the plasma membrane of a neighboring neuron, the intercellular space being diminished there from about 20 nm to 2 nm. At such synaptic contacts there exists a highly variable number of intercellular *junctional channels* made of transmembrane protein that bring the cytoplasms of the two coupled cells into contact. The junctional channels can be traversed by molecules of relatively large molecular weight (>1200 Da) such as the fluorescent dye lucifer yellow. After intracellular injection of the dye into a particular cell, its more or less widespread diffusion within the cell compared with its entry into neighboring cells connected to it by gap junctions gives a roughly quantitative picture of the permeability of these contacts.]

Interreceptor contacts via gap junctions have been described in many species, with differences between the lower vertebrates and mammals. In animals such as salamander, turtle, toad, and various teleosts, these tangential connections are via outgrowths called *teledendrites,* some being between cones but mostly between numbers of rods. In mammals, these interconnections are much more restricted: They exist between cones or between a cone and a small group of rods but not, it seems, between rods.

A most interesting phenomenon has recently been discovered (e.g., Steinberg et al. 1980) and concerns a process of renewal of disks in both R and C. Autoradiographic techniques show that new disks are permanently created at the base of the outer segment and are then progressively moved in a distal direction toward the summit of the outer segment. At this level they are separated and removed by phagocytes of the pigment epithelium. Histological research has managed to show exactly how at the base of the outer segment the plasma membrane folds itself to form an invagination and then a complete disk.

The above discussion was chiefly concerned with mammals. Within the whole population of vertebrates, there exists a tightly drawn line of phylogenetic development in both receptor morphology and in the nature of the pigments with which they are furnished, as we shall see later.

Limiting the present considerations to morphology, note that both rods and cones are normally encountered in vertebrates, apart from some exceptions that will be pointed out below.

Nonmammalian vertebrates, however, are distinguished by certain peculiarities (see Crescitelli 1972, 1977; figure 1.4). From fish to birds, passing via the batrachians and reptiles, *double cones* are encountered. These receptors, consisting of two cones tightly joined together without an interposed glial cell, are not found in mammals.

In all nonmammalian species optical and electron microscopy have shown several examples of a distinctive morphological differentiation. Groups of mitochondria occur in a structure below the outer segment called the *ellipsoid*. More proximally, there can exist an abundance of inclusions, generally of glycogen: These constitute the *paraboloid*. Finally, there is an even more proximal zone near the nucleus called the *myoid zone*, suggesting the possibility—probably real but not well established—that it is capable of extension or retraction depending on the light level.

In some amphibians (mainly the anurans) two distinct types of rods have been demonstrated called *red rods* and *green rods*, which contain a pigment different from rhodopsin (λ_{max} = 433 nm).

Finally, in reptiles and birds, between the OS and the ellipsoid of either single or double cones, inclusions of colored oil drops may be seen. Two such receptor arrangements are found, particularly in diurnal birds (such as the pigeon) possessing retinas with 80% cones:

• Single cones with oil-drop inclusions of variable color (yellow, orange, red, or sometimes colorless).
• Double cones (one principal receptor and one accessory) in which at least the principal contains an inclusion that is often yellow or orange, whereas the accessory, depending on its retinal location and the species, may or may not contain an oily inclusion.

In many species, notably in passerines, the distribution of cones and their inclusions is not haphazard. Thus the dorsolateral retina has predominantly single cones with red or orange inclusions ("red retinal sector"), whereas the medionasal retinal region contains double cones with predominantly yellow inclusions ("yellow retinal sector"). Rods are less numerous in these species and do not contain such inclusions (figure 1.4).

Attempts to relate these various forms to function suggest a color-filtering role for the oil drops. We will return to this suggestion later. It is possible that the ellipsoid and paraboloid provide light funneling that is probably related to directional receptive properties such as the Stiles-Crawford effect (see below).

4 TOPOGRAPHIC DIFFERENCES IN RECEPTOR DISTRIBUTIONS

Let us now look at certain structural differences between different zoological groups. While limiting the present discussion to the retinal level, we should note that some peculiarities persist all along the visual paths to the LGB and projection areas in the visual cortex.

4.1 THE PRIMATE RETINA

There are four *morphologically* distinct zones in the primate retina (figure 1.5; see Polyak 1941).

• The *optic papilla* (optic disk), the point of exit of the fibers of the optic nerve; at this place (the "blind spot"), which is nasal and inferior, there are no nerve cells, no receptors, and no pigment epithelium.
• The *area centralis* (macula lutea, yellow spot), a circular region 6 mm in diameter in humans, occupying 15° to 20° of the visual field, surrounding the point of impact (marked with an arrow in figure 1.5) of light that enters along the optic axis. The macular area is stained yellow with a xanthophyllic carotinoid pigment; in this region the retina attains its maximal thickness (500 μm) and has a high concentration of ganglion cells.
• The *fovea,* the circular depression in the middle of the area centralis and consequently the immediate surround of the visual axis. Here the retina attains its minimal thickness; there are no retinal blood vessels here which carpet the rest of the retinal surface. In humans its diameter is 1.5 mm (5° of visual field). In the very central and deepest part of the fovea (the *foveola,* or central fovea) the thickness of the retina is almost entirely taken up by the OS of receptors. The central fovea has a diameter of 500 μm (1° 20′ of visual field).
• The *peripheral retina,* comprising the regions beyond the macula,

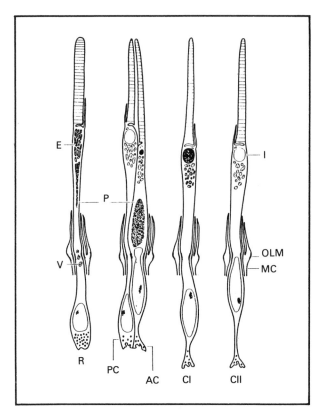

Figure 1.4
Diagram of chicken visual receptors, from EM studies. *Left to right,* Single rod: showing elongated mitochondria in the ellipsoid (E), the presence of a paraboloid (P),
containing glycogen, and also cytoplasmic vesicles (V) at the level of the outer limiting
membrane (OLM). The nucleus is near the synaptic base where numerous vesicles are
visible. Double cone: with principal (PC) and accessory (AC) components. PC contains
a large yellow oil-drop inclusion and AC a smaller inclusion reported as yellow-green.
Paraboloid (P) is large. There is no Müller cell (MC) between the two parts of the
double cone. Note positions of MC. Single cones, types I and II (CI, CII), also contain
oil-drop inclusions (I). (From Crescitelli 1972)

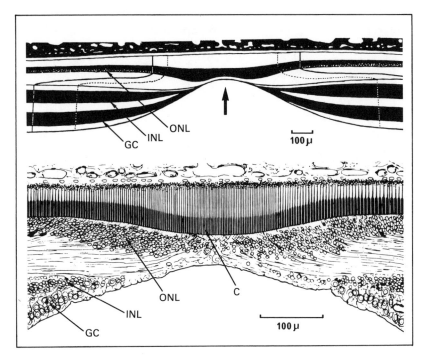

Figure 1.5
Human fovea. *Above,* The inner (INL), outer (ONL), and ganglion (GC) nuclear layers
are in black. The white dots in ONL show the extreme limit for rods, toward the
center. The vertical solid line delimits the region of photoreceptors where cones predominate. *Below,* Detail of the central fovea to a different scale (see bars). Notice the
length and thinness of the central cones (C). The ONL is formed entirely of cone
nuclei. Note that ONL is the only layer at the foveal center. The projection of the
visual axis is marked with an arrow. (From Polyak 1941)

has a relatively constant thickness with a certain loss of organization
toward the most peripheral parts, known as the *ora serrata.*

Differences in the *distribution of receptors* (C and R) accompany the
above morphological differences. Some global cell counts in primates
give the following orders of magnitude:

- Total number of C: 6.5×10^6
- Total number of R: 120×10^6
- Total number of optic nerve fibers: 10^6

These figures reveal an appreciable degree of convergence from the
receptors to the ganglion cells, of order 120/1.

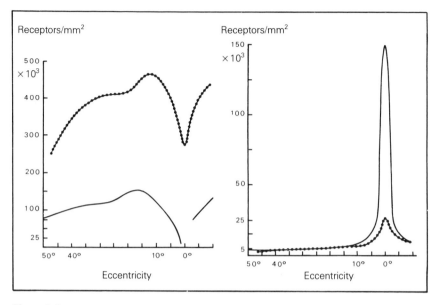

Figure 1.6
Distribution of rods (*left*) and cones (*right*) in the retina of cat (dotted) and human
(solid curve) as a function of eccentricity. (From Steinberg et al. 1973)

Ratios of the relative abundance of rods to cones in the human retina are shown in figures 1.6 and 1.7. Note that:

• Cones have a maximal density in the fovea (10^5 over 1.75 mm^2, or 57×10^3/mm^2; and 35,000 in a single foveola of 0.25 mm^2). They then become rapidly more rare toward the periphery (5000/mm^2 at 10° eccentricity).

• Rods have a zero density at the fovea, becoming maximally packed at 20° eccentricity (160,000/mm^2), decreasing in density again toward the periphery.

Cones have a special morphology in the fovea. Their OS is relatively elongated (see figure 1.5), and their thickness is about 1 to 2 μm, with their separation, center to center, being about 2.0 to 2.6 μm. Here the inner layers of the retina have suffered a lateral displacement, which explains the overall decrease in retinal thickness at the fovea. We shall see that in this region the cones make linear synaptic connecting paths.

At the macular periphery, cones are shorter with a thicker OS. Here the two REC types are already encountered with about one R

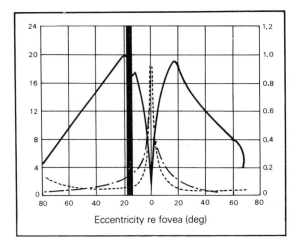

Figure 1.7
Receptor density and visual acuity. Density of rods (solid curve) and cones (dotted) in the human as a function of eccentricity, compared with photopic visual acuity (dotted/dashed curve). Measurements made along a meridian passing through the blind spot (vertical bar). Ordinate: (*left*) number of receptors of either type in 10^3 per unit area of 0.0069 mm^2; (*right*) relative visual acuity. (From Graham 1965)

for every two C. More peripherally still this becomes one C for two R, then one C for three or four R. Beyond the macular region the synaptic arrangements cease to be linear and become convergent instead (see below). This convergence becomes considerably greater in the retinal outer layers; for example, sensory units formed by 100 R converge on 17 Bi, with these converging on a single GC. This sort of arrangement continues far out into the periphery but eventually becomes much less well defined near the *ora serrata* (or *terminalis*), which marks the anterior limit of the retina.

4.2 RETINAS OF OTHER GROUPS

Apart from in primates, the fovea is found in many birds, lizards, and fish. The birds have the widest variety of retinal structure, often including two foveas, as we shall see below. In the majority of mammals apart from primates there is no fovea but only an *area centralis* (macula) around the entry point of the visual axis; such is certainly the case in carnivores, rodents, and the various classes of herbivore.

THE CAT RETINA

The cat retina (see figure 1.6), so much studied, merits a brief sketch of some of its quantitative aspects (see, e.g., Sternberg et al. 1973):

• The density of C is 4000 to 5000/mm^2 at the periphery, stays on that plateau toward the center, where it suddenly increases steeply to 26,000/mm^2 in the area centralis within 5° eccentricity.

• The density of R is higher throughout than that of C. From the periphery to 30° it increases from 250,000 to nearly 500,000/mm^2, reaches a maximum of 10° to 15°, and decreases abruptly at the center of the area centralis to 275,000/mm^2.

• The ratio R/C is about 10 at the center, increasing to 65 more peripherally and to 100 at the ora serrata. As a general rule, C are distributed at random among R.

SIGNIFICANT VARIATIONS IN THE VERTEBRATE LINE

Generally, both R and C receptors are recognizable in most vertebrate retinas; they are easily distinguishable in teleosts, mammals, and nocturnal birds but less so in lower fish, amphibians, reptiles, and diurnal birds. The old hypothesis of predominance of cones in diurnal animals and of rods in nocturnal still seems to be valid in essence, at least to a first approximation. Thus cones predominate considerably (80%) in diurnal birds but rods are also present; in nocturnal birds, rods are more abundant but cones are not absent.

Some retinas with homogeneous receptor content have been identified but only in limited numbers, because many originally specified as a purely cone or a purely rod retina have been found in detailed examination to also have a few rods or a few cones, particularly when classification rests on more subtle criteria such as their synaptic connections:

• *"Rod retinas"; R largely dominant:* guinea pig, rat, mouse, rabbit, Chiroptera, Cetacea, galago (bush baby), *Tarsius* (often considered "purely R" in spite of having a fovea), and lemur. [The last three species are in the Appendix.] *"Cone retinas"; C largely dominant: Tupaia* (tree shrew), certain teleosts, some snakes (colubrids), some lacertilians (lizard, chameleon), some chelonians (turtle), some squirrels (ground squirrel); (retinas of the last two classes are often considered to be "purely C," but this structural homogeneity is questionable).

5 DISTRIBUTION OF OPTIC NERVE FIBERS, VISUAL FIELDS, AND BINOCULAR VISION: PHYLOGENETIC ASPECTS

Important factors in vision are the extent of the visual fields of each eye (monocular field) and above all the degree of overlap between these two symmetrical fields, which assures the possibility, at least

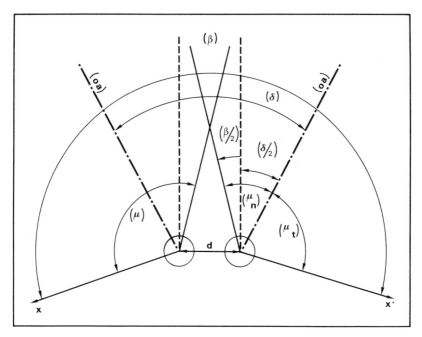

Figure 1.8
**Diagram illustrating the principal geometrical parameters that determine the arrange-
ment of visual fields.** d, interocular distance; oa, optic axes of the eyes whose angle
of divergence is δ; μ, the visual field of each eye with a nasal portion μ_n and a temporal
portion μ_t; xx′, the total visual field; β, the binocular field of vision. Two dashed
parallel lines, normal to the interocular line, have been drawn in the sagittal plane. A
few estimates and approximations are possible for quantities indicated here (β/2, δ/2,
$\mu_n = \mu_t$); see the text also.

in theory, of binocular vision in this overlapping area and of stereoscopy, vision in depth. It might be interesting to pursue this theme
briefly by following the types of binocular vision in the line of vertebrates, particularly in the birds and mammals.

To attempt a purely geometrical evaluation of visual fields we specify the following parameters in the medial horizontal plane (figure
1.8). [The term *monocular* refers to total visual field of one eye. *Unioru-
lar* refers to visual field seen by one eye in situ.]

- Total visual monocular field (μ)
- Divergence (δ) of the visual axes
- Linear distance (*d*) between the eyes' anterior nodal points
- Correlated with these, the angle of binocular vision (β)

• Where necessary, the lateral uniocular field of vision (λ) of each eye

• The total visual field (xx'), also called the *panoramic* field or traditionally, the *cyclopean* field

The difficulty in these estimates is to know the position of the visual axis in relation to the monocular field. Assume to begin with the most complex case where the nasal and temporal visual fields are not symmetrical with respect to the visual axis. Call these hemifields $\mu(n)$ and $\mu(t)$, respectively, such that

$$\{\mu = \mu(n) + \mu(t)\}.$$

We can then write the following simple equations, bearing in mind that the most accessible experimental data are δ, the divergence of the visual axes, and μ, the monocular field (and neglecting d, the separation of the anterior nodal points of the two eyes). Thus

$$\beta = 2\mu(n) - \delta$$

and

$$xx' = \delta + 2\mu(t).$$

In the case where the nasal and temporal monocular hemifields are identical $\{\mu(n) = \mu(t)\}$ these relationships become

$$\beta = \mu - \delta$$

and

$$xx' = \mu + \delta.$$

In these simplified conditions (which are not valid for primates, where $\mu(n) \neq \mu(t)$), measuring μ and δ is sufficient to determine the other two quantities, binocular field (β) and total field of vision (xx'), as well as the lateral monocular field. Also λ, the lateral uniocular field of vision, is $\mu - \beta$. Finally, a blind area, that space behind the head in which nothing is visible, can be specified by the angle (in degrees) $360 - xx'$.

[We have not specified in the above notes all the precautions necessary when measuring these parameters of spatial vision (see, e.g., Hughes 1977). Some are concerned with in vivo measurements, others with anatomical topography from studying cadavers. Both the optical parameters (refraction of rays entering the eye) and anatomical structure (what rays reach the retina and where) must be considered. Values given below, compiled from various sources, generally agree only approximately with the simplified theoretical considerations outlined above.]

5.1 NONMAMMALIAN VERTEBRATES

In fish, batrachians, reptiles, and birds the chiasm is entirely crossed; each retina projects to contralateral nervous centers and in particular to the dorsal midbrain optic tectum, which in mammals becomes the superior colliculus. In addition, in these diverse groups the eyes are either immobile with respect to the head or can be moved independently. There may occur some coordinated eye movements but not necessarily with the essential linkage that is present in all mammals, as we shall discuss below.

For this reason, specification of a binocular zone of vision β has no useful purpose, since independent movements of the eyes can change it. It is also clear in these groups, remembering the total crossing at the chiasm, that the "fusion" of images and vision in depth become possibilities. Indeed, as we shall see, stereopsis is effected by such fusion and it can only be accomplished by involving the central commissures in these animals.

That having been said, let us first consider *avian studies*. [In birds, the retina, unlike in most other groups, does not enjoy a circulatory supply spread over most of its area. But this absence of a widespread vasculature is to some respects compensated by the presence of a strange formation, the pecten (comb). This emerges from the place of exit of the optic nerve (which has an elongated contour) and projects for a variable distance into the vitreous humor in the ventro-lateral quadrant of the back of the eye. Essentially, it comprises a network of vessels and of pigmented cells. This structure has a varied morphology, depending on the type of bird, which has been carefully studied. Beside that, hypotheses are certainly not lacking concerning its possible function(s). Maybe there is a nutritional role; maybe it is concerned with the sensitivity of the retina to movements since given its position it could cast a shadow over the retina and improve motion detection; maybe it has a secretory purpose for regulating intraocular pressure or finally, maybe it helps orientation in space (see, e.g., Meyer 1977).]

Apart from the above considerations, there has nevertheless been some success in distinguishing different types of organization related fairly clearly to the way of life of the bird. From a neuroethological

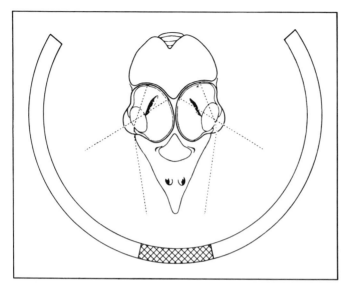

Figure 1.9
Projection of the visual fields of a bird (house martin). The eye of this animal has a double fovea and also contains a pecten. The central foveas are concerned with monocular vision and the lateral foveas with binocular vision (in the hatched area). (From Meyer 1977)

point of view, one might in fact suggest classifying the birds into three categories:

1. *Species with narrow heads and very laterally placed eyes.* The angle μ is of order 165° and δ is of the same order. From these facts, the binocular field is relatively poor (about 30°). However, the total visual field (xx') is, in contrast, rather large (about 300°). Domestic species such as the pigeon, the Passeriformes, and the Galliformes belong to this group.

2. *Diurnal predators* (swallow, kingfisher, and, above all, birds of prey). In these the diversion of the visual axes is much less (90° in the kestrel), and the total field of each eye remains high (about 140°). Thus the panoramic visual field also remains high (220°) (figure 1.9).

3. *Nocturnal predators* (owls). These animals have some peculiarities: The eyes are immobile in the orbit (absence therefore of any ocular movements); their rather tubular eyeballs reduce the total field of view of each eye (70°). The divergence of the optic axes remains large (50°), but the field of binocular vision is high (60°). The total visual field is reduced (160°). These data are summarized in table 1.1.

Table 1.1. Visual fields and distribution of optic nerve fibers

Species	Visual axes' divergence (δ)	Monocular Field (μ)	Binocular Field (β)	Uniocular Field (λ)	Cyclopean Field (xx')	Ipsilateral Fibers (%)
Mammals						
Rabbit	160	190	10–20	170	360	10
Rat	120	190	80	100	320	10
Horse	80	220	65	140	360	20
Cat	7	145	100	45	190	40
Monkey	Small	170	140	40	200	50
Human	Small	170	140	40	200	50
Birds						
Pigeons and pas-seriformes	160	165	<30	135	>320	0
Diurnal pred-ators	90	140	40–60	100	220	0
Nocturnal pred-ators	50	110	60	50	160	0

Note: Figure 1.8 explains the angles delta, mu, beta, lambda and *xx'*. (From data of Duke-Elder 1958; Vakkur & Bishop 1963; Hughes 1977; Meyer 1977).

The variation in the size of visual field and the laterality of the eyes in birds is accompanied by an interesting evolution of their retinal organization, in which everything seems to point to adaptations designed for high visual acuity. These retinas contain particular regions where the receptor density is heightened (and also the Bi and GC density) and where the receptors are also narrower. This increases visual acuity and in certain cases augments movement sensitivity also. These regions might be limited circular areas of the retina or bands that cross some or all of the retina.

The bird retina also shows central areas of thickening with depressions that typically constitute foveas, this structure being presumably destined to improve acuity even further (known to be very high in this class) by also exploiting the total morphology to act like a magnifying glass. In these foveas, there is really nothing but receptors, the other retinal nervous elements having been displaced sideways. Without going into any great detail, we must nevertheless mention a few correlations that have been established between retinal structure and behavioral necessity.

Thus, universally within the species in group (1) above, that is, those that are least specialized as predators, there is only one central fovea at the retinal point of impact of the eye's visual axis. These animals that have a wide lateral field of view but a small binocular field have essentially no common foveal vision. Their sharpest vision can only occur laterally for each separate eye, depending on the visual axis' position for each eye.

In fact, matters are a little more complicated than this in practice. In the pigeon, for example, there are *two* zones of greater cellular density, particularly in the inner plexiform layer. One is near the fovea centralis and "looks laterally"; it is situated in the yellow region of the retina (see above). A second, called the *area dorsalis*, is in the red retinal area; it occupies the dorsotemporal quadrant of the retina, which is precisely the small area in which binocular vision becomes possible. These double areas of retinal thickening presumably have a high visual acuity and can provide this species with a true frontal vision (for pecking) and also with a lateral (far) vision (Galifret 1968; Yazulla 1974; Martinoya et al. 1981).

The diurnal predators have *two foveas* in each eye, a typical central fovea and a second fovea laterally and temporally placed in the retina. With these four foveas the animal enjoys three types of sharp vision, two for lateral monocular vision and one for frontal binocular vision.

The former is presumably used for clearly detecting the prey and the latter for capturing it using frontal binocularity (figure 1.9).

Finally, it seems that in the nocturnal predators only the lateral temporal fovea has evolved: The animal's gaze is always ahead in front of its beak.

5.2 MAMMALS

In mammals, the extent of the binocular visual field varies greatly between different groups. Two sorts of eye movements occur that do not seem to be essential in lower orders:

• Eye movements that are effectively always *conjugate*, meaning that the rotation of one eye implies a similar movement in the contralateral eye, while retaining the same angle between the two visual axes of the eyes and equally, at least in the higher species, maintaining the parallelism of these two axes.
• *Convergent* movements between the two eyes with the visual axes intersecting at a fixation point; this effect makes too simplified estimates of the binocular field a little theoretical in real life (figure 1.10).

Thus our first area of concern is the *optical binocular field*, determined from purely geometrical considerations, taking account of purely physical measurements, such as the deviation of the visual axes of the eyes that are themselves assumed to be in a "rest position"; the shape of the head; the interocular distances, and so forth. [The ophthalmoscopic determination *in vivo* of characteristic retinal landmarks, on which the specification of a resting position depends, can present some difficulty, particularly when the retina comprises no special characteristic at the point of impact of the visual axis (e.g., in rodents). Nevertheless, the point of entry of the optic nerve (the blind spot) can always be used if its position with respect to other retinal parameters has already been established.] As the mammals have evolved, the binocular field has extended progressively, this being achieved by reduction in the divergence of the axes and by the eyes ceasing to be lateral.

Unfortunately, not all the necessary measurements are available for all animals (even laboratory bred); in particular, the differences between $\mu(n)$ and $\mu(t)$ are often lacking. However, we can roughly estimate the visual axes as bisecting the angle μ when these axes are very lateral and the eyes very divergent (which circumstances allow the use of the simplified equations above). However, a more exact

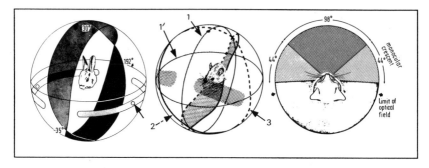

Figure 1.10
Visual fields determined ophthalmoscopically in rabbit, rat, and cat. The equatorial
cyclopean visual fields of the rat and rabbit are of the same order of size but the
binocular field is three times wider in the rat than in the rabbit. The binocular field of
the cat is scarcely any larger than that of the rat but its cyclopean view is much less.
(See text and table 1.1.) For the *rabbit*, the shaded zone represents the binocular field,
the black zone is the blind area, the lateral circle (arrow) is the blind spot. For the *rat*,
the shaded zone to the rear is the blind area; the two dotted lateral areas mark the
projections of the zones of high ganglion cell density (>6000/mm²). (1) Vertical and
(1′) horizontal central meridians; (2) anterior and (3) posterior boundaries of the uniocular field. For the *cat*, the central binocular field is 98° and the lateral monocular fields
44°; to the rear is the blind area. (From Hughes 1977)

knowledge of the visual axes becomes necessary in cases of small
divergence and in species where the nose, for morphological reasons,
interferes, making the angle $\mu(n)$ very different from $\mu(t)$. Such is the
case in the cat, where $\mu(t) = 93°$ and $\mu(n) = 50°$ (figure 1.10). In
primates, and humans in particular, even though the difference is a
little less marked, the two hemifields are similarly unequal, being 70°
nasal and 100° temporal.

  Those aspects apart, there are additional problems in determining
the binocular field because, as we have said, it is difficult to measure
the rest position of eyes, particularly in rodents (see below and also
figure 1.11). Table 1.1 shows some significant measurements of this
type of survey for common experimental animals, giving values of δ,
μ, β, and of the total panoramic cyclopean field xx'.

  It is difficult to avoid the obvious teleological conclusions when the
organizations of different mammalian receptive fields are compared,
for example, contrasting arrangements in that well-known predator
the cat to those in an animal like the rabbit that is permanently in
danger of being caught. In the latter, the binocular field (which allows
a very successful spatial precision in motor aiming) is particularly

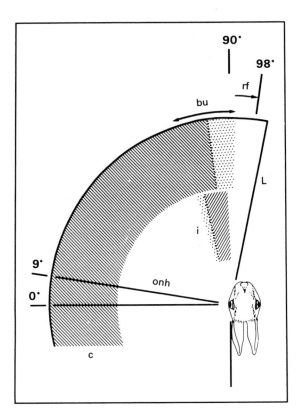

Figure 1.11
Diagram of the rabbit's visual field in the "freeze position." The zero vertical meridian
lies in the coronal plane passing through the anterior nodal point of the eye and the
blind spot is set at 9° more nasal (onh, optic nerve head). The oblique shadings show
the horizontal extent of the visual fields that project on to the contralateral (c) and
ipsilateral (i) cerebral cortex, measured by multi-unit or single unit recording. (The
dots show response areas that have been obtained from single unit recording only).
The limiting boundary (L) of the optical field is contralateral at 10° to 12° beyond the
sagittal plane and the retinal field (rf) embraces the first 8° beyond. The zone marked
(bu) shows that of "binocular units" where these sectors of both eyes overlap in the
freeze position. The contralateral projection is represented by the external hatched
ring. (From Hughes & Vaney 1982)

small, whereas the uniocular range of vision is very wide, with the result that the total field of view suffers a blind zone to the rear of only a few degrees (360 − xx'). This allows the animal to see the approach of an enemy from almost any direction. In contrast, the binocular field of view, so necessary for skilled visuomotor aiming, is much larger in predators like the cat, whereas their monocular field of view is considerably less than in the rabbit, with a relatively large blind area to the rear (Hughes & Vaney 1982).

This evolutionary development has been accompanied, in this class and this class only, by a second one concerned with neural arrangements. In particular, there is the emergence of a new trajectory for sensory afferents of the optic nerve that originate in the temporal retina. Significant numbers of these, instead of totally crossing the midline at the chiasm, can remain ipsilateral. Table 1.1 shows the relative proportions of ipsilateral and crossed pathway visual nerve fibers for different mammalian species.

A problem particularly pursued in the past ten to twenty years has been to determine how the increasing size of the binocular visual field in evolution, as determined by purely geometrical considerations, has been accompanied by changes in the type of separation of the ganglion cell outputs from the retina (Hughes 1972, 1976, 1977, 1979). Let us take two different species to illustrate the principles involved:

• In *cats* or in *primates* (which are similar in this respect) with the eyes in their resting positions, the visual axes diverge very little. Correspondingly, the ipsilateral optic nerve fibers come from the temporal retina and the crossed population from the nasal, with the fractions of ipsilateral and crossed being closely similar.

• In *rodents* (mouse, rat) and *lagomorphs* (rabbit) the situation is quite different. Assuming it is possible to define a resting position for the eyes, we can say that the visual axes are in fact very divergent (almost in line one with the other). The monocular fields are vast, exceeding 180° (190° in the rabbit). They overlap a little in the forward direction; each monocular field crosses the midline over at least part of its extent, though there are in fact differences in detail between rabbit and rat (see figures 1.10 and 1.11).

[In the rat the resting position of the eyes has only been determined indirectly (for the anesthetized animal or the cadaver). Under these conditions the binocular field begins at 40° below the horizontal in front of the head and spreads to 65° beyond the vertical behind the

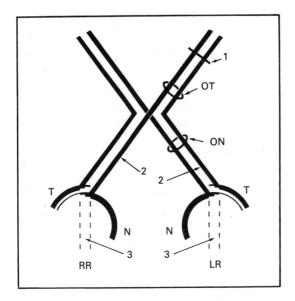

Figure 1.12
Ipsilateral and contralateral retinal projections in the cat. The thickness of the shading at each retina corresponds with the percent of ganglion cells going to each tract. (N), (T), nasal and temporal half-retina of the right retina RR and left retina LR; ON, optic nerve; OT, optic tract; (2) parts of ON degenerating after section of OT at (1). Regions of overlap (3). (From Stone 1966)

head (see figure 1.10). The invasion of the contralateral hemifield is greatest in the upper nasal quadrant and extends to 40° lateral, which results in a width of binocular field of about 85°.

In the rabbit it is possible to define a resting position of the eyes by the *freeze position,* a sort of hypnotic position that this animal takes up in certain behavioral states (figure 1.11). Under those conditions the binocular field begins at 30° below the horizontal to the front and stretches to 70° beyond the vertical to the rear in the mediosagittal plane. But in this case the invasion of vision into the contralateral field is more limited, being only 15°, thus limiting the maximal width of the binocular field to 30°.]

The distribution of the ganglion cells between crossed and uncrossed outputs (either side of a *line of decussation*) also needs to be addressed.

• In the *cat* (figure 1.12; Stone 1966, 1978; Stone & Campion 1978; Cooper et al. 1979) 100% of the axons from the nasal half-retina cross the midline and project to the opposite cerebral hemisphere. Only 75% of ganglion cells of the temporal half-retina send outputs ipsilaterally and 25% of the outputs from the temporal retina cross the midline. Therefore the retinal line of decussation is well defined for ipsilateral fibers but is more diffuse for the crossed population. Thus near the midline at the area centralis there is a region of *temperonasal overlap* (0.2 mm, 9°). From here about half the ganglion cell axons project ipsilaterally and half contralaterally.

• In the *macaque* there is also a ganglion cell overlap between crossed and uncrossed outputs from both sides of the fovea, within an area corresponding to about 1° of visual angle (Stone et al. 1973; Bunt et al. 1975).

• In *rodents* and *lagomorphs* different problems arise. At present it is agreed that the ganglion cell outputs in all retinal locations have a contralateral destination except for a certain limited number of ganglion cells sited in an inferior temporal crescent of the retina that have an ipsilateral projection.

6 INTERMEDIATE CELLULAR LAYERS

We now introduce a discussion of the cells of the inner nuclear layer and the inner and outer plexiform layers as well as of the ganglion cell layer (figures 1.13, 1.14, and 1.15); the ganglion cell layer is described in more detail in the next section. Our analysis will amplify certain aspects, not only descriptively but also concerning the study of the functional circuitry in which they are incorporated. That is essential for a proper understanding of retinal mechanisms. We preface this study with a few basic observations.

It would have been traditional and easy, as was customary even quite recently, to keep separate (as we do here to some extent) a chapter concerned with retinal histology from another concerned with retinal functional mechanisms. But visual research results are multiplying explosively at present, and so we will discuss the material in a less restrictive way that follows the methods of research used at present. There is now a somewhat revolutionary tendency in experimental approach both to identify cellular function (e.g., by unitary microelectrode recording, intracellular where possible) and simultaneously to exploit cell marking techniques (horseradish peroxidase, procyon yellow, etc.) to identify the type and connections of the cell. It has necessarily become very difficult from a tutorial point of view to separate purely histological parts of a text from others that

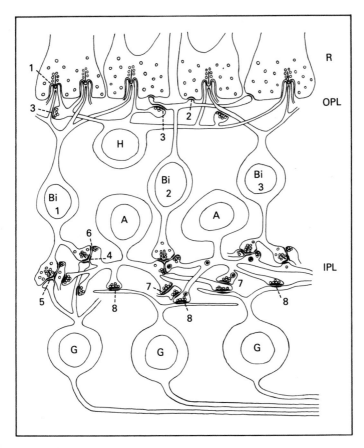

Figure 1.13
Diagram of synaptic connections in the frog retina. R, receptor cell pedicles; H, horizontal cell; Bi1, Bi2, Bi3, bipolar cells; A, amacrine cell; G, ganglion cell. The outer level of synaptic connections is in the outer plexiform layer (OPL) and the inner level is the inner plexiform layer (IPL). Note: in OPL the invaginating synapses R → Bi and R → H, marked 1, superficial synapses R → Bi, marked 2; "normal" synapses or dendrodendritic (?) H → Bi, marked 3. In IPL, synapses Bi → A (4); Bi → G (5); reverse synapses A → Bi (6); connections A → A (7), and A → G (8). Certain Bi, here Bi1, connect directly with G; others, here Bi2, Bi3, only make the connection via A. (From Dowling 1968)

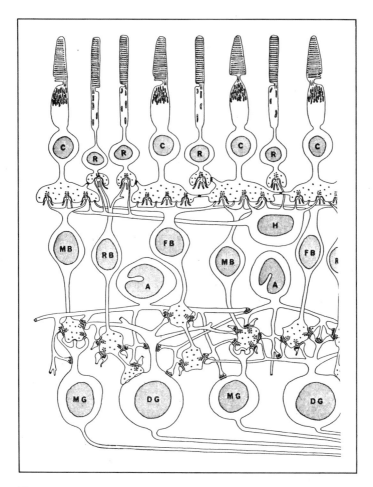

Figure 1.14
Interconnections between macaque retinal cells. C, cones; R, rods; FB, flat-topped
bipolars; RB, rod bipolars; MB, midget bipolars; MG, midget ganglion cells; DG,
diffuse ganglion cells. (From Dowling & Boycott 1966)

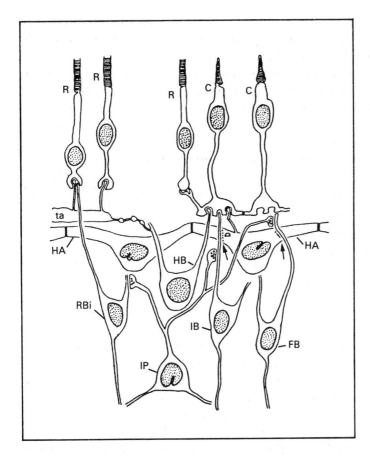

Figure 1.15
Outer plexiform layer organization in the cat. The basal regions of the receptors are interconnected by gap junctions; cone pedicles (C) make such junctions extensively with neighboring cones and singly with rods (R). Apart from these connections the pathways from cones and rods remain strictly separated. Rod bipolars (RBi) are connected only to rods (via an invaginating synapse with a synaptic ribbon). Some cone bipolars form invaginating synapses with cone pedicles (invaginating bipolar IB) and others make superficial synapses (flat-topped bipolar FB). Type B horizontal cells (HB) make invaginating connections with cone pedicles but their axonal connections (ta) are only with rods. Horizontal cells without axons (HA) connect with neighboring HA (by large gap junctions) and also with the dendrites of cone bipolars (dotted lines marked by arrows). An interplexiform cell (IP) extends its dendrites into the OPL contacting all the bipolars by chemical synapses.

concern purely functional properties. Some duplication of information will inevitably occur in the present chapter and chapter 4, which is devoted to retinal function.

Those who are tempted to summarize all data related to retinal circuits must be warned that there are dangerous reefs to be wrecked upon. Not only is it a question of trying to précis what is in any case complicated data even when it concerns only one species, but also of trying to incorporate the wide variations that occur among different mammals (e.g., rabbit, cat, and monkey) and to a greater extent among different vertebrate groups. It is tempting but nevertheless extremely hazardous to risk extrapolation from one species to another and to overgeneralize.

The intermediate cellular layers contain the cell bodies of two sorts of cells: the bipolar cells (Bi), which connect the receptors to the ganglion cells, and the horizontal cells (H), which are concerned with cross-connections (Dowling & Boycott 1966; Dowling 1968; Dowling & Werblin 1969).

6.1 BIPOLAR CELLS

Cajal distinguished two categories of bipolars, one being small and connecting with cones, the others larger and associated with rods. Recent data show the situation to be more complex, with many classes of bipolar cells being recognized: One criterion is the extent of their dendritic field, another is the receptor type, cone or rod, with which they are connected (see, e.g., Stell 1972; Kaneko 1983). These numerous types of bipolar cell have, by general consensus, been separated into three essential categories according to the receptors they serve:

• *Rod bipolars* (RBi), with large dendritic fields connecting with a large number of rods (and sometimes cones); they make *invaginated* synaptic contacts with the spherules of rods.
• *Midget bipolars* (MBi), which in contrast connect with a single cone and have a very narrow receptive field. The way they connect with the cone pedicle subdivides these into *midget invaginating* (M(i)Bi) and *midget flat-topped* (M(f)Bi).
• *Flat-topped bipolars* (FBi), which similarly only synapse at cone pedicles but without invagination and with a large field.

The axons of the bipolar cells terminate in the inner plexiform layer with their arborizations in either the outermost (a) or innermost (b) sublayers, depending on their connectivity: rod bipolars in (b), invaginating cone bipolars in (b), flat-topped cone bipolars in (a).

This classification into three types seems to hold quite well in monkey retina. In contrast, recent research in the cat, with precise individual categorization of each neuron and subsequent morphological identification (sometimes with a patient complete reconstruction of the cell) has led to results that are much more complicated than was expected (Kolb et al. 1981; Nelson & Kolb 1983; McGuire et al. 1984). In the light of such results, concentrated essentially on the pericentral regions of the retina, there appear to be the following classes of bipolar in this species:

• A single type of *rod bipolar* (RBi) making an invaginating synapse at the spherule and sending its axon to terminate in the sublamina (b) of the IPL.
• Not fewer than seven types of *cone bipolars* (CBi), distinguished by their dendritic field, narrow or wide, by the level of their terminations, and by their function. In detail, at least two types are invaginating and terminate in (b); two other types (flat-topped or semiinvaginating) terminate in sublamina (a). We will meet these CBi bipolars again in chapter 4 under the respective identifiers CBi b1, CBi b2, CBi a1, CBi a2.

6.2 HORIZONTAL CELLS

The stellar-shaped cell bodies of these cells are situated in the outer layer of the outer nuclear layer and their tangential (horizontal) processes synapse in the outer plexiform layer connecting with receptors and bipolars in complicated ways (Kolb 1970, 1979; Gerschenfeld et al. 1982; Hashimoto & Ueki 1982; Sakai & Naka 1982).

The first detailed studies on horizontal cells were made on *lower vertebrates* (teleosts, Urodela, and reptiles in particular). They showed the existence of (1) two categories of H, one type with an axon, the other with dendrites only; (2) gap junctions between REC and H, suggesting reciprocal connectivity such as REC → H → REC; (3) gap junctions between H cells, creating a veritable interconnected network in the outer plexiform layer; (4) a range and specialization of H cells according to the type of REC, rod or cone of one or other type (identifiable by their oil-drop inclusions and/or by their spectral response curve).

In mammals it is generally agreed that there are two types of H cells. Those called *HA* have no axon but a spread of thick dendrites that extends to the outer plexiform layer; those called *HB* have finer dendrites and notably a long, fine axon.

Studies in the cat (Kolb 1979) show that HA cells have electrical synapses and apparently no other. These are set up between their dendrites and three other types of structures: (1) in the recesses of cone pedicles; (2) on other neighboring HA cells, establishing a sort of horizontal network; (3) en passant junctions on the dendrites of cone Bi, whether they are invaginated or flat-topped.

HA cells make more complex connections, specifically in that their synapses (possibly electrical) are arranged with cone pedicles, yet they only send their axons to rod spherules. In contrast, HB cells apparently do not establish contacts with one another.

In summary, in the cat (but probably also in other species), HA are only in contact with cones and form a sort of superficial network, whereas HB do not make up such a network but establish C → R connections.

This having been said, EM studies of rod spherules and cone pedicles show typical invaginated structures with contacts both with bipolar dendrites and horizontal cell processes. Figure 1.16 shows the typical picture of the parafoveal region in primates: the rod spherule (R) with, in the center, the terminals of two RBi and laterally some H cell processes. The cone pedicle (C) comprises dendrite terminals of midget bipolars, M(f)Bi and M(i)Bi, and a bipolar Bi(f) that here is also associated with horizontal cell terminals (H) (Kolb 1970).

7 GANGLION CELL LAYER

This level contains not only ganglion cells but also horizontally interconnecting cells called *amacrines* (A in figures 1.13 and 1.14).

7.1 AMACRINE CELLS

These neurons, apparently lacking axons, and whose lateral processes seem to insert at the level of synaptic connections between Bi and GC, were named amacrines by Cajal. Their classification is not well defined at present. Many types have been distinguished, up to 15 by Cajal. Attempts to simplify this morphological complexity have included separating amacrines into two groups, *stratified* (As) and *diffuse* (Ad). This distinction rests on the fact that the tangential spread of their processes sometimes spreads in one or two horizontal planes (As), whereas others are no respecters of the horizontal stratification of the retina (Ad).

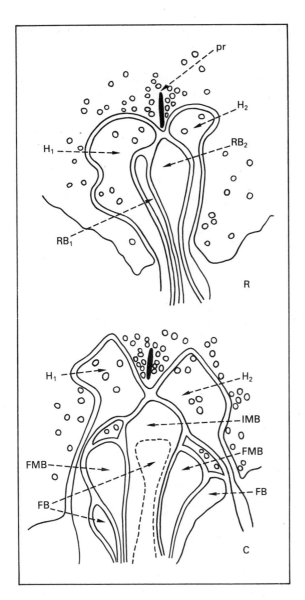

Figure 1.16
Connections between receptors, bipolars, and horizontal cells in macaque retina, based on EM. (R) Rod spherule with presynaptic ribbon (pr), contacting, within an invagination, two rod bipolar dendrites (RB_1, RB_2) and two axonal contacts with separate horizontal cells (H_1, H_2). (C) Cone pedicle, also invaginated, with a triad comprising two horizontal cell dendritic terminals (no doubt also separate, H1, H2) and also an invaginating midget bipolar cell dendrite (IMB) with noninvaginating terminals from cells described as flat-topped midget bipolars FMB and others called flat-topped bipolars FB, all of which contact the pedicle in a much more superficial way. (From Stell 1972)

Histological studies in the cat by Famiglietti and Kolb (1975) were rstricted to stratified amacrines, more specifically to those that have small dendritic fields and moreover are characterized by *two* layers of spread in sublaminas (a) and (b) of the IPL. These are classified as *A II* amacrine cells. A II amacrines set up two types of synaptic contacts: (1) electric synapses (gap junctions) with cone bipolars that connect with ON ganglion cells (i.e., GC that respond to the onset of a light stimulus) or (2) chemical synapses at other GC with an OFF physiological action (i.e., responding to extinguishing a light). A II cells also have a role in the intraretinal chain of rod signal transmission.

Golgi studies (Kolb et al. 1981) further divide amacrines into four groups in the cat: amacrines with narrow dendritic fields that include the A II just described; amacrines with small fields; amacrines with moderate fields; amacrines with large fields (> 500 μm). The classification is complex, and it is hard to find any clear guiding principle in this rather excessively detailed catalogue of cell types, except perhaps that some amacrines branch in the sublamina (a) and some in (b) and that neurochemical studies (see chapter 4) increasingly reveal quite a gamut of possible transmitter action in these cells.

7.2 INTERPLEXIFORM CELLS

Detailed study of inter plexiform (IP) cells is quite recent (figure 1.17). These neurons have their somata sited in the inner nuclear layer near A cells (to which class they probably belong), their processes extending laterally in the IPL but also directed toward EPL, where they synapse with the elements of that layer, namely, Bi and H cells (Dowling and Ehinger quoted in Dowling 1986).

Their discovery, first in the carp, then in the American *Cebus* monkey, and subsequently in other species, was initially achieved using fluorescence microscopy. This showed the cells to be catecholaminergic—more precisely still, dopaminergic, dopamine having been demonstrated to be their (or one of their) probable transmitters (Dowling 1986). They have since been shown by Golgi techniques to be present in other species; among these is the cat, whose IP cells show no histofluorescent reaction to dopamine.

[We will see below how morphological and histological studies have recently been supplemented by neurochemical and immunohistochemical techniques that have identified a whole range of transmitters that are probably active at the various different retinal levels.]

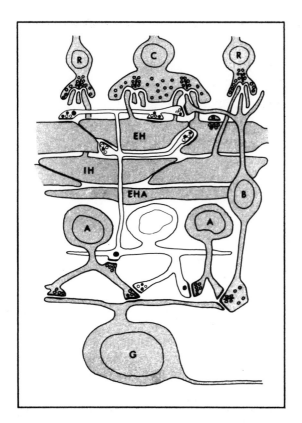

Figure 1.17
Synaptic connections of an interplexiform cell IP in carassius retina. Such a cell receives afferents at the level of the amacrines (A) of the inner plexiform layer. It makes no contact with ganglion cells (soma or dendrite). In the OPL, the processes of the IP synapse with the most external horizontal cells (EH) and with dendrites of bipolars (B). No contacts are observed with receptors, C or R, nor with the more internal horizontal cells (IH). (From Dowling 1986)

EM studies have identified in more detail the types of synaptic contacts at IP cells:

• They only receive synaptic influences in the IPL, where they are postsynaptic for amacrine cells and themselves make synaptic contacts with amacrines and bipolars.
• In the EPL they are presynaptic with (i.e., make synaptic contacts on) cone and rod bipolars and also (for other IP cells in some species but not cat) with H cells (Kolb & West 1977); in contrast, they do not seem to contact the REC. Apparently all synapses made by IP cells are chemical.

In summary, these cells seem to constitute a sort of feedback connectivity from IPL to EPL.

7.3 GANGLION CELLS

Here also, many varieties or subclasses have been described. Essentially, three subclasses have been categorized according to the horizontal spread of their dendritic field: *diffuse ganglion cells* (GCd), with a large field sometimes limited to one retinal plane (*stratified ganglion cells*, GCs) and *midget ganglion cells*, with a restricted field (MGC). Recent histological analysis of some retinas (notably cat and monkey) has gone much further in establishing functional correlations; we shall discuss this in chapter 4.

DENSITY

It is illuminating to consider the densities, high or low, of ganglion cell populations and to trace *isodensity contours* that are known to vary with species (see, e.g., Whitteridge 1973). Figure 1.18 shows:

• Retinas with a low GC density that changes little between center and periphery. This is found in nocturnal species, particularly in rodents.
• Retinas with higher GC density but with little spatial variation. Species such as squirrels and *Tupaiidae* are found in this class.
• Retinas with a very large spatial gradient from center to periphery, notably in the primates, where the isodensity contours are concentric around the fovea.
• A concentration along a horizontal band (*horizontal streak*) with, in addition, a higher density either in the center (e.g., cat) or in the temporal periphery (herbivores).
• Again, a band organization but with the GC concentration most accentuated in the temporal regions. This type is found in the rabbit.

While we are far from being able to establish absolutely tight correlations with ethological factors, the following relationship does seem to be clear. In rodents and lagomorphs but also in herbivores, which all enjoy frontal binocular vision only in the most lateral temporal regions of the retina (i.e., not along each eye's visual axis), there is a corresponding tendency for ganglion cells to be more concentrated in the peripheral temporal region of the retina. The correlation is certainly not absolute but is worth thinking about. Thus it has been noticed that in the rabbit the area of temporal binocular vision does

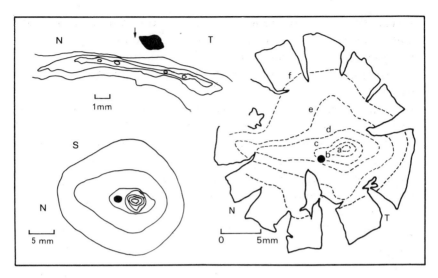

Figure 1.18
Distribution of ganglion cells in three mammalian species. *Upper left,* Rabbit: Isodensity contours in number of cells per 3000 μ²; from the periphery to the center, 10, 20, 30, and 40 cells/3000 μ². *Lower left,* Baboon: From the periphery inward, isodensity lines for 10, 15, 100, 200, 300, and 350 cells/5000 μ². *Right,* Cat: isodensity lines from periphery to center, contour f to contour a, respectively 125, 250, 500, 1000, 2000, 5000/mm². In black, the optic papilla, or blind spot. N, S, T, nasal, superior, and temporal retina. (From Wässle et al. 1983 and Whitteridge 1973)

not appear to coincide exactly with the area of highest GC concentration; another factor seems to be involved that is concerned with the distribution of GC soma size.

MORPHOLOGY AND DIFFERENT GANGLION CELL TYPES

Different ganglion cell types have been reported in different species. In *lagomorphs* the region presumed to be concerned with temporal binocular vision is particularly rich in large ganglion cells. This is clearly an example of specialization of cell type in a certain region being related to their function (in binocular temporal vision in this case; see Provis 1979, Provis & Watson 1981).

In the *cat* such distinctions have been pushed even further, to the extent of recognizing three types of ganglion cells (Boycott & Wässle 1974; Wässle et al. 1975, 1983).

• Type α has a large soma diameter (mean 33 μm), a wide axon, and a dendritic tree that is wide and tufted (180 to 1000 μm).

• Type β has a much smaller cell body (20 μm), a thinner axon, and a much more restricted dendritic tree (25 to 300 μm).
• Type γ has the smallest cell body (13 μm), the finest axon, and a dendritic field that is thinly spread but the extent of which is very variable.
• For the retina *in toto* the relative proportions of these different GC have been measured via a variety of convergent studies, starting with traditional histology and extending to retrograde cell marking and other techniques. Type α cells are about 4% of the population; β cells are a more numerous 55%; and the remaining class of α cells are both morphologically and, as we shall see, functionally diverse.

This type of GC classification points to several interesting conclusions: Small cells (β and γ) are the dominant classes in the area centralis with the α type being abundant in the immediately pericentral region. Both α and β types have dendritic fields which, although they are different in size, increase in diameter with increasing eccentricity according to a quasi-linear law, the slope of which (normalized for absolute size difference) is the same for the two categories of cells. In contrast, the dendritic field size of γ types remains the same, whatever the eccentricity of these cells (see, e.g., Shapley & Perry 1986).

Naturally, we can deduce that the cones would connect with the small GC and the rods with the large. In this species the quantitative convergence in the pericentral region is about 5.2 C per small GC and 600 R per large GC. In the periphery this ratio becomes multiplied by about 10 for C and by 3.5 for R. In other words, the convergence remains larger for rods than for cones at whatever part of the retina.

In the *macaque* there is not at present complete agreement about the classification of GC. Two nomenclatures have been suggested. One comprises two principal types Pα and Pβ and a final class of less abundant cells Pγ (Perry and Cowey 1981). On the other hand, Leventhal et al. (1981) designated these types respectively A, B, and C.

Cells Pα and A have large cell bodies with radial dendrites and wide axons; Pβ or B have small somata and short branching dendrites with a limited dendritic field and a thinner axon; Pγ or C have very small cell bodies, large dendritic fields and very fine axons. Their relative proportions in the whole retina are approximately A 8 to 12%, B 80%, and C 10%.

However, this classification has been recast by Kaplan and Shapley (1982) and by Shapley and Perry (1986), who propose the following groups:

• M ganglion cells (which were the Pα of Perry and Cowey). These GC have a dendritic spread which, though small at the fovea, increases with increasing eccentricity in a linear way like the α and β fields in the cat.
• P ganglion cells, which are much more numerous (Pβ in the former classification). Their dendritic spread, small at the fovea, remains so up to quite a large eccentricity (1.6 mm at the fovea, or 8°), which distinguishes these from the α and β GC of the cat and the M class in the macaque.
• Other much rarer ganglion cells that do not correspond with either P or M types but would formerly have been called Pγ.

What aspects of these monkey and cat organizations are homologous? From one morphological point of view it is true that P cells have a smaller dendritic field and finer axon (like β) and in a similar way the dendritic field and large axon of M cells suggest they may be homologous with α cells. Nevertheless, the rule of increasing extent of dendritic field with increasing eccentricity does not apply to P cells; in addition, the functional characteristics of the P and M types probably prevent them from being regarded as true homologues of the feline case.

CENTRAL TARGETS OF GANGLION CELL AXONS

The central destinations of mammalian retinal GC axons have been briefly discussed above; on the one hand, there is a thalamic destination (LGB, pars dorsalis) and alternatively, a midbrain destination (SC and pretectum); finally, there is a basal route to the nuclei of the basal mesencephalic tegmentum. We will discuss the first two routes here and the third in chapter 5.

In the *cat* a whole series of recent studies (Fukuda & Stone 1974; Illing & Wässle 1981) based on the retrograde transport of horseradish peroxidase (HRP) has allowed the tracing of α, β, and γ cell outputs to their two target levels, LGB and SC (figure 1.19).

• A total of 77% (of the 150 to 200 · 10^3) retinal ganglion cells reach the thalamus.
• The α axons (from 5% of the total number of ganglion cells) *all*

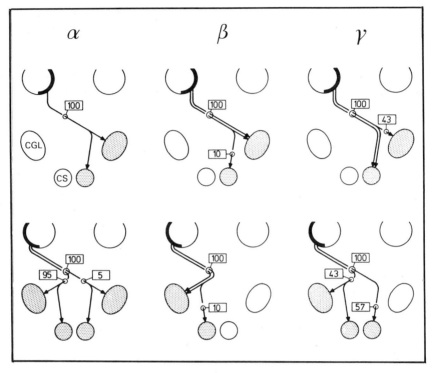

Figure 1.19
Comparison of retinotectal (i.e., to the superior colliculus, SC) and retinothalamic
(i.e., to the lateral geniculate body, LGB) projections in the cat. The numbers indicate
percentages for each of the three classes of ganglion cell α, β, γ. Distributions of
ganglion cells are shown above for the left nasal half-retina, below for the left temporal
half-retina. The total population of ganglion cells comprises 4.5% α, 56% β, 40% γ.
(From Illing & Wässle 1981)

divide to send one collateral to the ipsilateral LGB and the other to
the ipsilateral SC.
• This group of α axons contains all the fibers arriving from the con-
tralateal nasal retina but only 95% of those α fibers coming from the
ipsilateral temporal retina since 5% of these go off to the contralateral
LGB and SC.
• All the β axons (56% of all ganglion cells) cross the midline. There
are two groups; the larger (90%) has LGB only as its destination, the
minority group (10%) goes to both LGB and SC.
• The destination of γ axons is more complicated. All fibers from the
nasal retina cross the midline; 43% of them bifurcate to LGB and SC;

57% go to SC alone. Of the axons from the temporal half-retina, 43% divide to reach the ipsilateral LGB and SC, and 57% cross the midline to go solely to the contralateral SC.

To summarize, most of the information arrives at higher levels from the contralateral visual hemifield; nevertheless, LGB and CS receive 5% of the information from the ipsilateral visual hemifield via α ganglion cell axons and the SC receives 57% of information from the same field by γ axons.

In the *macaque* there is likewise a division of ganglion cell axonal distribution, particularly researched by retrograde HRP techniques. If we employ the latest proposed nomenclature—P cells, M cells, and "others"—we find that P cells have the (dorsal) parvocellular layers of LGB as their main target and the M cells the (ventral) magnocellular layers of LGB (perhaps together with a few axons to SC or the pretectum). As for the elements named (provisionally) Pγ, their principal destination seems to be the SC (Leventhal et al. 1981; Perry & Cowey 1984; Perry et al. 1984, Shapley & Perry 1986). We will return to these later when discussing function.

7.4 SYNAPSES AT THE LEVEL OF THE INNER PLEXIFORM LAYER

Here also, EM studies coupled with functional analysis have defined connectivities in IPL where IP cells (discussed above) are concerned as well as bipolar, amacrine, and ganglion cells.

To summarize, many sorts of junctions have been observed in various lower vertebrates as well as in primates.

• Bi cells synapse with a ganglion cell dendrite and with an amacrine cell A, the whole constituting a *diad*. At this level the Bi axon usually comprises a synaptic ribbon.
• Amacrine cells may form reciprocal and feedback synapses with a Bi axon. These have a normal structure with no synaptic ribbon.
• Amacrine cells may equally synapse with other A, thus creating a serial synaptic chain, each element being postsynaptic for the preceding one and presynaptic for the next.
• There are also synapses in the direction A → GC.
• Some Bi cells make axosomatic synapses with GC.
• In many species, the two functional types of GC, ON and OFF, show different levels of arborization of their dendrites; sublamina (a) for OFF and (b) for ON.
• Concerning the earlier mention of CBi bipolar cells (section 6.2),

it is tempting to conclude that ON channels are underpinned by invaginating CBi and the OFF channels by CBi with superficial (flat-topped) contacts.

The details have been elucidated further in the cat, not only by individual classification of GC as ON or OFF and as α or β, but also by detailed tracing of bipolar cell pathways and specification of amacrine types. Thus it should be noted that:

• Dendrites of both α and β GC branch horizontally in the inner plexiform layer. Two levels of branching exist: in the outermost zone of IPL, sublayer a, and the innermost, sublayer b. It appears that some α GC but also some β GC branch in sublayer a, and electrophysiological experiment has now shown that these are all OFF types (αOFF and βOFF). Other α and β GC branch in sublayer b; these are all ON cells (αON and βON).
• RBi cells practically never synapse with GC themselves but with amacrines, in particular type A II, which in turn contact a given category of GC.
• CBi cells make contact with both amacrines and GC; some synapse in sublayer b with ON GC, α or β, and others in sublamina a with OFF GC, α or β.
• A given GC (ON or OFF) enjoys connections with at least two different types of BiC. The principle enunciated above (invaginating CBi → ON GC in b; flat-topped CBi → OFF GC in a) does not seem to apply in this case. (See chapter 4.)

7.5 FUNCTIONAL UNITS OF THE RETINA

Given the morphological bias of this section, we should consider the resulting functional diversity of retinal units. It is clear, from differing dendritic spread and also degree of convergence, that the spatial acuity of different retinal areas must also be very different.

It has become traditional, in primates in particular, to distinguish two principal retinal trajectories:

1. *Linear* arrangements, in which one REC (typically one C) connects with a sole Bi (typically MBi), which contacts a MGC. This is a matter of "private lines for cones." Some researchers consider that there are also divergent lines for cones, such that one C output can be distributed to several Bi. Rods do not seem to give rise to such linear or divergent arrangements.

2. *Convergent* arrangements, in which a number of rods or cones (e.g., 10) make synaptic connections on one Bi with a more or less wide dendritic spread. Many Bi can in their turn converge on one GC. In addition, two suborganizations have been revealed:

• Numerous rods synapse with one RBi; then this connects with a diffuse GC (GCd).
• Several cones synapse with a flat-topped Bi, which also connects with a GCd.

An extra factor in this scheme, however, is that several horizontally interconnecting elements (H or A cells) generate lateral interactions between REC or Bi.

We shall see in chapter 4 how combining structural and functional data can better construct the major retinal circuitry. This has really only become possible by correlating results from a great variety of experimental investigations to establish the complex functional elements and their connectivities and relating them to specific aspects of visual function.

8 GLIAL CELLS

Mammalian retinas contain Müller cells, which are glial in nature (apparently related to astrocytes and oligodendrocytes). These align themselves radially throughout the thickness of the retina, between the outer and inner limiting membranes (see figures 1.1, 1.2, and 1.4). Questions concerning the glial nature of other elements are far from settled. These have arisen principally with respect to the nature of certain horizontal cells in the retinas of fish.

9 EFFERENT NERVE FIBERS

Centrifugal myelinated fibers in the retina of birds were described by Cajal and other workers (Maturana & Frenk 1965). These axons have been traced from the level of the optic nerve to terminal synaptic boutons on amacrines and certain ganglion cells situated at depth and known as *displaced ganglion cells*. These centrifugal axons comprise about 1% of the optic nerve fibers. They originate in the mesencephalic isthmo-optic nucleus. This structure lies medial to and also connects with the optic tectum, which is the essential visual sensory area in birds. There is thus a retino-tecto-isthmo-retinal loop, the function of which has yet to be determined (figure 1.20). If the existence of such fibers seems to be demonstrated in birds (see, e.g.,

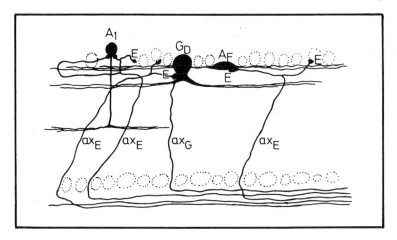

Figure 1.20
Efferent fibers in the avian retina. These axons (axE) make axosomatic synapses on amacrine cells (A_1), (A_F), and on a ganglion cell (G_D) the axon of which (ax_G) is also shown. (From Maturana & Frenk 1965)

Repérant et al. 1981), their presence in other vertebrate groups is not yet absolutely clear. Birds apart, some recent work has proposed the existence of a hypothalamic-retinal pathway in the dog (Terubayashi et al. 1983) and more recently still in a prosimian (Bons & Petter 1986).

The Physical Characteristics of Visual Stimuli

The study of what are conventionally called the *laws of visual sensation* is an ancient discipline that by the last century had attained a remarkable precision for the time. Then and thereafter a coherent and extensive set of data became established based solely on noninvasive analytical techniques, that is, by addressing the major functional characteristics of visual mechanisms by observing the sensations and visual skills of experimental subjects. This was all well in train before the modern introduction of more internal analyses using histological, physiological, or biochemical techniques.

Before discussing the laws of visual sensation, it is probably useful briefly to outline some of the fundamentals of the physics of light stimuli, and the laws of photometry and colorimetry.

1 RADIANT ENERGY: THE FUNDAMENTAL RADIOMETRIC UNITS

It is customary to describe the variables of light stimuli by using definitions that are generally applicable to all radiant energy whether or not it generates a visible stimulus. Let us therefore briefly examine some of the standard definitions of physics concerned with the geometrical and energetic characteristics of electromagnetic radiation (figure 2.1).

1.1 ENERGY FLUX AND IRRADIANCE

If radiation of whatever sort crosses a surface area S bounded by a closed curve, in a given direction, a radiant flux Φ may be defined by the radiant energy transported per unit time across S. Radiant flux has, therefore, the same dimensions as power and can be specified in watts (in the SI system).

The energy of illumination or irradiance $\mathcal{D}$ of S is defined as the element of flux $d\Phi$ per element of surface area dS (figure 2.1A).

$$\mathcal{D} = \lim_{\delta S \to 0} \; \delta\Phi/\delta S = d\Phi/dS \; [\text{watts/m}^2]. \tag{1}$$

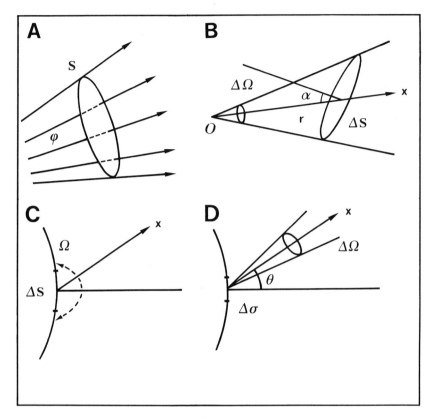

Figure 2.1
Definition of radiometric quantities. Diagrams illustrating the definitions of (*A*) irradiance $\mathscr{D}$; (*B*) radiant intensity $\mathscr{I}$; (*C*) source radiant emittance ϵ; (*D*) source radiance $\mathscr{B}$. See text.

1.2 SOURCES OF RADIANT ENERGY

A source of radiant energy can be a surface or a volume that emits radiation. The source is called *primary* if it emits radiation and *secondary* if it is limited to redistributing radiation by the total or partial reflection, whether diffuse or specular (i.e., directionally) of radiation emitted by another source.

Consider first of all the radiation from a *point source* (*O*) of negligible size compared with the observing distance (figure 2.1B). The energy emission from *O* in a given direction *Ox* can be described by the *energy* or *radiant intensity* of emission $\mathscr{I}$ in the direction *Ox* within an element of solid angle *d*Ω (expressed in watts/steradian, W/sr).

$$\mathcal{I} = \lim_{\delta\Omega\to 0} \quad \delta\Phi/\delta\Omega = d\Phi/d\Omega. \tag{2}$$

In general $\mathcal{I}$ varies according to the direction Ox; in the special case where $\mathcal{I}$ is constant for all Ox, the emitter is called a *uniform source*.

Purely geometrical considerations permit calculating the radiance of a surface δS receiving radiation from O within the solid angle $\delta\Omega$. If the angle the surface S makes with Ox is given by α and the mean distance $O–S$ is r, then from equations (1) and (2):

$$\mathcal{I} = \lim_{\delta\Omega\to 0} \quad \delta\Phi \cdot r^2/\delta S \cdot \cos\alpha = (d\Phi/d\Omega)\cdot(r^2/\cos\alpha) = \mathcal{D}\cdot(r^2/\cos\alpha). \tag{3}$$

Alternatively:

$$\mathcal{D} = \mathcal{I}\cdot(\cos\alpha/r^2). \tag{3a}$$

The irradiance thus varies inversely as the square of the distance from the source and directly with the cosine of the angle of incidence of the surface that intercepts the flux.

For a uniform source, equation (2) can be written (since $\Sigma d\Omega = 4\pi$)

$$\mathcal{I} = \Phi/4\pi \tag{4}$$

where Φ is the *total* flux emitted by the source.

In the case of an *extended source*, the idea of intensity becomes inapplicable and we can exploit two different factors, depending on the conditions.

First, let us consider a small area on the outer surface of the source (δS) and calculate the flux ($\delta\Phi$) emitted from it in all directions of a demi-space (i.e., in a solid angle 2π). This allows us to define the *energy or radiant emittance* (ϵ) of the source at a point O, central in the surface element δS (figure 2.1C). In the limit this can be written:

$$\epsilon = \lim_{\delta S\to 0} \quad \delta\Phi/\delta S = d\Phi/dS \tag{5}$$

To emphasize this, the emittance is again a surface flux density, but this time it is a question of *emitted* energy.

Alternatively, we can consider a point O on the surface of the source *together with* a direction of emission Ox. Consider the power radiated by an element of surface area ($\delta\sigma$) of the source in the element of solid angle in the mean direction Ox (figure 2.1D). This allows us to define an energy *radiance* as in equation (6) below. [The term radiance can often lead to confusion since it has sometimes been used to describe emittance and sometimes brightness.]

$$\mathcal{B} = \lim_{\delta\sigma\to 0} \quad \delta\mathcal{I}/\delta\sigma = d\mathcal{I}/d\sigma \tag{6}$$

where $d\mathcal{I}$ is the energy intensity in the direction Ox. We will not go into great detail concerning the relationships between ϵ and $\mathcal{B}$ in the general case where the brightness depends on the angle θ that Ox makes with the emitting surface. But we can show that for the special case of an *orthotropic* emitter for which $\mathcal{B}$ is the same in all directions (a source said to obey *Lambert's law*) the following applies:

$$\epsilon = \pi\mathcal{B} \tag{7}$$

The physical dimensions of these quantities are as follows:

• Energy or radiant flux (energy/time) [W].
• Irradiance (power/unit area) [W·m^{-2}].
• Energy or radiant intensity (power/unit solid angle) [W·sr^{-1}].
• Energy or radiant emittance (power/unit area) [W·m^{-2}].
• Radiance (power/unit area/unit solid angle) [W·m^{-2}·sr^{-1}].

Dimensionless factors are also exploited. One is the *transmission factor* or *transmittance* (τ), which is the ratio of the flux leaving a volume of a substance to the flux entering, related to the absorption of energy by the substance; another is the *reflection factor* or *reflectance* (ρ), which is the fraction of the flux falling on a surface that is reflected (either in a given direction or diffusely, depending on the nature of the surface).

1.3 SPECTRAL CONTENT OF ELECTROMAGNETIC RADIATION

An electromagnetic ray generally comprises different wavelengths that can be separated into a spectrum by dispersive devices (e.g., prisms, gratings). Such a spectrum can be either discontinuous or continuous.

The first case concerns *line spectra* in which the total radiation is composed of superimposed separate radiations that have been emitted from sources each of which produces a single radiation and is characterized by its own intensity, radiance, or brightness.

A *continuous spectrum* is defined by a smooth distribution of spectral energy. For this purpose one measures either an element of radiation $\delta\mathcal{R}$ or an element of radiance $\delta\mathcal{B}$ in a wavelength interval between (λ) and ($\lambda + \delta\lambda$). (See figure 2.2.) For this one might define either

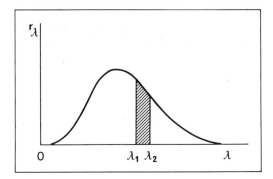

Figure 2.2
Hypothetical curve of a spectral distribution of radiant energy. (From Le Grand 1964)

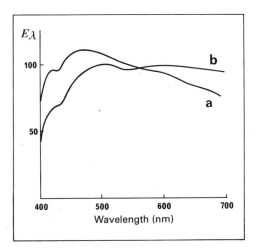

Figure 2.3
Energy distribution of solar radiation (a) before and (b) after passage through the atmosphere. (From Le Grand 1964)

the *spectral radiation* $r(\lambda)$ by the expression:

$$r_\lambda = \lim_{\delta\lambda \to 0} \delta\mathcal{R}/\delta\lambda = d\mathcal{R}/d\lambda, \tag{8}$$

or, better, the *spectral radiance* $b(\lambda)$ by the expression:

$$b_\lambda = \lim_{\delta\lambda \to 0} \delta\mathcal{B}/\delta\lambda = d\mathcal{B}/d\lambda. \tag{9}$$

Thus the spectral content of radiant energy can be specified by plotting the curve of r_λ or of b_λ as a function of λ (figure 2.2).

It has, however, become common practice (above all in the case of the visible spectrum) not to consider the absolute values of r_λ or of b_λ but to refer magnitudes to some particular value (say, the maximal magnitude). Thus a sort of relative value E_λ is obtained which (normally as a percentage) specifies the spectral energy distribution for the source (figures 2.3 and 2.4).

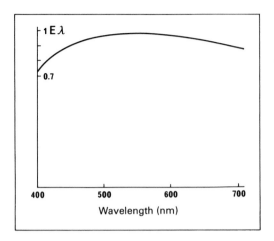

Figure 2.4
Spectral energy distribution
$\{E_\lambda = f(\lambda)\}$ for a black body at
5200°K. (From Le Grand 1964)

2 LIGHT ENERGY: FUNDAMENTAL PHOTOMETRIC UNITS

2.1 GENERAL CHARACTERISTICS

Light is a special class of radiant energy embracing wavelengths between 400 and 700 nm (or mμ), or 4000 to 7000 Å. [We will here use, interchangeably, mμ or nm (10^{-9} m); nm is recommended and the Å (1 Å = 10^{-10} m) is "forbidden" in the European Economic Community!]

A primary or secondary source emitting a single radiation in the visible spectrum (400 < λ < 700) is specified in terms of (1) its radiant energy, measured sometimes in a particular system of units that properly applies only to visual characteristics; these units are called *luminosities;* and (2) its color; a single radiation comprises *monochromatic* light.

Most light sources emit a continuous spectrum, thus a mixture of single wavelengths; others emit line spectra. For certain combinations of radiation that will be specified later, color disappears completely and the light is white (neutral, achromatic, colorless).

2.2 LUMINOSITY: UNITS AND MAGNITUDES

Here we discuss the measurement of visual luminosity, not only in energy units but nevertheless independently of the idea of the color perceived.

THE VISIBILITY CURVE

To measure the amount of radiant energy in general, the fundamental notion is that of flux, a measurement of power which, as we have seen above, also brings with it a whole series of other units deduced from flux by essentially geometrical considerations. Such a system is not very suitable for specifying the *visual* action of light. Consider, for example, one radiant source with a wavelength in the visible spectrum and another one outside those limits. The radiant energy units we have considered take no account of the effect of the radiation on the eye. But it is evident that a source for which $400 < \lambda < 700$ nm will be visible, but one with the same energy radiance for $\lambda < 400$ or > 700 nm will be quite invisible. Thus it is necessary to look for units of radiation that take the characteristics of vision into account. In such a photometric system a *luminance* or *visual brightness* is specified and is related to radiant energy magnitude.

Consider two sources, $S1$ and $S2$, emitting monochromatic radiation at λ_1 and λ_2, with energy radiances $\mathscr{B}_1$ and $\mathscr{B}_2$. If $\lambda_1 = \lambda_2$ the human eye matches $\mathscr{B}_1$ with $\mathscr{B}_2$ with no difficulty by comparing them. If $\lambda_1 \neq \lambda_2$ the problem of comparing them becomes more difficult and the more so the greater the difference in λ_1 and λ_2 becomes.

Supposing, however, that the practical difficulty in visually matching these sources (heterochromatic photometry) has been overcome (see, e.g., Pokorny & Smith 1986), we can then introduce a dimensionless coefficient of relative visibility V_λ for the wavelength λ such that after equalizing the brightness of λ_1 and λ_2 we could write:

$$V_1 \mathscr{B}_1 = V_2 \mathscr{B}_2.$$

Having determined the ratio V_1/V_2 for different pairs of wavelengths one could plot the curve of $V_\lambda = f(\lambda)$ step by step. We could find that it passes through a maximum at around 500 to 550 nm (figure 2.5), depending on the conditions under which it is measured, to be specified below. Thereafter, we are able to relate all values of V_λ to their maximal value taken as a unity (1.0) reference.

Thus a monochromatic (λ) visible source having an energy radiance $\mathscr{B}_\lambda$ will have a *visible brightness (luminance)* defined by

$$\mathbf{B}_\lambda = K_0 V_\lambda \mathscr{B}_\lambda \tag{10}$$

where V_λ depends on λ and where K_0 is a coefficient related to the choice of units. We will return to this point.

PHOTOMETRIC MEASUREMENTS AND UNITS

In principle, it should be sufficient to specify visible light by taking some photometric quantity, as in dealing with radiant energy, and from that deduce a number of other quantities by using the same fundamental relationships as were deduced above. Thus: the *(visual) luminous intensity* I of a point source would correspond to a radiant energy intensity $\mathcal{I}$, in such a way that dI is the visual intensity of an element $d\sigma$ and we could write:

$$dI = B \cdot d\sigma, \tag{11}$$

just in the same way as in equation (6) above.

Luminous flux F, corresponding to an energy flux Φ could be deduced by using the equation analogous to equation (2) above:

$$dF = I \cdot d\Omega \tag{12}$$

where I is the intensity and $d\Omega$ is the element of solid angle.

The (visual) *illumination or illuminance* D would be the surface density of the luminous flux received. Thus:

$$D = dF/dS \tag{13}$$

as in equation (1).

But it is in practical applications of this idea that the problems arise. To some extent the difficulty is concerned with the multiplicity of light units which, in the course of history, have been defined empirically in a variety of ways, often before their relationship with energy units had been clearly established. First of all, units were defined in relation to *luminous intensity*, using three units that were slightly different: the international candle, the Hefner candle, and now (in the SI system) the "new candle" or *candela* (cd). [The present definition of the candela (cd) is: "Luminous intensity in a given direction, of a source that emits monochromatic radiation of frequency $540 \cdot 10^{12}$ Hz, of which the energy intensity in that direction is $1/683$ W·sr^{-1}" (Sixteenth General Conference on Weights and Measures 1979).]

Starting with the candela, or other units of intensity in earlier days, it was possible to derive other practical units (by using equations (11), (12), and (13) above):

- The unit of luminous flux
  the *lumen* (lm): 1 lm = 1 cd·sr
- Units of illuminance
  the *phot* (ph): 1 ph = 1 lm·cm^{-2}
  the *lux* (lx): 1 lx = 1 lm·m^{-2} = 10^4 ph

the *foot-candle* (ft-cd): 1 ft-cd = 1 lm/sq foot
(which, since 1 lux = 0.0929 ft-cd) = 10764 lx
The *milliphot* has sometimes been used (= 10 lx).

Units of *luminance* have been defined in two ways: (1) by taking the *source intensity per unit surface area*. Thus the *stilb* (sb) corresponds to 1 cd·cm^{-2} and the *nit* to 1 cd·m^{-2}. Apart from these there are the English units of the *candle/sq foot* (cd·ft^{-2} and the *candle/sq inch* (cd·in^{-2}). (2) Alternatively, starting from an *illumination D* falling normally on a surface of reflection factor (ρ), we can say that its luminance is of the form $B = \alpha \cdot \rho \cdot D$ where α is a coefficient determined by these units. Supposing ρ ≈ 1 (for a perfect diffuser) and the source is orthotropic, these units of luminance can be defined thus:

• An equivalent phot, *lambert* (L), analogous to the ph
• An equivalent lux, *blondel* or *apostilb* (asb), analogous to the lx
• An equivalent foot-candle, *foot-lambert* analogous to the ft·cd

The relationships between all these systems of units are of a somewhat awesome numerical complexity [Agreed!—Translator] because of (1) conversions of English units into metric and (2) the introduction into calculations of the factor π (or its reciprocal) that is needed by the hypothesis of a uniform source.

In practice we will be content to stay with the following SI units:

• Luminous flux: lumen (lm)
• Luminous intensity: candela (cd) = lm/sr
• Illumination (brightness): lux = lm/m^2
• Luminance: (nit) = cd/m^2 = lm/sr/m^2

As units of luminance, we might add (not SI, but still used) the lambert (L) and its submultiple (mL) with the following conversion factors: 1 L = 1/π·10^4 nits = 3183 nits (1 mL ≈ 3 nits).

2.3 SOME LUMINANCE VALUES

Table 2.1 gives some actual luminance values, in mL, ranging between sunlight, viewed directly, to the overcast night sky. In this scale of luminance, a distinction is indicated between two ranges of vision: that between *diurnal* or *photopic* vision and, on the other hand *twilight* (nocturnal) or *scotopic* vision. This boundary was established long ago, and we will return to it in the following chapter. The boundary occurs in practice near 1 mL. The transition between one

Table 2.1 Some luminance values

Source	mL	Range
Solar surface at midday	10^9	
Tungsten filament	10^6	
Snow in sunlight	10^5	
White paper in sunlight	10^4	Photopic range ("diurnal vision")
Overcast sky	10^3	
Light level for reading	10	
White paper in moonlight	10^{-2}	
White paper in starlight	10^{-4}	Scotopic range ("twilight vision")
Overcast night sky; no moon	10^{-5}	
Absolute threshold, order of	10^{-6}	

range and the other is where the *Purkinje effect* is observed (figures 2.5 and 2.6).

2.4 SOME CHARACTERISTICS OF PHOTOMETRIC QUANTITIES

A certain number of fundamental rules apply to the photometric properties flux, luminance, and illumination. They arise from systemic observations made on human subjects and constitute no less than the basic factors concerned with the perception of light. The laws are as follows:

• *Transitivity:* If the luminances, respectively B_1 and B_2, of two fields appear identical and if fields B_2 and B_3 do also, then the two fields B_1 and B_3 will be equally identical.

• *Proportionality:* If two fields are equally bright, then they will remain so if the brightness of each is increased by the same factor.

• *Additivity:* For a collection of lights of different colors $B_1\lambda_1$, $B_2\lambda_2$, . . . , $B_i\lambda_i$, Abney's law states that the total luminance resulting from the superposition of all these lights is obtained by adding the luminances of the individual components:

$$B = \Sigma_1^i B_\lambda \delta\lambda, \tag{14}$$

or

$$B = K_0 \Sigma_1^i V_\lambda \mathscr{B}_\lambda \delta\lambda, \tag{14a}$$

taking into account the considerations mentioned above when $\delta\lambda$ is the elementary interval. [In principle, the elementary interval should

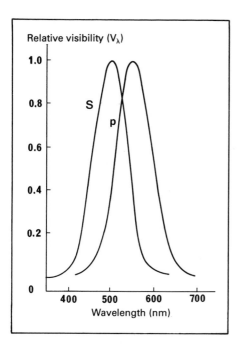

Relative visibility (V_λ)

Wavelength (nm)

Figure 2.5
Curves of the visual effectiveness of radiant energy in the scotopic (S) and photopic (p) ranges. (From Graham 1965 after Wright 1958)

be vanishingly small: in practice $\delta\lambda$ = 5 to 10 nm will suffice]. Notice that the above three properties, applied to luminances are equally valid if applied to luminous flux or to illumination.

2.5 RELATION BETWEEN RADIANT ENERGY AND PHOTOMETRIC UNITS

The interconnection of photometric units with energy units is made via the coefficient V_λ, which by definition is 1 for the wavelength for which it is maximal.

Systematic measurements of V_λ have been made as a function of λ for the whole visible spectrum and the essential, well-established result is that the curve $V_\lambda = f(\lambda)$ is different if it is measured in photopic, or diurnal, visual conditions with luminances > 1 mL than when in contrast scotopic, or twilight, vision is in action at luminances < 1 mL. In the first case V_λ is maximal at λ = 550 mμ and in the second at λ = 510 mμ (this for human subjects; see figure 2.5).

Another way to illustrate this frequency dependence is to plot *curves of equal luminance* perception at a series of different luminance levels; 1 mL and above, then 10^{-1}, 10^{-3}, 10^{-4}, and 10^{-5} mL (figure 2.6). The minimum of these curves, the most efficacious wavelength, is clearly at 550 mμ for the uppermost curve and moves progressively to 510 mμ as the luminance level is reduced. [This sort of experiment

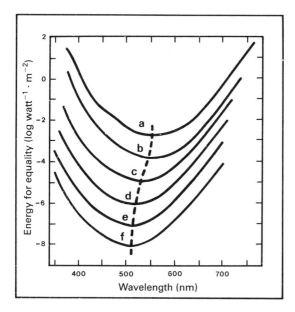

Figure 2.6
Contours of perception of equal luminance for sources as a function of λ, measured in subjects adapted to given luminance levels. Each curve is for a given level of adaptation of the subject; moving from one to the other curve represents a step of 10 dB (a to f respectively: 1.0, 10^{-1}, 10^{-3}, 10^{-4}, 10^{-5} ft-L). The dotted line marks the minimum for each curve. Its inflection clearly shows the Purkinje effect, a movement of sensitivity toward longer λ on passing from rod to cone vision. (From Judd 1951)

needs a certain number of precautions. As we shall see below, the experiment can only be satisfactorily carried out after the subject has adapted to each working luminance level.]

Alternatively, we can determine the significance of the K_0 coefficient that appears in equation (10). Working at the place of maximal V_λ (i.e., unity), at 550 mμ for photopic vision, the equation becomes:

$$B = K_0 \cdot \mathcal{B},$$

in other words, K_0 is a measure of the equivalent energy in the luminous flux. Measurements at 555 nm give $K_0 = 683$, that is, at 555 nm a flux of 1 lm is equivalent to 1/683 W. [For monochromatic radiation of frequency $540 \cdot 10^{12}$ Hz the spectral efficiency equals 683 lm/W (value adopted by the International Commission; see above).] From the above, the equation for the addition of brightnesses becomes:

$$B = 683 \sum V_\lambda \cdot \mathcal{B}_\lambda \cdot \delta\lambda \qquad (15)$$

Thus over the total extent of the spectrum the luminous flux can be written:

$$F = 683 \sum_{0}^{\infty} V_\lambda \cdot \Phi_\lambda \cdot \delta\lambda$$

where Φ_λ is the corresponding radiant flux at wavelength λ.

2.6 ILLUMINATION AT THE RETINA

Before continuing, we need to examine essential details of the interface between the physical stimulus' characteristics and the retinal receptors, in other words, the relationship between the luminance of a source and the brightness of its image on the retinal surface.

The factors concerned in determining the illumination of the retina are essentially two: the effective area S of the pupil and the transmittance of the transparent media of the eye, τ_λ.

The diameter of the pupil varies with the illumination by an expression of the form $d = f(\log B)$ (figure 2.7), whereas the factor τ_λ increases from 0.1 at 400 nm to 0.7 at 700 nm (figure 2.8). [Le Grand suggests, among other possibilities for $d = f(\log B)$, the expression $d = 5 - 3\,\mathrm{tgh}\,(0.4\log B)$.]

Consider, then, an extended source of luminance B illuminating the retina. By the simple laws of geometrical optics and photometry one can show that the retinal illumination D_r is given by:

$$D_r = 0.36\,B \cdot S \cdot \tau_\lambda \tag{16}$$

Therefore the luminance of the source and the corresponding illumination of the retinal image are proportional, independent of the dimensions of the object and its distance. This justifies the idea that luminance is a fundamental factor in the vision of extended sources.

The expression above is easily applicable if coherent units and values are available for B and D (lux and nits, for example, and S in cm^2). However, in the absence of an exact value for τ, a unit of retinal illumination D_r, called the *troland*, has been defined as follows:

$$D_r\,\text{trolands} = S \cdot \mathrm{mm}^2 \cdot B\,\mathrm{cd} \cdot \mathrm{m}^{-2} \tag{17}$$

One troland is the retinal illumination provided by a surface of luminance 1 cd·m^{-2} seen through an artificial pupil of area 1 mm^2. [An artificial pupil is typically a circular aperture, e.g., in a metal plate, of 2 to 4 mm diameter, placed in front of the eye which makes any possible changes in pupil diameter negligible: vision with this arrangement is often referred to as a Maxwellian view.]

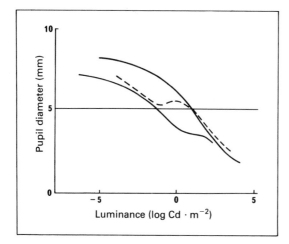

Figure 2.7
Changes in average pupil diameter with luminance. Results from three different authors. (From Le Grand 1964)

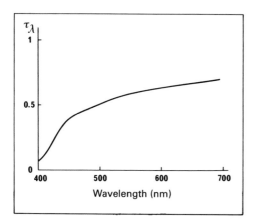

Figure 2.8
Transmittance τ_λ of the transparent media of the eye as a function of wavelength. (From Le Grand 1964)

2.7 THE STILES-CRAWFORD EFFECT

Another factor that influences the retinal illumination is the direction of entry of light rays with respect to the plane of the pupil.

Consider (figure 2.9) two light rays directed along a and b carrying the same light flux and reaching the same place on the retinal surface but entering the eye at two different points A' and B' on the pupil. Comparing the relative effectiveness of a and b by alternating the paths, Stiles and Crawford (1933) and Stiles (1939) established that the more oblique ray is *less effective* than the more orthogonal ray. Measuring a ratio in visual efficacy η with respect to that at the maximal point of entry, taken as unity, shows that η varies with a symmetry of revolution around the optimal point of entry, which is,

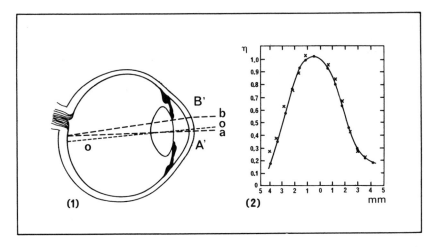

Figure 2.9
The Stiles-Crawford effect. (1) Horizontal section of the eye: oo, optic axis; a, b, rays entering the eye through A′ and B′ at the pupil. (2) Variation of the coefficient η (see text) as a function of the place of entry of the pencil of light in the horizontal plane (in mm) with respect to the optic axis′ point of entry, nasal and temporal. (From Graham 1965)

however, not necessarily the center of the pupil. Taking d as the distance between $A′$ and $B′$ on the pupil, an expression of the following form applies:

$$\eta = \exp\left(-2.3\,k{\cdot}d^2\right)$$

with d in mm and the coefficient $k \approx 0.05$, which varies somewhat with wavelength (figure 2.10).

It is convenient when studying the Stiles-Crawford effect to use the visual condition of a *Maxwellian view*: A lens focuses the image of a light source in the plane of the pupil such that the lens is seen as a uniform source. In this way, by employing a point source it is possible to use entry points at different places on the pupil aperture without changing the retinal illumination.

The existence of this effect necessitates a correction factor in the calculation of retinal illumination. Above a certain intensity, I, one must use an effective pupil area S_e that is smaller than the actual S because of the reduction in the efficacy of the pencil of light relative to its maximal efficacy.

Rather than go into great detail about such calculations, we give one example. Consider a source of 1 cd·m^{-2}; if the pupil is 5 mm in

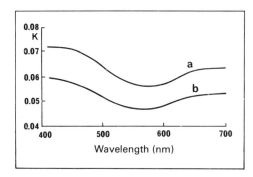

Figure 2.10
Variation with wavelength of the factor k in the Stiles-Crawford effect (see text). After Stiles' own measurements of 1937 (a) and 1939 (b). (From Le Grand 1964)

diameter its area is 19.7 mm², but the effective pupil due to the directional effect will be only 15 mm². In these conditions, the retinal illumination ($B{\cdot}S$) will be 15 trolands, not 19.7 (see also Stiles and Crawford 1934, 1937).

The Stiles-Crawford effect is still not very well accounted for. It is certainly not a property of an absorption in the eye media but a property of the retina itself, which must be more sensitive to rays incident on it normally rather than obliquely. It seems possible that the physical structure of the receptors themselves might account for their acting as directional wave guides on the incoming light pencil.

3 COLORIMETRIC UNITS AND QUANTITIES

A *monochromatic* light is entirely defined by two quantities, its wavelength (λ) and its luminance (B) or a quite different quantity related to the latter, for example, its luminous flux (F). In these conditions the eye behaves as a *bivariant* receptor, a knowledge of (B) and (λ) being necessary and sufficient to determine the visual effect generated.

3.1 VISUAL TRIVARIANCE: TRICHROMACY

Consider a source containing several single sources that form either a line spectrum $B_1\lambda_1$, $B_2\lambda_2$, . . . , $B_i\lambda_i$, or a continuous spectrum with an energy distribution $E(\lambda)$. How does the whole assembly summate?

ADDITIVITY OF LIGHT FLUX AND THE DEFINITION OF WHITE

In the experiment diagrammed in figure 2.11, the subject O observes a screen E, supposed to be a perfect diffuser, through a sheet D pierced by an aperture. An opaque barrier C separates the screen into two parts. Different pairs of sources illuminate each half-screen, S_1 and S_2 for one side, S_3 and S_4 for the other. Each source is defined by its luminance B (or its flux) and its color λ.

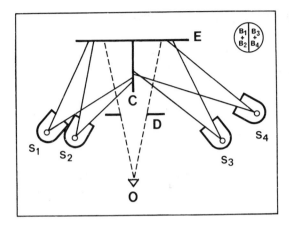

Figure 2.11
Diagram (schematic) of arrangements for light matching using different sources with different luminance values. See text. (From Le Grand 1964)

It is possible to demonstrate several essential facts with this arrangement. When monochromatic lights are mixed, the eye cannot distinguish the separate components in the resulting color. This observation has a general consequence in that, unlike the ear, the eye cannot separate the different components (e.g., of frequency) in a complex stimulus.

With an appropriate range of luminances and also completely different wavelengths, $B_1\lambda_1 + B_2\lambda_2$ on the one hand and $B_3\lambda_3 + B_4\lambda_4$ on the other, it is possible to match the two half-screens in *luminance* and in *color*. When such a match has been made, *Abney's law* (14) allows us to write:

$$B_1 + B_2 = B_3 + B_4. \tag{18}$$

However, given that not only the luminances of the two sides have been matched but also the colors, it must be true that a colorimetric relationship also applies, which we will distinguish by using an identity symbol:

$$B_1 + B_2 \equiv B_3 + B_4. \tag{18a}$$

The mixing of certain pairs of (monochromatic) colored lights can, provided that their luminances are appropriately adjusted, produce a new perception, one of *white light*. These two colors are then called *complementary*.

For every light (λ_1) outside the range 190 to 570 nm there exists a complementary (λ_2); see figure 2.16 (page 75). In contrast, all lights within that interval have no complementary color in the (monochromatic) visible spectrum but in the *purple*, which is not a spectrally pure color but one that can have a series of nuances from violet to red.

When the luminances B_1 and B_2 of two complementary colors (λ_1) and (λ_2) have been appropriately adjusted to give white, we can write:

$$B_1 + B_2 \equiv B_w, \tag{19}$$

where B_w is the luminance of the resultant white light.

If the luminances B_1 and B_2 of (λ_1) and (λ_2) have not been adjusted to an appropriate ratio we obtain a pastel color that is referred to as *unsaturated* (see below). By applying the additivity law we can write in this case:

$$B_1 + B_2 \equiv B_w + B_{2'}, \tag{20}$$

with $B_{2'}$ being the additional light needed in source (2) to give white.

To generalize, we can show that the addition of two colors λ_1 and λ_2, *whether they are complementary or not*, will produce a new nonsaturated color (λ_r) and:

$$B_1 + B_2 \equiv B_w + B_r, \tag{21}$$

where B_r is the luminance corresponding to a wavelength λ_r. This color λ_r will be intermediate between colors λ_1 and λ_2 if these are closer together in the spectrum than the complementaries; otherwise it will be either outside the interval or will correspond to one of the purples (a case we will not discuss here).

In this way the principle of the *trivariance* of color vision arises. The first part of the colorimetric equation has a variance of four, B_1, λ_1, B_2, λ_2, whereas the second has a variance three, B_r, λ_r, B_w.

This proposition is the more important since the equation can be generalized to a mixture of n colors. Grassmann's laws enunciate the additivity, multiplicativity, associativity, and transistivity of a mixture of colors and in the end one arrives at the conclusion that a mixture of any number i of colors λ_1, λ_2, . . . , λ_i is the equivalent of the addition of a flux B_w of white light to the flux B_r of a resultant color λ_r. This again becomes a matter of *three variables:*

$$\Sigma\, B_i\,(\lambda_i) \equiv B_w + B_r \tag{22}$$

All that we have just discussed relies on a theoretical standard white light (W), which is defined to have an equal energy at all wavelengths. This condition is in practice satisfied by a black body at a color temperature T_c, approximately 5200°K (see figure 2.4). Nevertheless the theory is still valid for lights as different as those from an incandescent lamp and from the blue sky.

The C.I.E. (Commission internationale de l'Éclairage) has defined three standards A, B, and C of white light. A: A tungsten filament lamp at 2850°K. B: The same lamp viewed through a filter made of specified solutions containing Cu and Co, representing a color temperature T_c of 4800°K. C: As B but filtered to be equivalent to a color temperature T_c of 6500°K. B is like sunlight and C like light from a thinly overcast sky.

A given color, instead of being defined by three quantities B_w, B_λ, and λ, can be specified by the dominant λ, by the total luminance of the mixture $B = B_w + B_\lambda$, and by a ratio called the *colorimetric purity* p, defined as:

$$p = B_\lambda/B \tag{23}$$

This factor equals 1 for a saturated monochromatic light and 0 for white light; it is counted negative for the purples (see figure 2.18). This definition of a color operates therefore with one luminosity variable and two chromatic variables.

Finally, we can say (e.g., from the well-known Newton's disk experiment) that a large number of colors mixed together eventually lead to white light.

DEFINITION OF A COLOR IN TERMS OF THREE PRIMARIES

Consider three monochromatic lights which we specify as *primaries* with wavelengths λ_1, λ_2, and λ_3. The problem is to determine to what extent it is possible—starting with these three colors—to effect a *trichromatic synthesis*, that is, to match any colored light according to quantitatively valid rules.

Consider the energy fluxes Φ of these primaries; their corresponding chromatic luminous fluxes F are given by:

$$F_1 = K_0 \cdot V_1 \cdot \Phi_1,$$
$$F_2 = K_0 \cdot V_2 \cdot \Phi_2,$$
$$F_3 = K_0 \cdot V_3 \cdot \Phi_3,$$

with $K_0 = 663 \, \text{lm/W}$ and the V values being the coefficients of relative visibility of the primaries.

It is convenient for this discussion not to use the absolute energy fluxes (Φ) but to relate the fluxes to three arbitrarily chosen units (Φ′)

called *primary energy units*, chosen so that the coefficients of visibility are automatically eliminated and the fluxes are expressed as relative quantities. The values of these ratios are, respectively:

$$\Gamma_1 = (\Phi)_1/(\Phi')_1,$$
$$\Gamma_2 = (\Phi)_2/(\Phi')_2, \qquad (24)$$
$$\Gamma_3 = (\Phi)_3/(\Phi')_3,$$

and are called the *chromatic fluxes of the primaries*.

Luminous flux can be introduced in expressions such as:

$$\Gamma_1 = F_1/L_1,$$
$$\Gamma_2 = F_2/L_2, \qquad (25)$$
$$\Gamma_3 = F_3/L_3,$$

where L_1, L_2, and L_3 are the *reference luminous fluxes* of the primaries defined by the equations:

$$L_i = K_0 \cdot V_i \cdot \Phi'_i$$

with $i = 1$, 2, and 3.

We can now introduce an alternative formulation for visual trivariance.

Let the three primary wavelengths be λ_1, λ_2, and λ_3. There are two cases to consider when one examines the addition of the three fluxes (see equation [21] above) according to the position of the extremes λ_1 and λ_3 in the spectrum: First, λ_1 and λ_3 are closer than the complimentaries, when the colorimetric equation can be written:

$$\Gamma_1 + \Gamma_3 \equiv \Gamma_2 + \Gamma_w, \qquad (26)$$

or

$$\Gamma_1 + \Gamma_3 - \Gamma_3 \equiv \Gamma_w, \qquad (26a)$$

since the matching of them to an intermediate wavelength (which λ_2 is by definition) is possible. In this equation Γ_w is a flux of white light.

Second, λ_1 and λ_3 are further apart than the complimentaries. In this case the color resulting from their admixture (see equation [21] again) is outside the range $\lambda_1 \rightarrow \lambda_3$ ($<\lambda_1$ or $>\lambda_3$ or purple). Thus the adjustment for white has to be made not with respect to λ_2 but with respect to its complimentary λ_r as in equation (19):

$$\Gamma_r + \Gamma_2 = \Gamma'_w \qquad (27)$$

It is easy to see that this time we must write:

$$\Gamma_1 + \Gamma_2 + \Gamma_3 \equiv \Gamma''_w. \tag{27a}$$

In summary, on condition that the possibility of taking negative fluxes into consideration is accepted, *the perception of white light can be achieved by an algebraic sum of three monochromatic primary fluxes* and the two equations share the common form therefore:

$$\Gamma_1 + \Gamma_2 + \Gamma_3 \equiv \Gamma_w. \tag{28}$$

Now consider monochromatic light of whatever wavelength λ. One can always achieve a white of the same flux by using a new flux combination of the colors λ_1, λ_2, and λ_3. Equation (28) remains true so that:

$$\Gamma'_1 + \Gamma'_2 + \Gamma_\lambda \equiv \Gamma_w. \tag{29}$$

Rearranging Grassmann's law allows us to rewrite each component thus:

$$\Gamma_\lambda \equiv (\Gamma_1 - \Gamma'_1) + (\Gamma_2 - \Gamma'_2) + \Gamma_3, \tag{30}$$

which shows that a *monochromatic light of whatever wavelength can be reproduced by the algebraic sum of three appropriate fluxes of primaries.*

Consider any light S. It can be regarded as a sum of monochromatic lights, and adding these equations according to Grassmann's law we finally have:

$$\Gamma_s \equiv \Gamma_1 + \Gamma_2 + \Gamma_3. \tag{31}$$

Every light S will have a luminous characteristic L_s expressed by the ratio between the luminous flux and the corresponding chromatic flux of that light:

$$L_s = F_s / \Gamma_s$$

and

$$\Gamma_s = F_s / L_s$$

The Abney law allows us to write

$$F_s = F_1 + F_2 + F_3$$

and therefore

$$L_s\Gamma_s = L_1\Gamma_1 + L_2\Gamma_2 + L_3\Gamma_3$$

which (as equation [25] above) gives:

$$L_s = L_1(\Gamma_1/\Gamma_s) + L_2(\Gamma_2/\Gamma_s) + L_3(\Gamma_3/\Gamma_s). \tag{32}$$

Note the following:

• It is important to understand, from the use of the terms "algebraic sum" and "negative flux," that this trichromatic synthesis does not apply in the general case to a projection screen with λ_1, λ_2, and λ_3 in one half and λ in the other but rather with λ_1 and λ_2 in one half and λ_3 and λ in the other; matching will not necessarily be possible except under these conditions.
• If the resultant light flux in question is not *saturated* monochromatic radiation (i.e., if $\Gamma_\lambda = \Gamma'_\lambda + \Gamma_w$), a *true trichromatic match*, that is, by the addition of three positive fluxes on the same screen, may or may not be possible.
• The choice of primaries is arbitrary, but for convenience in calculation it is sensible to adopt three different wavelengths as distant as possible from each other; in practice they are chosen to be in the red (R), green (G), and blue (B).

3.2 SPATIAL (GRAPHIC) REPRESENTATION OF COLORS

The above facts enable us to define a whole series of procedures for specifying spectral colors in a two-dimensional graphic color space, the object being to represent a given color as a mixture of parameters referring to the primaries. This task, very much peripheral to our major interests here, will only be discussed superficially and limited to two or three factors.

TRICHROMATIC COORDINATES: THE COLOR TRIANGLE

Consider a light of any color whatever. The problem in practical colorimetry is to define, in relative values, the three chromatic fluxes Γ_1, Γ_2, and Γ_3 of the primaries that match it. To this end we define three numbers γ_i, proportional to Γ_i for which the sum is equal to unity. This leads to:

$$\gamma_1 + \gamma_2 + \gamma_3 = 1, \tag{33}$$

and, from equation (31):

$$\gamma_1/\Gamma_1 = \gamma_2/\Gamma_2 = \gamma_3/\Gamma_3 = 1/(\Gamma_1 + \Gamma_2 + \Gamma_3) = 1/\Gamma_s$$

that is,

$$\gamma_i = \Gamma_i/\Gamma_s \tag{34}$$

These numbers are called *trichromatic coordinates* or *trichromatic coefficients* (figure 2.12).

Any light can be defined under these conditions by two of these coordinates, the other being deduced from equation (33). Also, from equation (32), we can specify its luminosity factor L_s as:

$$L_s = L_1\gamma_1 + L_2\gamma_2 + L_3\gamma_3. \tag{35}$$

From this one can imagine a variety of representations of these three values in one plane to represent a light by its trichromatic coordinates. For example, *Maxwell's color triangle* is an equilateral triangle p_1, p_2, p_3, the height of which is taken as a unit of length and the γ_i values as the distances of the characterizing point M from its three sides: $\gamma_i = MN_i$ (knowing that the sum of the MN_i in such a triangle is equal to the height). The corners of the triangle represent the primaries. Unfortunately, this representation is not very convenient and it is preferable to use the *chromatic coordinates* of Wright, which exploit an isosceles right-angled triangle in which the coordinates γ_1 and γ_2 are taken as abscissa and ordinate (c_1, c_2 in figure 2.12) and the coordinate γ_3 is deduced from equation (33).

DISTRIBUTION COEFFICIENTS

Suppose that for *each monochromatic light* λ in the spectrum, the corresponding trichromatic coordinates $\gamma_{1\lambda}$, $\gamma_{2\lambda}$, and $\gamma_{3\lambda}$ had been determined experimentally. Consider a uniform source of light S defined by its spectral energy distribution $E_\lambda = f(\lambda)$. How can we represent the coordinates of this source in a graphic spatial representation of color?

Accepting that $\Gamma_s = \Gamma_1 + \Gamma_2 + \Gamma_3$, the problem becomes to determine the flux Γ_i, knowing E_λ and $\gamma_{1\lambda}$, $\gamma_{2\lambda}$, and $\gamma_{3\lambda}$. Calculation, which we will not present here, leads to three expressions of the form:

$$\Gamma_1 = \Sigma(\alpha \cdot \gamma_1 \cdot V_\lambda \cdot E_1 \cdot \delta\lambda)/L_1 \cdot \gamma_{1\lambda} + L_2 \cdot \gamma_{2\lambda} + L_3\gamma_{3\lambda} \tag{36}$$

where α is a constant factor depending on the physical nature of E_λ; V_λ is the luminosity factor already defined above for light of the wavelength λ; $\delta\lambda$ is the elementary wavelength interval; L_1, L_2, and L_3 are the luminance factors corresponding to the three primaries from which one can write, as in equation (35), the luminance factor for the wavelength λ as $L_1 \cdot \gamma_{1\lambda} + L_2 \cdot \gamma_{2\lambda} + L_3\gamma_{3\lambda}$.

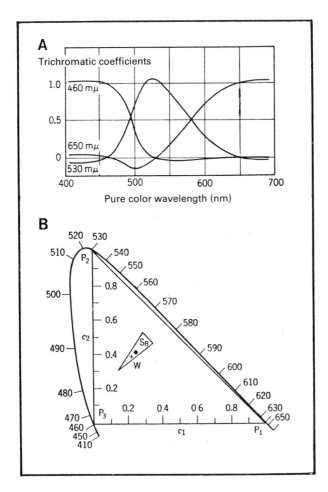

Figure 2.12
Trichromatic coordinates and Wright's color chart. (*A*) Mean trichromatic coordinates for 10 subjects: $\gamma_1 = 650$ nm; $\gamma_2 = 530$ nm; $\gamma_3 = 460$ nm. The curves cut the axes at the position of the primaries. As any one coefficient passes through the value 1, the two others pass through zero. (*B*) Wright's color chart constructed from the above data. At the center, scatter of the white, *W*, value for 36 subjects. (From Le Grand 1964)

To simplify all of this we introduce new magnitudes called *distribution coefficients* defined by three expressions of the form

$$\bar{\gamma}_1 = (\gamma_{1\lambda} \cdot V_\lambda)/(L_1 \cdot \gamma_{1\lambda} + L_2 \cdot \gamma_{2\lambda} + L_3 \cdot \gamma_{3\lambda}). \tag{37}$$

Determination of the chromatic fluxes constituting the light S thus becomes the three summations of:

$$\Gamma_i = \Sigma\, \alpha \bar{\gamma}_i \cdot E_\lambda \cdot \delta\lambda, \tag{38}$$

the trichromatic coordinates being deduced using equation (34). *Note:* The distribution coefficients $\bar{\gamma}_1$, $\bar{\gamma}_2$, $\bar{\gamma}_3$ are numbers proportional to the chromatic fluxes, like the chromatic coordinates. However, their sum is not unity but they obey the following equation (from equation [35]):

$$L_1 \cdot \bar{\gamma}_1 + L_2 \cdot \bar{\gamma}_2 + L_3 \cdot \bar{\gamma}_3 = V_\lambda \tag{39}$$

Rigorously, Γ_1, Γ_2, and Γ_3 should be integrals:

$$\Gamma_i = \alpha \int \bar{\gamma}_i \cdot E_\lambda \cdot d\lambda.$$

In practice, measurements in a limited number of spectral "bins" are made, thus reverting to equation (38) above.

PRACTICAL PROCEDURES

From the above it is clear that the basic need is to determine experimentally the trichromatic coordinates for every monochromatic spectral light. The distribution coefficients can be deduced from these if the relative visibility functions are known and this then provides the solution for specifying lights of whatever spectral composition.

We will not describe all the methods used in detail but rather point out the steps involved: (1) the choice of the primaries λ_1, λ_2, and λ_3; (2) the determination of the trichromatic coordinates γ_1, γ_2, and γ_3 for pure colors (essentially for every 10 nm spectral interval); (3) the evaluation of the relative luminance factors for the primaries L_1, L_2, and L_3; (4) calculation of the distribution coefficients, taking into account the relative visibility function V_λ (for the average subject). In practice (based on the work of Maxwell, Wright, and Guild, among others), this consists essentially in matching two fields, one formed by the three chosen primaries and the other by the monochromatic light that is being studied, to which we may add one of the primaries (negative flux).

Another basic factor concerns the choice of primaries. As we have said, this is essentially arbitrary, but as we shall see, certain selections can lead to more convenient answers than others. The main point is that because of the linear nature of the relationships that are applicable in colorimetry, transformation from one system of primaries to another can be resolved by a series of linear equations relating the one set of chromatic fluxes to the other:

$$\Gamma'_i = \Sigma_j \, a_{ij} \cdot \Gamma_j.$$

THE RGB AND XYZ SYSTEMS

We will now briefly discuss two systems of representation that have been used in recent times. These different spatial plots of color, derived from each other are based on numerical data obtained from measurements on what is customarily defined as a *standard observer* as specified by the Commission Internationale de L'Éclairage (values adopted in 1939).

One system that more or less chose itself is based on three monochromatic primaries found in the mercury discharge (whence their choice) and situated at red **R** (700 nm), green **G** (546.1 nm) and blue-violet **B** (453.8 nm). This is the RGB system (figure 2.13). Thus the quantities determined for this system are: the trichromatic coordinates, typically r, g, b; and the luminance factors for the three primaries (on the condition that a certain white light source *W* for which E_λ is constant throughout the spectrum will fall at the center of the diagram). Thus it is found that: $L_r = 1$; $L_g = 4.5907$; $L_b = 0.0601$. Following the above, the distribution coefficients need to be determined.

From this, the specification of a pure color can be determined completely. Thus, for example, to obtain a light matching 500 nm, the respective values of the chromatic fluxes for r, g, and b (given by tables) are -1.1685, 1, and 0.7780; the luminous fluxes (*F*) comprising it are therefore, from equation (35), respectively, F_r: -1.1685; F_g: $1.3905 \times 5.5907 = 6.3834$; F_b: $0.7780 \times 0.0601 = 0.0467$.

Figure 2.13 shows the standard chromatic diagram for the RGB system. Each primary is situated at the corners of a right-angled isosceles color triangle. All real stimuli are situated within the hatched area. The monochromatic colors extend around the border of the diagram (*spectral locus*), whereas a complex light and *a fortiori* white light (*W*) are situated within the boundary. Finally, we may, some-

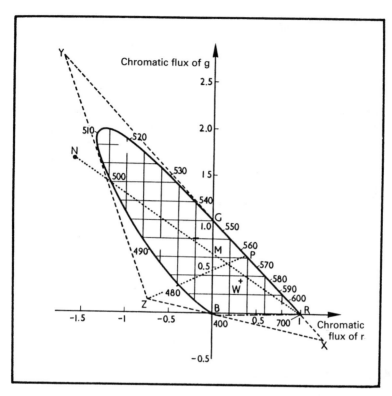

Figure 2.13
The CIE RGB color chart. Point W represents the uniform spectral energy white. The points X, Y, and Z are imaginary stimuli. The line XZ is the line for zero luminosity. See text. (From Le Grand 1964)

what theoretically draw in this diagram a straight line on which are sited all "nil luminosity stimuli" $L_s = 0$. Thus, the equation for this line is $L_r \cdot r + L_g \cdot g + L_b \cdot b = 0$, and it is found that this is satisfied by $0.93\ r + 4.53\ g + 0.06 = 0$. In practice this line passes close to scarcely visible colors like dark red and deep violet.

However, it has become clear that this system has some practical disadvantages. First, because of the choice of primaries, one of the trichromatic coordinates is always negative for monochromatic lights, which inconveniences calculations, and second, because there is a risk of attributing a physiological significance to primaries called red, green, and blue which, since their choice was arbitrary, is not necessarily true. Therefore, another system of precise color specification has been devised that is called the *international XYZ system*, based on the following rules (figure 2.14):

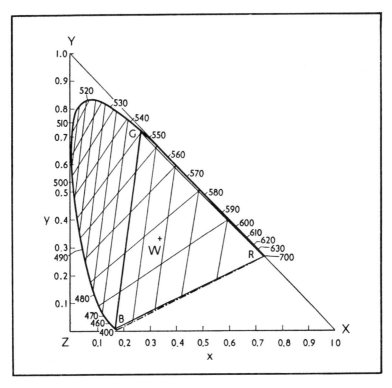

Figure 2.14
The XYZ color chart. The meaning of points R, G, B, and W is explained in the text.
(From Marriott 1962)

• Each of the primaries is not a pure color but a linear mixture of the monochromatic lights **R, G,** and **B**: $X = a\mathbf{R} + b\mathbf{G} + c\mathbf{B}$ and similarly for Y and Z.

• The points representing the primaries X and Z are on the "line of nil luminosity," that is, the chromatic fluxes of X and Z correspond to zero luminous flux ($L_x = L_z = 0$).

• The luminance unit $L_Y = 1$ lm.

• The sides XY and YZ of the triangle of primaries are tangent to the monochromatic spectral contour, XY in the extreme red at 700 nm and YZ at a fixed point 504 nm.

• The white source W, with equal spectral energies, remains in the center of the new diagram.

In this system the following data are assembled starting from the **RGB** data and applying linear transformations:

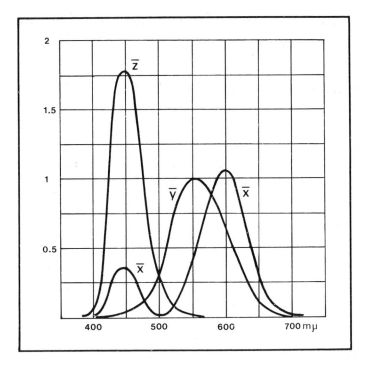

Figure 2.15
Distribution coefficients in the XYZ system. Ordinate: Quantities of the selected primary stimuli needed to match pure color of wavelength λ. Abscissa: wavelength λ (nm). (From Judd 1951)

- The three primaries X, Y, and Z starting from the **R, G, B** fluxes
- The trichromatic coordinates, here called x, y, and z and defined as above in equation (34):

$$x/X = y/Y = z/Z = 1/(X + Y + Z) \qquad (40)$$

- The distribution coefficients

$$\bar{x} = x/y{\cdot}V_\lambda,$$
$$\bar{y} = V_\lambda, \qquad (41)$$
$$\bar{z} = z/y{\cdot}V_\lambda.$$

However, as in figure 2.15, which shows the values of these coefficients, it will be noticed that in the x curve there is a (zero) minimum at 504 nm separating two bell-shaped peaks. This is not due to any special characteristic of the visual system but arises because in the color diagram, by an arbitrary choice, this wavelength is at the location of the tangent between the (monochromatic) spectral locus and the side YZ of the triangle (see above and figure 2.14 and 2.15).

PRACTICAL APPLICATION OF THE XYZ SYSTEM

There are a variety of applications for the XYZ system; here are a few examples.

Specification of Light Sources
A light source is characterized by its spectral distribution E_λ, which can be defined by the three chromatic fluxes that match it. These are calculated, as in equation (38) above:

$$X = \Sigma\ \alpha\cdot\bar{x}\cdot E_\lambda\cdot\delta\lambda,$$
$$Y = \Sigma\ \alpha\cdot\bar{y}\cdot E_\lambda\cdot\delta\lambda,$$
$$Z = \Sigma\ \alpha\cdot\bar{z}\cdot E_\lambda\cdot\delta\lambda.$$

The summation is carried out for all equal intervals $\delta\lambda$ throughout the whole visible spectrum (in fact for 79 intervals of 5 nm between 380 and 770 nm). The factor α that we have met before has a value depending on what is being measured. If E_λ represents an energy flux in the interval $\delta\lambda$, and X, Y, and Z are the chromatic fluxes, then α is equivalent to K_0 (see equation [15]). If, as is more often the case, E_λ is given in relative values, we can simplify matters by writing $\alpha\cdot\delta\lambda$ = 1 and the expressions become

$$X = \Sigma\ \bar{x}\cdot E_\lambda,$$
$$Y = \Sigma\ \bar{y}\cdot E_\lambda,$$
$$Z = \Sigma\ \bar{z}\cdot E_\lambda.$$

The magnitudes of X, Y, and Z no longer represent the fluxes but in fact their *relative* trichromatic component values, the *tristimulus values*. These tristimulus values allow the specification of any source, the spectral distribution of which is known and from which the trichromatic coordinates x, y, and z can be calculated according to equation (40) above.

For the white source **W** where E_λ = 1, we find that X = 21.36; Y = 21.37; Z = 21.35 and thus $x = y = z = 0.33$.

For a *black body*, the coordinates can be calculated for different $T°K$ and plotted on the XYZ color chart along a curve called the *black body locus* (figure 2.16). [A "black body" is a body or surface that absorbs all radiation falling upon it; it emits radiation with the wavelength of maximal emission decreasing as its temperature increases.]

We can proceed in the same way for the white light standards *A*,

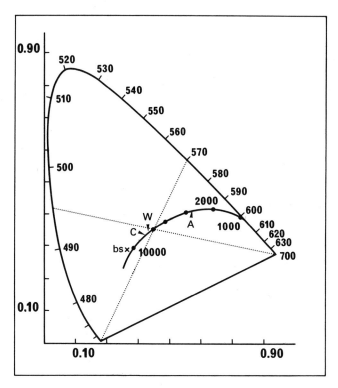

Figure 2.16
Position of various light sources in the CIE XYZ color chart. The standard light sources
A, C, and *W* are shown on the black body temperature curve together with that
corresponding to blue sky, b.s. Shown also is the existence region for complementary
colors: given a defined white, here *W,* complementary colors must lie on straight lines
through *W.* Thus only the regions 410 to 495 nm and 500 to 570 nm have complementary colors with one another (see dotted boundaries and figure 2.14). (From Le Grand
1964)

B, and *C* and on this one curve you can see the coordinates marked
for two of these standards (A: 2850°K, and C: 6740°K) and also for
W: 5500°K.

In the special case of pure colors, namely, those on the (monochromatic) spectral locus, we can evaluate *x, y,* and *z* by taking $E_\lambda = 1$
for the single wavelength under consideration and the value 0 for all
the others. Thus we can write:

$x = \bar{x}/(\bar{x} + \bar{y} + \bar{z})$,
$y = \bar{y}/(\bar{x} + \bar{y} + \bar{z})$,
$z = \bar{z}/(\bar{x} + \bar{y} + \bar{z})$,

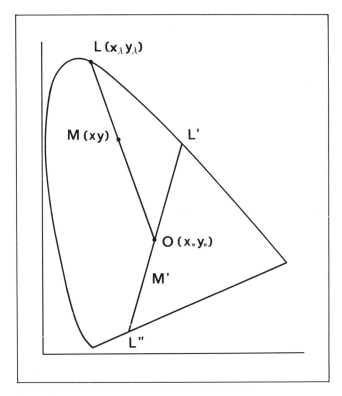

Figure 2.17
Definition of a dominant wavelength in a color. O represents the defined white light (x_0, Y_0) and M the color in question (x, y). The dominant wavelength is defined as L (x_λ, y_λ) such that all the points OML are aligned. M' is situated in the purple region. (From Le Grand 1964)

and in this way arrive at a curve upon which are represented the coordinates x and y for each λ, z being deduced of course from $[1 - (x + y)]$.

Complementary Colors
The complementary of a given color can easily be specified by extending the straight line joining λ to the reference white W until it reaches a point on the opposite boundary of the color chart. It can in fact be shown that for any two colors to be complementary with respect to a specific white light, then the points must be so aligned. We can easily see (figure 2.16) that having chosen the point W as a white light source, then only wavelengths outside the interval 495 to

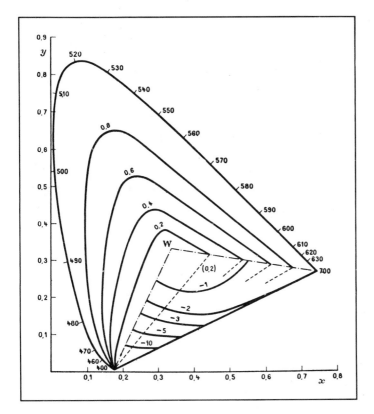

Figure 2.18
Contours of equal color purity factor, with W defining (white) achromatic light. (From Le Grand 1964)

---

570 nm have a spectral complementary; the wavelengths situated within this interval have their complementary in the purple.

The Dominant Wavelength and Color Purity
Instead of defining a source by its tristimulus values, we can specify a dominant wavelength λ_D and a certain *stimulus purity factor* p_e, where $p_e = OM/OL$ (figure 2.17), on condition that a standard reference white (e.g., light W) has been defined. [p_e must not be confused with the colorimetric purity $L/(L + L_w)$ that we have seen before. But in practice the use of one or other p factor allows a light to be specified (more simply than with the XYZ system) by its dominant wavelength and its saturation; see figure 2.18.]

Consider therefore (figure 2.17) the points M (x, y) representing the light source and $O(x_0, y_0)$ representing the coordinates of the standard white chosen. The dominant wavelength will be given by the point L, the intersection of the straight line OM with the XYZ boundary. The color will be the more and more saturated the closer M approaches L and is further from O.

THE COLORS OF OBJECTS

After these varied considerations concerning the color of lights we can discuss some interesting factors concerning the colors of objects. Consider an object illuminated by some particular incident light. It will absorb part of the light and reflect the rest. However, there are two ways that this can happen; by *specular* (i.e., directional) reflection and by *scattering* of light in all directions. In the first case the object appears shiny and glossy, and in the other case, matte.

Suppose an object is illuminated by an incident monochromatic light B_λ. To an observer it will have a luminance $B'_\lambda = \rho_\lambda \cdot B_\lambda$ with the reflection factor ρ_λ depending on λ. The factor ρ_λ is 1 for perfect diffusers and zero for surfaces that are perfectly black at this wavelength.

Suppose now that the incident illumination is from a complex source of the type $E_\lambda = f(\lambda)$. The color of the object will depend on the variation of the reflectance with wavelength, on the function $\rho_\lambda = f(\lambda)$, that is, on the relative reflections (and absorptions) in the various regions of the spectrum. Thus the spectral composition of the reflected light is given by expressions of the type $X + \Sigma \bar{x} \cdot E_\lambda \cdot \rho_\lambda \cdot \delta\lambda$ and similarly for Y and Z.

Again, in white light an object that scatters all visible radiation without absorption will appear white, whereas a black body will totally absorb all radiations.

A body will appear to be colored if it has a *selective absorption* in some dominant spectral range. We can estimate this for such an opaque body by calculating the total reflected flux:

$$F = 683 \Sigma \Phi_\lambda \cdot \rho_\lambda \cdot V_\lambda \cdot \delta\lambda.$$

We can show that if there is a dominant wavelength (called a *centroid*), we can write:

$$\lambda_c = 683 (\Sigma \Phi_\lambda \cdot \rho_\lambda \cdot V_\lambda \cdot \lambda \cdot \delta\lambda)/(\Sigma \Phi_\lambda \cdot \rho_\lambda \cdot V_\lambda \cdot \delta\lambda) \text{ nm.}$$

Essentially, a body will appear *red* if it absorbs the short wavelengths, *yellow* if it absorbs wavelengths up to about 530 nm, *green* if it selec-

Table 2.2 Physical units and colorimetric factors

Energy Units	
Radiant flux	Φ
Irradiance	$\mathcal{D}$
Radiant intensity	$\mathcal{J}$
Radiant emittance	ϵ
Radiance	$\mathcal{B}$
Spectral distribution	E_λ
Spectral transmittance	τ_λ
Spectral reflectance	ρ_λ
Luminosity Units	
Luminous flux	F
Illuminance	D
Luminous intensity	I
Luminous emittance	R
Luminance	B
Luminosity factor	V_λ
Luminous transmittance	τ
Luminous reflectance	ρ
Luminous efficiency	F/ϕ
Colorimetric Factors	
Primary stimulus	
Trichromatic coefficients	x, y, z
Distribution coefficients	$\bar{x}, \bar{y}, \bar{z}$
Tristimulus values	X, Y, Z
Dominant wavelength	
Subjective Attributes	
Brightness	
Luster	
Hue	
Saturation	

Partly after Yves Le Grand (1964). For subjective attributes see also chapter 3.

tively scatters light in the middle of the spectrum, and *blue* if it absorbs the long wavelengths.

Finally, depending how the substance absorbs and/or scatters light, the object will have a higher or lower luminosity (bright or dark) and its color will be more or less saturated (saturated or pastel). The two groups of variables luster and saturation, being more or less independent, lead to such distinctions as a "lively" or "strong" color; bright and saturated "pale"; bright but unsaturated "deep"; saturated and dark with "jet-" and "grey-" qualifying the appearance of a black color (see chapter 3).

COLOR FILTERS

A few words now on the opposite of reflection of light from opaque bodies, namely, the *transmission* of light through a color filter. A filter can be defined by its transmission factor τ_λ, which is wavelength dependent. In this way the resulting transmitted light will be modified in its composition according to expressions of the type:

$$X = \Sigma\, E_\lambda \cdot \bar{x} \cdot \tau_\lambda \cdot \delta\lambda,$$

and similarly for Y and Z. As with the reflecting objects just considered, the dominant color λ_c of a filter of transmission factor τ_λ can be expressed as:

$$\lambda_c = (\Sigma\, \Phi_\lambda \cdot \tau_\lambda \cdot V_\lambda \cdot \lambda \cdot \delta\lambda)/(\Sigma\, \Phi_\lambda \cdot \tau_\lambda \cdot V_\lambda \cdot \delta\lambda).$$

The major physical units and colorimetric factors that have dominated our discussion in this chapter are listed for reference in Table 2.2.

3

The Psychophysical Laws of Visual Sensation

This chapter discusses the basic laws of visual sensation that have been discovered by psychophysical experiments on human subjects. Certainly, it is not always easy to separate psychophysical studies in humans from neurophysiological investigations in animals, since the latter often follow as a direct consequence and elaboration of the former. That is why the present chapter contains, as an adjunct and sometimes necessarily, some of the data obtained from animals.

1 PROBLEMS CONCERNED WITH ABSOLUTE THRESHOLDS

1.1 ABSOLUTE THRESHOLDS THROUGHOUT THE SPECTRUM

The aim is to determine absolute visual detection thresholds between 400 and 700 nm. Experiments are made by using a narrow (1°) pencil of monochromatic light, projected as a brief stimulus (40 ms) either on the cones of the central fovea or on the periphery where rods predominate, notably in the perifoveal regions (at 8° to 10°). Examination of such curves (figure 3.1) illustrates the following (Bartley 1951; Pirenne 1962; Barlow & Mollon 1982): The absolute thresholds, expressed as (relative) log-light energies in either the foveal or peripheral retinal region, are minimal in the range 500 to 550 nm. At either side of the minimum, the sensitivity decreases and becomes relatively feeble at the extremes of the visible spectrum (deep red and violet). The absolute threshold in the perifoveal region is significantly lower than that in the fovea. At maximal sensitivity the difference is 2.5 log units. The deduction from this is that the sensitivity of the rods is greater than that of the cones. The wavelengths for maximal sensitivity also differ, being at 510 nm for the peripheral region where rods predominate and at 555 nm for the cones of the central foveal location.

The observer's perceptual impressions are also different in the two regions. A liminal peripheral stimulus is achromatic whatever its wavelengths, whereas the liminal foveal stimulus, as well as being perceived merely by its presence, is also preceived as colored. This

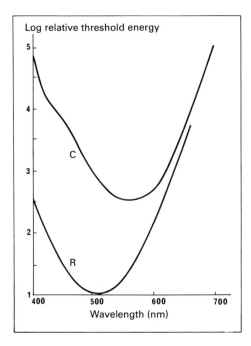

Figure 3.1
Spectral sensitivity curves for rod vision (R) and cone vision (C). The distance between the two curves is the photochromatic interval. (From Bartley 1951)

points to one of the fundmental facts of retinal physiology, which is that the quality of color is limited to cone (C) sensations, whereas the rods (R) only generate achromatic effects.

Determining the absolute threshold value systematically along a diameter of the retina passing through the fovea, using a briefly exposed narrow pencil of light as stimulus, also clearly confirms the variation of threshold with retinal position (figure 3.2). In photopic conditions the highest sensitivity is found in foveal regions. In contrast, in conditions of twilight vision, the lowest threshold is only obtained by fixation on a point at 10° to 15° eccentricity. [Naturally, the threshold so obtained goes to infinity if and when the chosen diameter crosses the blind spot.]

1.2 EFFECTS OF THE DURATION AND EXTENT OF THE STIMULUS

The absolute threshold varies with both the duration and the spatial area of the stimulus, according to well-defined laws that are to some extent homologous (see, e.g., Le Grand 1964; Barlett 1965).

EFFECTS OF DURATION

Bloch's law describes how, in humans, the duration of a given constant narrow-beam light stimulus affects its luminance threshold B_1.

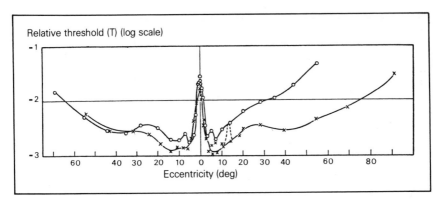

Figure 3.2
Spatial variation of the absolute threshold (T) for white light. The test field is 0.072°
diameter (4.3 min arc) presented for 0.05 s to a totally dark-adapted subject along a
meridional axis passing through the fovea. The two curves relate to two different
directions in which the measurements were made: crosses, along a staight line inclined
at 10° to the horizontal to avoid the blind spot; cicles, along the vertical meridan. (From
Pirenne and Marriott 1962)

This law, which owes much to the Bunsen-Roscoe laws of photochemistry, states that below a certain critical duration t_c the threshold
B_l depends on the time of exposure t according to the relationship
$B_l \cdot t$ = constant. In other words, for very brief exposures there is a
summation of the amount of light energy; the threshold decreases
with prolonged exposure, until a critical exposure time t_c is reached,
which according to the experimental conditions, in particular according to the type of receptor involved, ranges between 30 ms for
cones to 100 ms for rods. Thus, if $B_l \cdot t$ is plotted on the ordinate as
a function of t on the abscissa, the curve is, in this range, a straight
line parallel to the abscissa and, for $t >> t_c$, then becomes a straight
line at 45°, showing that B_l has then become independent of duration
(figure 3.3, top).

Discussions of this sort of research often envisage certain transitional stages, such as an intermediate duration range within which
B still depends on t but only partially, and enters a region governed
by a more complex relationship that continues to include a certain
duration dependence.

The results of the Blondel and Rey (1911) experiments are described
by

$$B_l \cdot t = B_\infty (t + t_0)$$

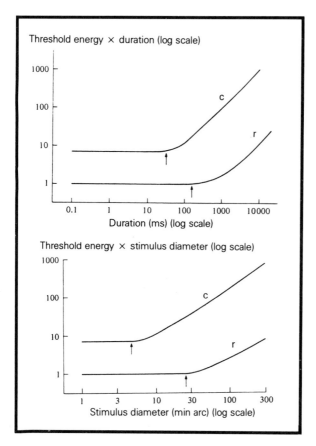

Figure 3.3
**Variation of the threshold luminance as a function of duration and extent of the
stimulus.** *Above,* Thresholds as a function of stimulus duration. In this experiment the
area of the stimulus is kept constant. *Below,* Thresholds as a function of stimulus area
for constant stimulus duration. Note that in each case the product of the liminal
stimulus by the independent variable (duration and diameter, respectively) is constant
up to a certain critical value (the summation time and the summation area, respectively, see arrows). r, rods; c, cones. (From Barlow & Mollon 1982)

where t_0 is a time constant characteristic of each subject and, depending on experimental conditions (notably whether peripheral or central vision), is in the region of 0.2 s. B_∞ is the threshold for long duration stimuli. This gives, for example, $B_1 = 3\,B_\infty$ for $t = 0.1$ s and 11 B_∞ for $t = 0.02$ s.

Other expressions have been proposed, for example, as a power law (Bt^n = constant) with $n = 2/3$ (Galifret & Piéron 1946). In any case, B becomes independent of duration beyond about 1000 ms.

EFFECTS OF STIMULUS AREA

When the area of a stimulus is increased for a constant duration, researchers have found essentially very similar results to those concerned with duration. A certain area, having a certain critical diameter δ_c, defines a limit below which for small visual angles the absolute threshold B_1 is related to the diameter δ by expressions of the form $B_1 \cdot \delta^n$ = constant.

In the fovea, it is agreed that Ricco's law applies, in which the exponent 1 is unity; thus B_1 is inversely proportional to δ and ($B_1 \cdot \delta$ = constant). This law applies for angles less than 5 minutes of arc (min arc). Beyond that n falls to zero, which corresponds in the case of wide stimuli to B_1 = constant (figure 3.3, bottom).

Here again there exists an intermediary zone of stimulus size (between approximately 7′ and 5°) for which n takes values between 0.3 and 0.5 (according to Piéron 1945): $B_1 \cdot \sqrt[3]{\delta}$ = constant.

In the peripheral retina another law was proposed by Piper with $n = 0.5$. In fact n decreases after 30′ and δ ceases to be a limiting factor beyond a few degrees.

The significance of these laws of temporal and spatial summation are evident in that they define the resolving powers of each of the two receptor systems. Clearly, also, these effects have found their parallel, at least in part, in the processes of neural interactions shown in either the retina or, depending on the particular effect, in the more central processing stages.

1.3 QUANTITATIVE MEASUREMENTS OF ABSOLUTE THRESHOLDS

Over the years, numerous investigations have been devoted to the quantitative measurement of absolute thresholds in the most favorable conditions, that is, for perifoveal vision (around 10°) and after maximal dark adaptation. Given how remarkably small the values obtained are (in luminosity units or energy units), it becomes absolutely necessary to consider these energies in terms of light quanta.

PRINCIPLES OF EXPERIMENTATION

Let us first examine the questions arising in measuring a *threshold*. The problem is a quantitative one: What is the minimum energy, in terms of absolute energy units, necessary for a stimulus to be seen? The variety of methods employed has led to results that have been presented differently depending on the type of measurement used. The following experimental arrangements have been used:

• A large visual field is illuminated for relatively long times, say several seconds. In these experiments the eyes are allowed to wander freely within the field. The method allows a figure for the *absolute threshold retinal illumination* to be calculated.
• Alternatively, a field of very small solid angle is presented, again with a long exposure. The gaze is again left free and the measurement is generally made in peripheral vision. In this case the threshold is made in terms of *minimal total radiant flux.*
• A very small angle field is presented for a very short time (10^{-3} s). In this case the eye clearly cannot have moved significantly during the exposure. When the measurements are made in the most sensitive part of the retina, the result specifies the *minimal (absolute) energy* needed to stimulate the retinal receptors.

These experiments need to incorporate carefully selected controls. One of these consists in applying different stimuli randomly at various light intensities. The subject is generally obliged to make some "forced choice" response (yes or no, sometimes including perhaps). The threshold is generally taken as the value that gives 55% to 60% positive answers on the sigmoid curve that describes the probability of response as a function of light intensity (Barlow 1956). [One might be tempted to select not 55% or 60% but 50%. In fact, the choice is made on the theoretical basis that the sigmoid obtained is not symmetrical with respect to the 50% level. It is a question of its being a Poisson function in which the most significant point is, practically and for the type of curve obtained in experiments, that which corresponds precisely with 55% positive responses.]

EXPERIMENTAL VALUES FOR THE ABSOLUTE THRESHOLD

Let us examine some representative values found by each of the methods just outlined (see, in particular, Pirenne 1962).

Minimal Retinal Illumination
A certain number of studies have been made in white light; the mean value of the just-perceptible luminance in a large area visual field is equal to $0.75 \cdot 10^{-6}$ cd $\cdot$ m^{-2}.
We can recalculate this luminance, given the energy units of white light, into that for a given wavelength, normally 507 nm, as:

$B = 5.08 \cdot 10^{-7}$ erg $\cdot$ s$^{-1} \cdot$ sr$^{-1} \cdot$ cm^{-2},

which (by exploiting the formula $D = 0.36 \cdot \tau \cdot S \cdot B$ where $\tau = 0.5$ and $S = 0.5$ cm^2) corresponds to a retinal illumination (in energy units) of:

$D = 0.45 \cdot 10^{-7}$ erg $\cdot$ s$^{-1} \cdot$ sr$^{-1} \cdot$ cm^{-2}

or

$D = 0.45 \cdot 10^{-14} = $ W $\cdot$ cm^{-2}.

Minimal Energy Flux
For extrafoveal vision of white light the mean value is $4 \cdot 10^{-9}$ lm $\cdot$ m^{-2}. From this remarkably small value it can be deduced that during conditions of maximal atmospheric transparency a source of 1 cd can be seen at a distance of 16 km (in dark adaptation).

Minimal (Absolute) Light Energy
For this sort of study, the viewing conditions for maximal retinal sensitivity need to be arranged: dark-adapted subjects, light of 510 nm, projected at 15° to 20° eccentricity on the retina (the place of maximal retinal sensitivity). Using a flash avoids any effects of temporal summation (*duration laws*) as well as of any significant eye movement. By exploiting a small solid angle stimulus (10 min arc) effects of spatial summation are also circumvented. Under these conditions, magnitudes of around 2 to 6 $\cdot$ 10^{-10} erg are obtained.
     In this way it becomes clear that the system can be activated by an extremely small amount of energy and, remembering the particulate nature of light stimuli, numerous researches have been designed to determine the minimal number of quanta needed to excite the rods.

PROBLEMS IN DETERMINING MINIMAL NUMBERS OF QUANTA

The Case of Total Retinal Illumination
Recall that in this case the stimulus is wide and long lasting and is thus not confined either spatially or temporally. At 507 nm, as we

have seen, the liminal power reaching the eye is 0.45 erg $\cdot$ s^{-1}. The energy of a 570-nm quantum being $hv = 3.92 \cdot 10^{-12}$ erg, we can estimate the effective number of quanta. To this end it is also necessary to take into account an extra factor f, which describes the amount of light reaching the retina that is effectively absorbed by rhodopsin. Using an estimate of 0.2, this leads to a number of quanta absorbed by all the rods of 2300 s$^{-1} \cdot$ cm^{-2}. Since the density of the rods is $13.4 \cdot 10^6 \cdot$ cm^{-2} at this eccentricity, we arrive at the conclusion that on the average one quantum is absorbed in a population of 5800 rods per second or, in other words, on the average each rod absorbs a quantum every 5800 s (100 minutes!) or that $1.72 \cdot 10^{-4}$ quanta are absorbed per rod per second. Given the indivisibility of a quantum, this also means that, at the 50% threshold, less than 0.3% of the rods can have been affected by light during a 15 s exposure and that 97.7% are not.

Again, as we shall see below, apparently a single quantal absorption does not suffice for a visual effect. The wide field will therefore only be perceived when a finite number of quanta have been absorbed by a receptor unit within the limits of temporal and spatial summation. It is generally considered that a receptive *unit* at this eccentricity must contain about 11,000 rods, with a possible summation time of 0.1 s. In other words, the field will be seen only if the several quanta fall on the same spatial receptive field (*summation pool*) within a short time, ≤ 0.1 s (the *summation time*). However, this method of wide area stimuli does not lend itself very well to more detailed estimates of the quantal excitation threshold of the rods.

Methods Using Narrow-Beam, Short-Duration Stimuli
In this case, having taken all necessary precautions (see above), we find a range of thresholds quoted between 2 to $6 \cdot 10^{-10}$ erg at 510 nm, 54 to 148 quanta. These estimates need to be qualified as above by the two coefficients τ_λ and f_λ, the one related to absorption in the transparent eye media and the other to the fact that only part of the light entering the eye activates the rods. After these corrections, values of 9 to 14 quanta are obtained for the light intensity corresponding to 55% positive responses.

Then estimating, as above, the number of rods r likely to have been affected by these quanta, we arrive at a figure of around 500. From these data it is possible to make a few statistical hypotheses.

First, we might ask whether a given receptor in the 500 might absorb more than one (i.e., at least 2) quanta. We can estimate that if a number a represents the mean number of quanta absorbed, the probability that a single rod must absorb at least two quanta, $a(a-1)/2r$, is about 10% for $a = 10$ and $r = 500$, a figure that is much less than the fixed threshold of 55%. In contrast, the probability that different rods will absorb a total of 9 to 14 quanta is very high.

In other words, (1) any single rod is capable of excitation by effectively absorbing one quantum, (2) the absorption of two or more quanta by a rod is not a *necessary* condition for reaching threshold, but (3) the absorption of a single quantum is not a *sufficient* condition for attaining threshold.

We are still confronted with the problem of specifying an exact quantal number for effective stimulation, it being understood that we only know the total number a. In other words, we are in the classic position of trying to determine the probability of an event happening when the total mean number of events is very small. Thus given a number a the probability that x quanta will be effectively absorbed simultaneously will be given by the term in the Poisson function:

$$\pi_x = (e^{-a} a^x)/x!$$

Postulating the simplest case that the signal will always give rise to perception if $x \geq n$ and never if $x < n$, where n is considered to be the true threshold, then the probability that at least n quanta will be absorbed by the retina is the sum of the probabilities for $x = n$, $x = n + 1$, $x = n + 2$, etc. This is a matter of the Poisson summation $p_n = \Sigma_{x=n}^{\infty} \pi_x$ that can also be written

$$p_n = 1 - \sum_{x=0}^{n-1} \pi_x,$$

or as

$$p_n = 1 - e^{-a}\{1 + a + a^2/2! + a^3/3! + \ldots + a^{n-1}/(n-1)!\}.$$

A selection of Poisson curves for $p = f(\log a)$ can thus be drawn for various values of the parameters n, the threshold for seeing. The curves comprise a family in which each curve has a different slope, depending on n. For each value of n the slope is maximal at a certain point corresponding to $a = n$ (figure 3.4).

To these maximal slopes there can be assigned a representative probability ranging between $p = 63.2\%$ for $n = 1$ to $p = 52.7\%$ for

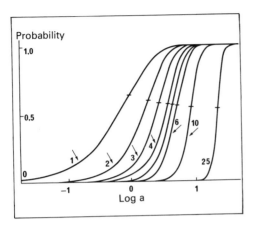

Figure 3.4
Family of curves of the summed probability (Poisson integrals) that a stimulus will contain *n* quanta if *a* is the average number of quanta acting on the retina. The curves are drawn for different values of *n* between 1 and 10 and for *n* = 25. The point *a* = *n* is marked on each curve: This corresponds to a probability of 63.2% for *n* = 1 to 52.7% for *n* = 25. (From Pirenne and Marriott 1962)

n = 25. In practice, in the range that concerns us (*n* between 5 and 10), it is near 55%; thus 55% is used in practical threshold estimation (Pirenne 1962).

We are now in a position to start considering the experimental data, using the results from subjects stimulated under the conditions defined above. Curves are drawn of the %*p* for positive perception of the energy content of the stimulus, expressed as quanta incident on the retina (figure 3.5). These experimental curves for *p* = log *a* have a certain slope that can be compared with the theoretical curves by translation along the x axis. This comparison (justified since the coordinates have the same dimensions) finally led to the conclusion (Hecht et al. 1942) that the actual number of effective quanta is 5, 6, 7, or 8. There is thus some disagreement between the calculated values and the experimental data when using this ingenious method. The disagreements have a variety of origins.

Some authors, including Barlow (1956), have emphasized that the curve which serves as the reference to estimate the number of quanta may not in fact correspond with the Poisson integral of quantal events. In fact, the intervention of factors peculiar to the subject are far from being excluded. The positions of response probability curves can differ depending on whether forced choice criteria ("seen or not

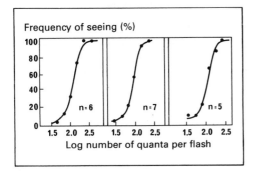

Figure 3.5
Frequency-of-seeing curves for a light flash as a function of its luminous energy (number of quanta ($h\nu$) incident on the cornea). Fifty estimates for each point on three subjects. Stimulus diameter: 10 min arc, presented 20° peripheral, duration 1 ms, wavelength 510 nm. The curves correspond to Poisson sums for $n = 5, 6,$ and 7. (From Pirenne and Marriott 1962)

seen") have been used or whether the possibility of answering "probably seen" is introduced (figure 3.6).

The curves are clearly different, the probability being greater for a given mean intensity (abscissa) if the third possible reply is included. But they are parallel and with a less steep slope than the theoretical curve calculated with only the quantal catch as a factor. Therefore we must, for the want of better knowledge, estimate that the real number of necessary quanta will be a little greater than that predicted by the experimental curves.

Discussion of this problem has also led to comparing the probability curves for one eye, for the other, and for the two together. It is interesting to note that the binocular absolute threshold is lowered by 0.1 log unit, a factor of 1.6, with respect to the monocular, for the same probability of seeing. This value is quite close to that to be expected if the two eyes belonged to different individuals; this probability is calculated from the probability of seeing the stimulus with one eye, of seeing it with the other, and of seeing with both eyes without any interaction between them, whether summatory or inhibitory. In that case the probability is 75%.

Another aspect of the same question concerns the case of several narrow-beam stimuli striking the retina simultaneously. The effects differ according to the separation of the visual fields of the stimuli.

Consider k adjacent localized fields, each narrow-beam (0.1°), with a total spread of 1°. The threshold is found to be reduced by a factor

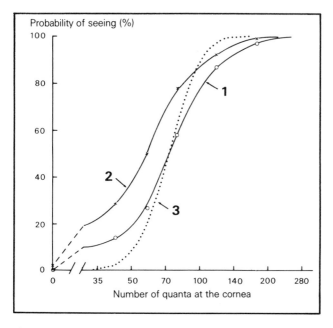

Figure 3.6
Absolute human threshold of perception. Subject observes flashes of five different intensities in random order. The total number of stimuli in each class is 100; in addition, 300 "blank" stimuli of zero intensity are delivered. The subject is asked to report "seen" or "not seen," or in addition "perhaps seen." Curve 1. Open circles, frequency of seeing when answers confined to "seen" and "not seen"; Curve 2. crosses, when "perhaps seen" allowed also. Note that the second arrangement lowers the threshold (defined as 50% seen) from 73 to 50 quanta. This number corresponds to about 15 photoisomerations. The calculated frequency-of-seeing curve (dotted) for a probability of absorption of 15 quanta or more (assuming a "seen"/"not seen" method is used) is steeper than the experimental curve and implies a lower variability than the real curves. Therefore extra sources of variability must exist. (From Barlow & Mollon 1982)

k. A physiological summation by neuronal facilitatory interaction between the adjacent fields is the most likely explanation.

However, if the fields are separated more widely, for instance, by 3°, the probability of seeing is again increased, but by a smaller factor. It becomes the *summation of the probabilities of individual, separated events.* In this case, for two spots, as above in considering two eyes, the probability will be 75%. [Let 0.5 be the probability of seeing one patch (A) and 0.5 the probability of seeing another (B). The probability of seeing something will be that of seeing A, or B, or A and B. The probability of not seeing A is $(1-0.5)$, of not seeing B is $(1-0.5)$ also. The probability of not seeing either A or B will be $(1-0.5)^2 =$

0.25. Thus the probability of seeing something will be $(1-0.25) = 0.75.$]

Between these extremes, at intermediate stimulus separations, the stimuli will demonstrate an improvement in the threshold probability of seeing intermediate between that appropriate for mutual interactions and that characteristic of a combination of independent probabilities.

[In brief, it was tempting to treat the retina as a system comprising a large number of independent units and on this basis some authors (Bouman 1955) constructed a "two quanta" theory. We will not go into detail but the main ideas were that the peripheral retina is made up from independent functional units of about 10 min arc diameter. Each of these needs two quanta to be excited and vision takes place when at least one of them is so excited. This theory encounters a whole series of objections that we have no space to embark upon here.]

All the factors just discussed are concerned with rod mechanisms in peripheral vision. The equivalent situation for cone vision is somewhat more complicated. Essentially, it seems that the probability curves for the fovea are steeper, corresponding therefore to a greater number of quanta being needed for vision. In addition, the values are varied, depending on the researcher. Thus Marriott (1959) found that $n = 8$ to 10 for a red field with 0.1-s exposure and central fixation. However, Pinegin (1958), using a field of 1 min arc, found $n = 15$ for central vision compared with $n = 8$ for peripheral vision; and for a 22' field found 31 at the central and 12 in the periphery.

Such studies on the quantal nature of liminal visual perception have given rise to quite a series of investigations at the level of single receptors and their liminal excitation mechanisms. These will be discussed later.

2 ADAPTATION IN THE RETINA

The retinal receptors are subject to modifications in their absolute threshold that are linked to ambient light conditions or to previous light exposure. When a subject moves from a bright environment and suddenly enters a darkened room, it takes several minutes before he or she can see objects with low luminance. On the other hand, a subject who moves from a dim room to a bright environment is at first dazzled but after a short interval can once more appreciate visual contrasts in the environment.

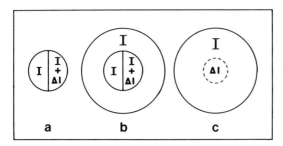

Figure 3.7
Different experimental arrangements for studying detectability of light intensity changes (ΔI) at suprathreshold intensity levels (I). (From Pirenne and Marriott 1962)

These common experiences show two retinal adaptation phenomena that have quite different time courses: *dark adaptation*, which is a slow and progressive lowering of visual thresholds as a function of the time spent in the dark, and *light adaptation*, which is a very rapid increase in thresholds when the general level of ambient light rises. This rapid increase in light adaptation is to some extent like any classic receptor adaptation, whereas the slower dark adaptation, as we shall see later, is related to the rate of regeneration of visual pigments, particularly of rhodopsin, in the dark.

2.1 LIGHT ADAPTATION

To analyze how retinal sensitivity varies with the ambient illumination, *I*, requires measuring the differential threshold, δ*I*, as a function of one of two controlling parameters: the baseline intensity level *I* and the time for which the subject has been exposed to that level of illumination. In other words, the experimental arrangements are very like those used for measuring differential intensity thresholds (Pirenne 1962; Barlett 1965; Barlow 1972). Various experimental arrangements are suited to these studies, and figure 3.7 shows some of the most frequently used.

EFFECT OF INTENSITY IN LIGHT ADAPTATION

The fact that the visual contrasts within an object and its general appearance remain rather constant in spite of changes in the luminance level (within wide limits up to 10 log units) is well explained by studying how differential thresholds vary with ambient illumination. Figure 3.8 shows the results of an experiment in which, for various baseline illumination values *I* presented as a parameter 20° field, de-

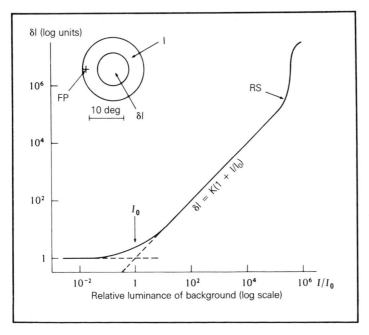

Figure 3.8
Effect of background illumination on the detection of a superimposed stimulus. The subject's fixation point (F.P.) is the cross *(inset, upper left)* and an adjacent uniform field to the right is viewed. A patch of light appears in the center of this visual field and its threshold detectability (δI) is measured as a function of the background illumination I. To ensure that the threshold depended on rods, the stimulus was blue/green, relatively peripheral, and of long duration. This light is considered relatively ineffective for cones. In contrast, the surround field was orange with the aim of fully adapting the cones and thus excluding them. In these conditions, the first part of the curve is horizontal, i.e., the differential threshold is constant, thereafter, over a further increase in I of 10^6, Weber's law is obeyed (Log $\delta I \approx \log (1 + I/I_0)$. Beyond that still, the curve rises more steeply because the rods saturate (RS); yet further, the cones start to take part. (From Barlow & Mollon 1982)

tecting the introduction within this field of an added 9° test field δI for a short time (0.2 s) is studied in terms of δI. The liminal increase in luminance δI is plotted as a function of the baseline luminance I, here on log/log coordinates.

Rod mechanisms predominate at low illumination, but when the light level exceeds 2 or 3 log units, the cones become involved. In order to maintain the effects of rod involvement as long as possible, Aguilar and Stiles (1954) used a blue-green test stimulus favoring rod absorption and a red adapting field "switching off" the cones (cf. figure 3.1).

In conditions of low luminances (-4 to $+4$ log units) only involving rods, the curve shows three ranges (figure 3.8):

• An initial horizontal plateau corresponding to a range of ambient light intensity in which the incremental threshold δI is independent of I.
• A wide zone of linear increase of log δI as a function of log I. The point where the increase takes off is represented by an intensity value I_0 (point of intersection of the increasing straight line with the plateau). Beyond I_0 the straight line has a slope of unity which, since the abscissa is expressed as log I/I_0, represents a relationship of the form $\delta I = K(1 + I/I_0)$.
• Beyond that zone (beyond $+4$ log units), the curve steepens abruptly, the differential threshold increases significantly and the rods can then be considered as having become saturated, doubtless because their individual responses have all attained their maximum. It is only beyond this point that another plateau begins that this time involves cone mechanisms.

There are two important factors to note in these discoveries. Weber's law, which established a relationship between the incremental change and the existing stimulus level (here the adapting field), is shown to be valid over a wide intensity range: The existence of an I_0 value proves the existence of a retinal "dark light" ("lumière intrinsique," "Eigengrau") which although its magnitude is small is nevertheless responsible for the just-perceptible luminance difference only beginning to increase beyond about 3 log units luminance. [With smaller test fields or for shorter test exposure times, the slope of the linearly rising part is no longer unity but tends toward 0.5, leading to a curve of the form $\delta I = K \sqrt{(I/I_0)}$.]

Considering a wider intensity range leads to assessing the involvement of cones. There also a large part of the plot is linear with a slope close to unity (Weber's law), but the intercept marking its origin I_0 is at a much higher intensity. The "dark light" noise of cones is much greater than that of rods, this no doubt being one reason for the cone's low sensitivity at low light intensity.

TIME COURSE OF THE δI RESPONSES

We now attack the dynamics of the light adaptation phenomenon by discussing the time course of adaptation. We will concentrate on two observations that embrace the essentials of this question.

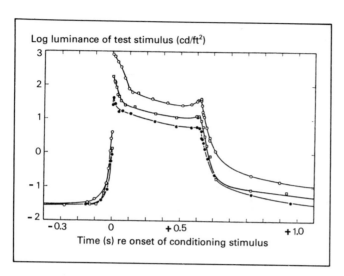

Figure 3.9
Time course of the threshold during a short-term adaptation to a light stimulus. Each conditioning stimulus lasts 0.5 s. The parameter is conditioning luminance: open circles, 10 cd/ft²; open squares, 30 cd/ft²; dots, 100 cd/ft². (From Graham 1965)

First of all, consider those *short-term effects* that follow an adapting stimulus. Crawford (1947) used an adapting (conditioning) stimulus at 12° and a central test stimulus of 0.5°. The conditioning stimulus is applied at time zero and cut off at time 0.5 s. The test stimulus is a flash of 0.1 s (figure 3.9). Essentially, an immediate increase in the liminal test stimulus is seen on application of the adapting light but—surprisingly—this is *preceded* by an increase in test threshold before the onset of the adapting stimulus (time zero). The interpretation of this remains to be finalized; it is, in any case, a proof that light adaptation is not solely a photochemical process but involves retinal neuronal mechanisms that alone might be capable of such apparently retrograde actions.

Another study focuses on a much longer time scale and analyzes the establishment of an *adaptation level* during a maintained light stimulus (Baker 1949). The subject is dark adapted for 10 minutes before the experiment starts. At zero time the adapting field is switched on at a level of retinal illumination between 5 and 5000 Td (troland), subtending 12 degrees of arc. The test stimulus is concentric and lasts for 0.02 s. The liminal δI is measured during 1000 s of adaptation at that level. The results show that the differential threshold changes

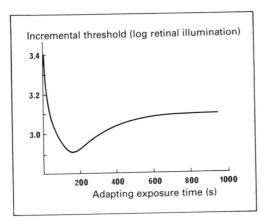

Figure 3.10
Variation of the incremental threshold for a foveal stimulus on the background of a
wide adapting light field, as a function of the time of exposure to the background.
The subject was dark-adapted until time zero, then exposed to a 5000-Troland adapting
field for the time (in seconds) indicated in the abscissa. (From Graham 1965)

with time, being higher to begin with, then decreasing during about
100 s, and again rising a little and settling to a plateau value at around
10 minutes (figure 3.10).

In this second type of experiment, as in the first, the time course
of the initial drop in sensitivity is rapid and during that interval the
pigment concentration will presumably not be much changed.

2.2 DARK ADAPTATION

Much slower processes accompany a protracted exposure of the eyes
to darkness (see Pirenne 1962; Bartlett 1965; Barlow 1972, Barlow &
Mollon 1982).

GENERAL EFFECTS

Consider a typical experiment. The subject is exposed for 3 minutes
(time −3 to 0) to white light from a 35° field at 1550 mL. At time zero
the light is switched off. The subject is required to fixate on a point
of red light, and the absolute threshold is determined every minute
or so for an 0.2-s test stimulus at 3° to 7° eccentricity at a wavelength
around 460 nm.

Under these conditions the threshold is first seen to decrease rapidly to reach a first plateau in about 7 minutes. During that phase
the stimulus retains a certain chromatic quality (in this case blue-
violet), but later a new threshold lowering begins, lasting for 20 to

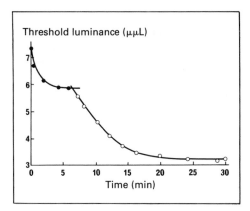

Figure 3.11
Time course of human dark adaptation. Dark adaptation following a 3-min exposure to white light of 1550 mL luminance. Test field: uniform flash of 3° diameter at an eccentricity of 7° with respect to the fixation point, duration 0.2 s, short wavelength (violet). Natural pupil. All points from one subject. For the first four points (black dots) the subject sees the stimulus as violet or blue, even at threshold. For the other points, threshold stimuli are perceived as colorless. (From Pirenne and Marriott 1962)

25 minutes, and now the light is not perceived as colored. In all, the threshold falls by about 4 log units (10,000 times) between time 0 and 25 minutes. The first phase comprises a lowering of 2.7 log units, that is, 500 times (figure 3.11).

FACTORS AFFECTING DARK ADAPTATION: CONES AND RODS

A whole collection of well-established observations agree in attributing the first phase of dark adaptation to the cones (a more rapid, limited, effect) and the second phase to rods (slower and more extensive). Here are some of the essential data underpinning this idea of cone/rod duality.

Color Effects
During dark adaptation a colored, slightly suprathreshold, stimulus appears with its normal color saturation if it is presented during the first phase (when only the cones are involved). The same stimulus will be perceived as pale, bluish, and unsaturated during the second phase when practically only the rods are excited.

Directional (Stiles-Crawford) Effects
Another reason for attributing the first phase to cones and the second to rods is provided by using two pencils of light entering the pupil

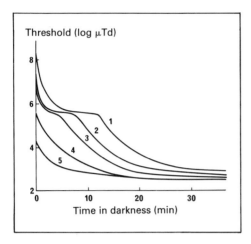

Figure 3.12
Dark adaptation curves as a function of time at different preceding light adaptation luminances: (1) 400,000 Td; (2) 38,900 Td; (3) 19,500 Td; (4) 3800 Td; (5) 263 Td. (From Bartley 1951)

at different places but touching the retina only in the fovea. The visual efficacies of these two pencils on the fovea (i.e., on the cones) is normally different (see chapter 2, section 2.7). Note also that during the *first part* of dark adaptation (when vision is cone dominated) the thresholds show large differences between a central and peripheral entry to the pupil during the first 5 minutes. However, thereafter the values become the same. In fact the effect is negligible for the second part of the curve, which is attributable to rods, since rods show little of the Stiles-Crawford directional effect.

Initial Level of Illumination
If dark adaptation is measured following previous exposure to different light levels of successively lower intensity, the relative duration of the first phase (cones) becomes progressively less, and when the pre-adapting light levels are low the time course of the lowering of the threshold, not surprisingly, resembles that for the rods (figure 3.12).

Duration of the Adapting Stimulus
The time course of dark adaptation scarcely changes when durations of exposure to the adapting light have been greater than about 10 minutes. In contrast, after short exposures to given intensities of adapting light, a reciprocity is observed between the time of exposure d to the adapting light and its luminance B. This reciprocity between d and B continues for up to 100 s for the later segment of the curve. The operating characteristics, in this range, suggest that the energy supplied to the receptors $(B \times d)$ determines the adapting effect of the light and the later dark adaptation's time course.

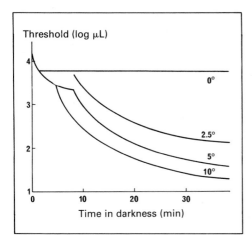

Figure 3.13
Dark adaptation at different parts of the retina. Dark adaptation explored with 2° pencils of light directed to different parts of the retina at eccentricities 0°, 2.5°, 5°, and 10°. (From Bartley 1951)

Retinal Position and Area of the Test Stimulus
The shape of dark adaptation curves also changes when a small area test stimulus is moved to different parts of the retina at different eccentricities. Figure 3.13 shows the results for a 2° test field at the fovea and at 2.5°, 5°, and 10° eccentricity. Notice a confirmation of the cone rod duality in the passage of the shape from a foveal to peripheral type.

A complementary result is obtained when the stimulus diameter, this time staying central on the retina, is increased in diameter. It would be expected that for small-area stimuli the cones would be most concerned and as the size of the test stimulus increases both types of receptor would become involved. This is again shown to be so by a change from a foveal type of response to the more complex response (for cones plus rods).

Spectral Composition of the Stimulus
Some already long-established experimental results have shown the influence of color of the test stimulus on the shape of adaptation curves. The family of curves obtained after changing the stimulus color from deep red to blue, always located in the parafoveal retinal region, clearly shows that in the red it is the cones that are involved at threshold, whereas the shorter wavelengths stimulate rod responses (figure 3.14).

Special Cases
There are also special cases in which a known anomaly in peripheral vision affects the dark adaptation curves in a predictable way. First,

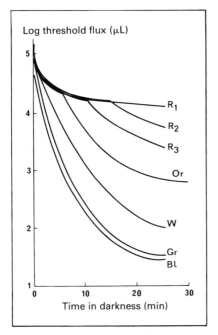

Figure 3.14
Dark adaptation at various wavelengths. Dark adaptation explored with a 1° pencil of light directed at 5° above the fovea. R₁, dark red; R₂, R₃, lighter reds containing more and more orange; Or, orange; Gr, green; Bl, blue; W, white. (From Pirenne and Marriott 1962)

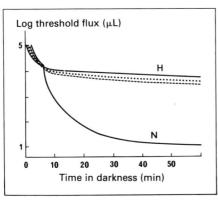

Figure 3.15
Dark adaptation for three "night-blind" subjects. Compare these, *H*, with the normal curves, *N*. (From Pirenne and Marriott 1962)

night-blind people, whose deficit is linked to vitamin A lack or is congenital, have poor night vision because of rod dysfunction. This is seen clearly in their dark adaptation curve which is purely foveal, that is, the lowering of threshold in darkness is rather small and rapid (figure 3.15).

Monochromats, who cannot perceive colors, are presumed to be lacking cones. They have a visibility curve that coincides with that for rods (λ_{max} = 520 nm) and, even in photopic conditions, show a

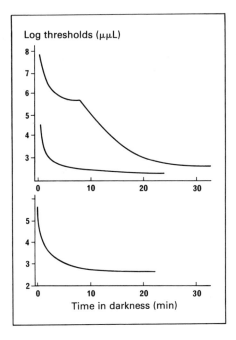

Figure 3.16
Dark adaptation in a (rod) monochromat. *Above,* Curves for a normal subject, light adapted at 1600 mL (*upper*) and 3 mL (*lower*). *Below,* Curve for monochromat. The (rod) monochromat presents a "rod type" curve even when he is adapted at 1600 mL. Thresholds for violet light (450 nm) for a 3° field projected at 7° from the fixation point. Initial light adaptation 4 min. (From Pirenne and Marriott 1962)

dark adaptation that lacks the first limb of the normal adaptation curve which is linked with cone excitation (figure 3.16). [Notice, however, that the dark adaptation in monochromats is relatively faster than that for the rods in the normal retina. It traces a curve much more like that of a normal subject who has been exposed to a light of low intensity, such as we have described above].

2.3 RELATION BETWEEN DARK ADAPTATION AND SENSITIVITY REDUCTION
IN THE LIGHT

Apart from phenomenological studies, the analysis of adaptation processes has led to interesting insights into the mechanisms concerned.

RHODOPSIN LEVELS AND DARK ADAPTATION

This is a matter of research results (discussed in more detail later) concerned with the correlation between rhodopsin content and the level of dark adaptation. For the moment, two basic factors will suffice: (1) during dark adaptation, rod thresholds decrease together with increasing rhodopsin amount. (2) However, the relationship is far from linear but rather is logarithmic and is such that the threshold is still at + 2 log units above its minimum when 90% of the visual purple has been regenerated.

NERVOUS AND PHOTOCHEMICAL FACTORS IN RECEPTOR THRESHOLD CHANGES:
SUMMATION POOLS

Given the nonlinear relationship that exists between rhodopsin amounts and dark adaptation level, the question arises as to whether the threshold elevation of a group of rods exposed to light is solely due to their desensitization by rhodopsin loss or whether intrinsic mechanisms in the retinal neuronal network also play a part. This problem has been particularly addressed by Rushton and Westheimer (1962).

These authors measured dark adaptation curves after exposure to a light flash (avoiding the complication of eye movements) calculated to decompose (bleach) about 50% of the rhodopsin. The bleaching (conditioning) stimuli comprised a 3° field; the test flashes for measuring the absolute threshold were of the same size and projected on exactly the same place on the retina. Two separate arrangements were then devised. In the first the bleaching field was projected after passing through a grafting of spatial frequency 2 cycles/degree, creating alternate light and dark stripes and therefore sparing 50% of the receptors in the total field. The time course of the resulting dark adaptation was then tested with a uniform field. In a second experiment, the situation was reversed, adapting with a uniform field of the same total luminance in the grating pattern (obtained by reducing the initial light intensity by a neutral filter of optical density 0.4) and testing with a grating pattern.

This experiment allowed the assessment of the relative contribution from photochemical and neuronal factors (taking stringent experimental precautions). The dark adaptation curves should not be the same for bleaching by the grating (when 50% of the rods are spared) and bleaching by the uniform field (when no rod is spared) if the adaptation is solely a photochemical matter. In fact, the result is quite the contrary: The adaptation curves are identical for the two conditions (figure 3.17).

The researchers concluded that the increase of threshold due to the effect of light must incorporate postreceptor nervous interactions within an area that Rushton called a *summation pool*. It is the level of excitation in this pool that is modified by exposure to light, the cause of the change being some signal related to pigment decomposition. This type of experiment also led to the idea of a *bleaching signal* and that the general excitation in the pool is conditioned by the sum of

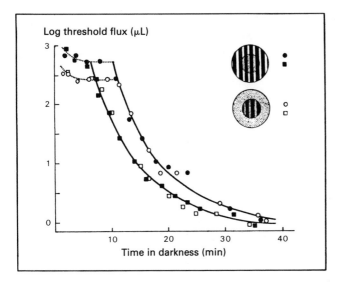

Figure 3.17
Human dark adaptation in a limited area of the retina. Prior bleaching by illumination from a banded field and subsequent threshold test with a uniform patch (*upper inset,* and filled symbols in the curves), then prior bleaching by illumination from a uniform field and subsequent threshold test with a banded field (*lower inset,* and open symbols in the curves). In two experiments (circles and squares), curves for the open and closed symbols coincide; the thresholds therefore depend on the total bleaching, not on its retinal distribution (see text). (From Rushton and Westheimer 1962)

such signals originating in the receptors that absorbed the quanta of light needed to bleach their pigment.

EQUIVALENT BACKGROUND ILLUMINATION

In 1947, Crawford had emphasized that the time course of dark adaptation is not invariable with the size of the test stimulus used. However, if he introduced as a dependent variable not the threshold but the background illumination of the Weber differential threshold curve that corresponded with the threshold precisely ("equivalent background illumination"), the time course of the adaptation became independent of the size of the test spot. [This was known as Crawford's transformation.] The experiments were taken up again by Blakemore and Rushton (1965), who were able to use a rod monochromat as a subject, which allowed a very large range (7 log units) of intensity to be explored without cone mechanisms complicating the issue.

Figure 3.18 illustrates one such experiment. To the left of the top

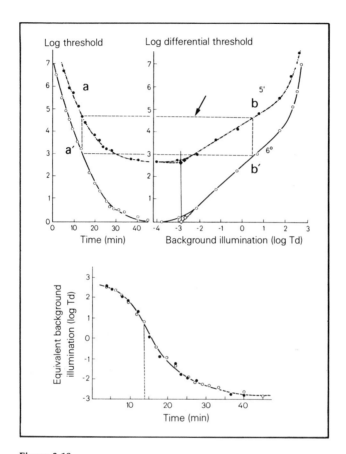

Figure 3.18
Crawford's transformation. *Above,* Crawford's transformation for a rod monochromat.
Left, Dark adaptation curves; log threshold as a function of time in the dark, following
an exposure to intense light. *Right,* Differential thresholds; log threshold as a function
of background illumination. Filled circles, curves a and b: test flashes 5 min arc; open
circles, curves a' and b': test flashes 6°. The dark adaptation is different in the two
cases *(left)* but the same difference is found when a desensitization is generated by
background illumination *(right). Below,* A curve, derived from the above curves, representing the equivalent background illumination as a function of time in the dark. A
horizontal line drawn from whatever value of log threshold (arrow) cuts the curve to
the left in the upper diagram at a certain time in the dark and the curve to the right
at a certain background luminance. In this lower curve, corresponding pairs of time
and background luminance are plotted for both the 5 min arc test flash (filled circles)
and the 6° test flash (open circles). They coincide; therefore the equivalent luminance
does not depend on the size of the stimulus. (From Blakemore & Rushton 1965)

graph are drawn the dark adaptation curves after an intense retinal illumination that bleached approximately 50% of the rhodopsin. Two test stimuli are used, one subtending 5 min arc (a), the other 6 degrees (a'). The adaptation curves (a, a') are different, as expected. To the right, from the same two test stimuli, are the curves (b, b') for the differential threshold (b, b') (ordinate: log) as a function of background light (abscissa: log trolands). These two curves are also different. However, we can also plot, for each size of test stimulus, a new relationship (derived as described in the caption to figure 3.18) in which the abscissa is time and the ordinate is the background illumination that produces a differential threshold of the same magnitude as the absolute threshold measured at each particular time during dark adaptation (Crawford's transformation). The observations then all lie on a single curve, whatever the size of the stimulus.

The total adaptation occurs as if the desensitizing signals generated by the amount of bleached pigment in the receptors in the summation pool are equivalent to the desensitizing signals that would have been generated by the presence of a real background light.

THE BLEACHING SIGNAL

Has it been possible to relate this assumption of a bleaching signal to any concrete event? Observations on pupillary diameter seem to support the suggestion. Alpern and Campbell (1962) submitted subjects to a monocular exposure to intense light and then observed the pupillary diameter of the opposite eye when the subject was left in darkness. The opposite eye demonstrated a strong contraction as if signals to light were being transmitted from the bleached eye and acted on the other by means of the consensual nature of the pupillary reflex to light exposure. This contraction diminished progressively in a way that essentially agrees with time course of regeneration of visual purple, being complete in 20 minutes. If a temporary blindness of the bleached eye is engendered by pressure on the eyeball, the pupillary contraction of the opposite eye is interrupted.

It has been suggested that the bleaching signal might well be simply the resulting afterimage (the image of a bright fixated object that persists after the eyes are closed). The problem was that to quantify the intensity of the consequent afterimage could only be done by comparing it with another real image stabilized on the retina: The afterimage is itself stabilized on the retina and one can only compare the comparable. By arranging such a real stabilized image by transmitting a small image of a real source via optical apparatus firmly connected to the cornea by suction, Barlow and Sparrock (1964) were able to compare the afterimage with the real stabilized image by photometric comparison and to show that: (1) the luminance of the afterimage decreases progressively, to disappear after 30 minutes, with a time course that agrees very well with dark adaptation; and (2) during the dark adaptation, the equivalent background luminance, determined by the Crawford transformation, is effectively equivalent to the luminance of the afterimage.

From all of this, we can conceive the afterimage to increase the threshold by its luminance during dark adaptation. The afterimage luminance decreases with time and the amount of rhodopsin that has been resynthesized increases. These factors make the summation pool increasingly excitable by real images and hence lower the absolute threshold. The reality of this scheme still needs to be proved physiologically. It seems at present that no appropriate objective signal at the level of the retinal receptors has yet been found.

3 SIMULTANEOUS CONTRAST, VISUAL ACUITY, AND SPATIAL FREQUENCY RESOLUTION

Psychophysics has addressed a variety of complicated phenomena concerned with the power of the visual system to discriminate stimuli of different luminance presented simultaneously. Traditionally, these have been reported either in terms of simultaneous contrast (interaction between neighboring visual fields of different contrast), or of visual acuity of the visual system (power of separating images). Recently, a whole range of research has been developed concentrating on the discrimination of grating patterns, leading to the specification of the transfer function of visual analyzing systems in the spatial frequency domain.

3.1 SIMULTANEOUS CONTRAST

The term *contrast* is applied to a variety of different situations. It might be in reference to the simultaneous contrast, which we will discuss here, or between two neighboring regions in a visual field that have a different luminance and/or color; but it is also applied to successive contrast when there is a temporal juxtaposition of different luminances or colors. We will only consider the simplest case of simultaneous luminance threshold contrast, taking into account the importance it has assumed in the analysis of retinal mechanisms (see chapter 4).

Consider two juxtaposed fields of different luminances, one high (I_{max}), the other low (I_{min}). By convention the contrast is expressed as:

$$C = (I_{max} - I_{min})/(I_{max} + I_{min}),$$

or, in terms of the mean luminance $\{I_m = 0.5\,(I_{max} + I_{min})\}$, as:

$$C = (I_{max} - I_{min})/2I_m$$

In practice this contrast (*Michelson's contrast*) will vary between 0 (nil contrast, luminance identity) to 1 (or 100%), when $I_{min} = 0$ and $I_{max} \neq 0$.

One of the well-known luminance contrast effects is that a field of a given luminance appears to be more or less bright if it is placed adjacent to a field that has a lesser or greater luminance. To study this type of interaction of contrasts, a *test field* is observed in isolation or with a contiguous (spatial-) *inducing field*, which generates the subjective change in luminosity of the test field. The effect is measured by comparing the appearance of the test field in each situation with another *reference field* placed at a short distance away to avoid interaction with the inducing field. When the contrast of the reference field (the dependent variable), must be reduced to match the test field during spatial induction, then the effect of the contrast is to diminish the relative luminance of the test field.

To make quantitative estimates it is usual to employ an annular inducing field surrounding the test field. The luminance (L_i) of the inducing field is systematically changed until the central test luminance (L_r) matches that of the far reference (L_t). Log (L_r) is plotted against log (L_i); see figure 3.19 (Heinemann 1955).

For a given L_t it is found under these conditions that when L_i is less than L_t, then the latter is little changed with respect to its true value (test field alone). In addition, the curve rises very slightly, indicating a subjective impression of increased luminance of the test field when the inducing field is less bright. Conversely, when L_i becomes greater than L_t, the contrast effect is very evident, L_r decreasing rapidly. In other words, the test field becomes rapidly less bright in appearance than it really is. Repeating the experiments for a series of different L_t generates a family of similar curves.

The conclusion is essentially that an increase in the inducing field luminance reduces the apparent luminance of the test field when $L_i > L_t$. When the inducing field has a lower luminance ($L_i < L_t$), the inverse effect but a much more limited one is produced.

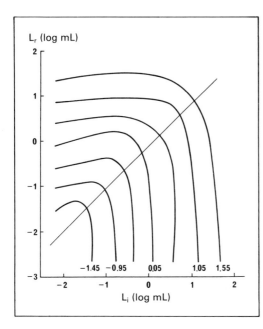

Figure 3.19
Luminance contrast. The apparent luminance of a test field (L_t) (measured by matching it to a variable reference luminance [L_r]) that results when the test field is surrounded by an inducing field of luminance L_i. Each curve is for a given L_t (parameter indicated beside each curve). (From Graham 1965)

Among other parameters that could affect the apparent luminance, the spatial relationships between the test and inducing fields lend themselves to an infinite variety of combinations. We will mention only a few of them that have a reasonable interpretation in terms of well-identified retinal mechanisms.

Let us first consider *Mach bands*. The simplest way to view this phenomenon is to examine the boundary between a bright edge and a dark edge. Figure 3.20 illustrates this (Fiorentini 1972). Examination will convince the reader that near this border differences of luminance are seen such that on the bright side there appears a yet brighter strip and on the dark side a yet darker strip. Thus while the objective luminance contour is a more or less steep step (depending on the individual case), the subjective brightness at different places (evaluated, for example, by comparing it with a view of the middle of the test field through a slit as a reference luminance) has a hump near the bright side of the border and a trough near the dark side. More careful measurements show, in addition, that the two reinforcements of bright and dark are not symmetrical, the bright hump being more prominent than the dark trough. We shall see below how neurophysiological measurements have pointed to a likely interpretation of this phenomenon created by the boundary between different luminances (see figure 4.65).

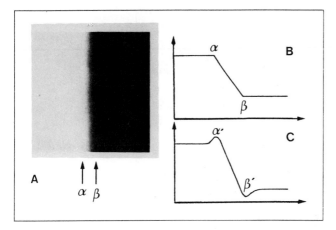

Figure 3.20
Contrast in Mach bands. *A*, Figure showing a boundary between a bright zone and a dark zone. *B*, Actual luminance variation between α and β. *C*, Subjective perception of the same (by matching the perceived luminances with a test strip). The corresponding positions of α and β are marked in each of the three diagrams. (From Fiorentini 1972)

We shall now indicate other phenomena linked to simultaneous contrast but even more briefly and purely descriptively. One class concerns *area contrast*. Craik (1966) and Cornsweet (1970) have demonstrated that of two circular fields of the same luminance, one will appear brighter than the other if the former has a lower bordering luminance than the latter.

Other topographies show somewhat complex border illusions, such as *Hermann's grating*, which comprises a series of black squares separated by white strips. The intersections of these lines appear to be relatively gray, with the exception of those that are centrally visually fixated (figure 3.21).

Finally, there is *Ehrenstein's contrast*, in which centrally interrupted black crosses show enhanced white at the interruption and white crosses an enhanced black. This is more easily seen in figure 3.22 than described (Jung 1978).

3.2 VISUAL ACUITY

Visual acuity is defined as the capacity to discriminate the fine details of an object in the visual field. In principle, the just-separable distance between two points, or other details of an object, can be expressed in a variety of ways: their absolute linear distance, or the angle subtended by them at the eye, or the linear separation of their two im-

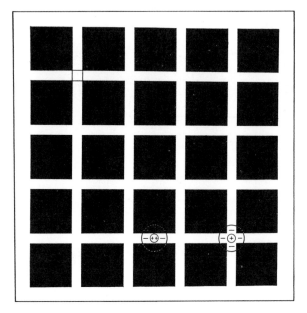

Figure 3.21
Hermann's contrast illusion, with a white grating. Note the apparent reductions in brightness at the intersections. These can be to some extent explained by the existence of circular concentric antagonistic ON-OFF neuronal units. A unit detecting a white line between intersections might have its ON center relatively more stimulated (leading to an increase in perceived luminance contrast) than when the ON center coincides with an intersection, where the OFF surround may receive relatively more illumination, leading to poorer contrast there (see inset diagrams). Refer also to chapter 4, section 5.1 and chapter 5, section 2.2. (From Brooks & Jung 1973)

ages on the retina. In fact, the only conveniently manipulable factor is the angular separation of the two points. That is one possible measure of acuity. The other, more usually adopted, is its reciprocal. This number is larger the smaller the angle and so increases with increasing acuity. In practice, acuity is expressed by the reciprocal of the angle in minutes of arc. As an indication, the retinal images of two points of apparent angular separation 1 min arc are, neglecting all aberrations and diffractions, separated by 4.9 μm.

METHODS FOR MEASURING ACUITY

Acuity can be measured in a variety of ways that cannot always be considered equivalent. Essentially there are three ways of proceeding:

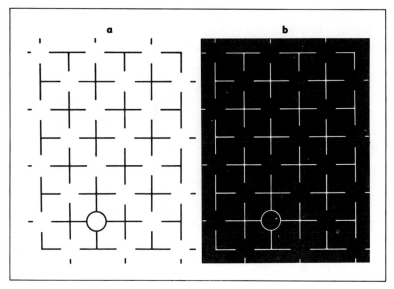

Figure 3.22
Ehrenstein's brightness illusion. In *a* the black lines and in *b* the white lines increase the relative contrast of the open centers to which they converge. These more contrasty centers themselves induce the impression of brighter (in *a*) and darker (in *b*) diagonal lines. These illusions disappear where the center is surrounded by a circle with the same contrast as the straight lines. (From Brooks & Jung 1973)

• *Detection* of a black point on a white background, for example, or of a fine opaque wire or crosshair against a white background.
• *Recognition of objects or shapes* (such as letters) or the localization of a gap in an O (called a *Landolt's C*). These methods are very common in ophthalmological clinics. They, as well as other optotypes that have been proposed are undeniably of practical interest; however, they do not always lend themselves easily to quantitative measures because of their complexity (figure 3.23).
• *Resolving* the separation between two punctate stimuli or between the parallel lines or, above all, between the lines of a grating (*Foucault's disk*). This sort of test is usually discussed in terms of a *spatial frequency domain,* unlike the others which represent *detection of a single spatial feature.* It is convenient to discuss distinguishing an individual feature and resolving gratings separately.

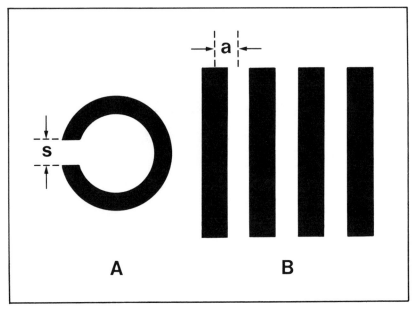

Figure 3.23
Arrangements for studying visual acuity. *A,* Black Landolt C annulus. The thickness
of the ring and the width of the gap (*s*) are each fixed at 1/5 the external diameter of
the ring. *B.* Grating of dark and light bars of equal width (*a*). In this case the distance
between the centers of the dark and bright stripes is also equal to *a*. Other arrangements are also used. In either case, acuity is defined as the reciprocal of the minimal
angle (in minutes of arc) subtended by *s* or *a* when they are just perceptile. (From
Pirenne and Marriott 1962)

VISUAL ACUITY IN PERCEPTION OF SINGLE SPATIAL FEATURES

Influence of Peripheral Optics
Before attacking the problems purely neurophysiologically, we need
to note a number of peripheral optical factors influencing the retinal
image that might be involved. An important consideration in this
respect is clearly the pupillary diameter. Rigorously, this can determine three parameters of visual reception: retinal illumination, aberrations, and diffractions.
    Obviously the *retinal illumination* depends on pupillary diameter.
Experimentally, however, a tenfold increase in luminance causes a
reduction in pupillary area of only 35%, representing an increase in
retinal illumination of only 0.8 log unit, which in turn generates a
minimal increase in acuity of 0.2 log unit.
    Optical aberrations linked with pupillary diameter are of many types,

all due to differences in real lenses from the simple laws of geometrical optics that incorporate the Gauss approximations. Thus all rays from the same punctate source will not converge on a single point and the image of a plane surface will not be a plane surface. Generally, these aberrations increase with pupillary diameter. However, in practice this factor does not seem to enter until the pupillary opening is very large indeed (i.e., in night vision) and has very little effect in normal mesopic or photopic conditions.

As for *chromatic aberrations*, which clearly depend on wavelength, in monochromatic light acuity is best for the mid region of wavelengths (blue or red light being less favorable), and we must not neglect these factors in constructing acuity theories. But here again, the practical effects seem to be somewhat unimportant.

Finally, *diffraction* of rays also has its effect. When the aperture of an optical instrument is diminished, its acuity is limited in a way precisely linked to this reduction. In fact, visual acuity does decrease when the pupillary diameter is diminished below a certain value.

The cost of these various interacting aberrations is such that the power to separate details in a visual field by the eye depends on pupillary diameter at very small apertures, increasing with increasing diameter up to 1.5 to 2 mm but, in contrast, does not seem to be affected by the pupillary aperture for greater diameters (2 to 4 mm), when the eye is thus working on a plateau value within the normal bounds of mesopic and photopic vision.

Acuity Variation with Luminance and Color
Turning now to consider factors concerned with the nature of the stimulus, we will again consider acuity of a single feature and of a grating separately. The variables that have some significant effect on acuity are, in this case: luminance of the target and its contrast with respect to the background, duration of presentation, eccentricity on the retina, and the level of dark adaptation. We will only give a few examples.

First consider an *opaque line* (wire or crosshair) crossing the visual field with a contrasting luminance. Here, we might expect its perception (i.e., the acuity) to increase with the background luminance (figure 3.24). Notably, this curve always shows two limbs: One corresponds to the cones with their high spatial resolving power, and the other corresponds with, as we already know, the poor resolution of rods (Hecht & Mintz 1939).

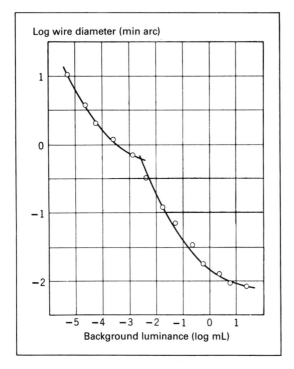

Figure 3.24
Relationship between the intensity of the background and the visual angle of a
just-perceptible opaque wire. (From Bartley 1951)

Another experiment concerns the visibility of an *illuminated slit* presented for a short time. The subject is required to judge its orientation
correctly. The luminance of the slit is varied and the minimal slit
width needed for a correct perception is estimated (Niven & Brown
1944). Note (figure 3.25) that the brighter the slit the less wide it
needs to be for a correct response. On log/log coordinates this decreasing relationship is surprisingly linear. When the duration of presentation is restricted, the function suffers a translation but its slope
does not change. Such results show, like others above, a certain
equivalence ("trading") between the area of the stimulus and its duration for a liminal performance.

In every way, the liminal angular magnitudes for detectability in
optimal conditions are astonishingly small, for example:

• Black spot on a white background, 20'' to 30''
• Illuminated slit on a black background, 30''

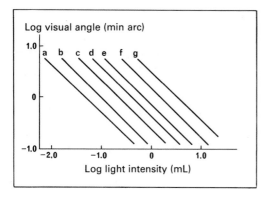

Figure 3.25
Vision of an illuminated slit. Relationship between the visual angle subtended by an illuminated slit, exposed briefly, and the intensity of the slit for which the orientation is correctly perceived. The various straight lines correspond to different exposures, becoming shorter and shorter from left to right (in ms): $a = 189$, $b = 87.1$, $c = 42.3$, $d = 20.9$, $e = 10.7$, $f = 6.27$, $g = 4.13$. (From Bartley 1951)

- Black line on a white background, 1″ sometimes less
- Two white dots on a black background, about 1′
- Two black dots on white background, 2′
- Two bright parallel lines on a black background 40″ to 1′

Black Landolt C's have been another very useful way to determine acuity (in this case the reciprocal of the angle subtended by the opening in the annulus). Variables explored include luminance, background color, and position of the image on the retina.

Thus in figure 3.26 Mandelbaum and Sloan (1947) demonstrate how rapidly acuity decreases with eccentricity in photopic conditions (luminances > 1 mL). In twilight vision this does not occur except for a small maximum near 5°. (In night vision this corresponds with the familiar need to fixate a little *to one side* of a dim star to see it.)

Figure 3.27 shows how acuity varies as a function of intensity depending on whether the image is on the fovea or more peripheral, also whether the color of the image is blue or red, and whether or not the subject can see the background color.

Every measurement made away from the retinal regions where there are both receptors emphasizes the duality of receptor systems.

Immediately below we will deal with the use of grating images to explore the transfer of spatial information but note here their use in determining acuity. Figure 3.28 compares acuity values determined

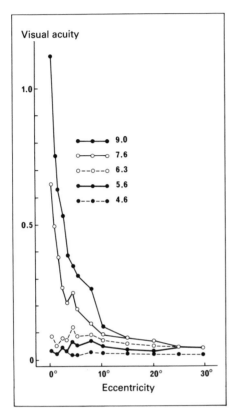

Figure 3.26
Visual acuity as a function of the eccentricity in the horizontal meridian. Measurements using black Landolt Cs viewed in the temporal retina for five intensities of white light (from 4.6 to 9.0 log units in μL). Peripheral measurements made with 0.2-s exposure, central measurements with exposures of several seconds. (From Pirenne and Marriott 1962)

by broken annuli (curve b) and by a visual spatial grating (i.e., a series of dark and bright strips, equidistant and of high contrast) for which the maximal detectable spatial frequency is determined. In general, an acuity increase with increasing luminance is observed together with the two successive limbs in the curves representing that increase and showing the successive interventions of rod and cone mechanisms. Typically, for constant luminance the grating is more easily discriminated than the "C" at low luminances (<30 Td), but at high luminances the "C" is better discriminated than the grating.

Another grating observation (figure 3.29) shows that the acuity of its perception in a monochromat varies much less with illumination and only in one continuous curve, presumed due to rods, without the separate branch that in other experiments has indicated a duality of receptor operation in acuity.

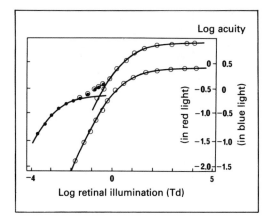

Figure 3.27
Variation of visual acuity with retinal illumination of the field in red and blue light. Measurements using black Landbolt Cs: lower curve for measurements in red light and upper curve for measurements in the blue. Filled circles, measurements for the periphery of the visual field, on a field subjectively colorless and attributable to rods; open circles, measurements made at the fovea and only involving cones. The half-filled circles refer to points obtained for the parafoveal region attributable to both cones and rods acting (the background appears colored). In these experiments, exposures were of long duration. (From Pirenne and Marriott 1962)

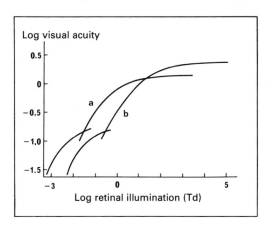

Figure 3.28
Variation of visual acuity with retinal illumination, using two different test objects: (a) a grating and (b) interrupted annulus (Landolt C). (From Bartley 1951)

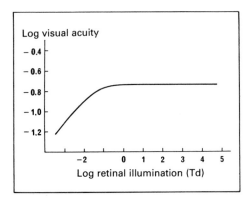

Figure 3.29
Visual acuity for a (rod) monochromat. Test object: gratings of equal width bright and dark lines illuminated with blue light (dominant wavelengths 490 nm); 3-mm diameter artificial pupil. The curve is single and corresponds to the curve normally attributed to rods. (From Pirenne and Marriott 1962)

Other Measures of Visual Acuity in Clinical Practice
Apart from the above detailed acuity studies, current clinical practice has introduced less sophisticated, and also less precise, methods that nevertheless allow a rapid estimate of the visual capacity of a subject. As a general rule these comprise a table of letters of the alphabet (after Snellen 1862). By convention, an angle of 1 min arc is taken as the "limiting" value for acuity. The agreed unit of acuity, $A = 1$ is the recognition of a letter subtending a 5 min arc total visual angle with lines or gaps of 1 min arc. In France the letters are viewed at about 5 m; the letter corresponding to $A = 1$ will therefore be 7.3 mm high. Another convention is to use a decimal notation, A being a fraction with a denominator 10 and a numerator m defined by $m = 50/v$ where v is the liminal angle in minutes needed by a subject to recognize a letter (e.g., an acuity of 6/10, 4/10, etc).

In the English-speaking countries the reading distance is 6 m, (20 ft) and the fraction A is expressed with the normal viewing distance as numerator (6 m or 20 ft) and the denominator being the distance (in meters or feet) at which the (5 min/1 min) letters just recognized by the subject being tested would have been recognized by a normal subject (e.g., 6/18 = 20/60). [But this will probably change to the other method in the EEC.—Translator] Note that the conventional choice of 5 min arc letters is sensible, otherwise "supernormal acuities" could be encountered (>10/10 or > 6/6 or >20/20).

3.3 DETECTION IN THE SPATIAL FREQUENCY DOMAIN

Recently, studies of the visual system's operation by analyzing its performance in terms of spatial frequency have been vigorously pursued. Gratings of alternating bright and dark stripes, the contrast and the spatial frequency of which can be varied, are exploited. This type of investigation has a dual importance. First, it goes far beyond merely using acuity as a measure of the spatial performance of the visual system by yielding information on behavior in the whole gamut of visual spatial frequency detection rather than only in the limited conditions of acuity thresholds. Second, it can determine the transfer function of the system to spatially periodic stimuli by well-established methods of harmonic analysis; in particular, the linearity of the system can be well investigated in these experiments.

Depending on the case, the grating spatial luminosity variation will either be sinusoidal or square wave, spatial contrast changing smoothly in the former and abruptly in the latter but with the stripes in either case being of the same width. Often the stripes are fixed in the subject's visual field and the subject is required to fixate on a given point. The stimuli are either switched on and off upon a mean luminance background or are instantaneously exchanged, dark stripes for light stripes, with this *grating contrast alternation* introducing a basic temporal variation. Relevant variables are the following:

• *Spatial frequency,* the number of luminosity alternations per degree of visual angle (cycles/degrees)
• *Level of retinal illumination,* which is the mean luminance level (L_m), or level of light adaptation, at which the measurements are made
• The *contrast,* namely, the difference between the maximal luminance of the bright stripes (L_{max}) and the minimal luminance (L_{min}) of the dark stripes, alternating throughout the experiment, and expressed as $C = L_{max} - L_{min}/ 2Lm$
• The *spatial frequency waveform,* the variation of luminance along the grating (e.g., sinusoidal or square or sawtooth)
• The *stripe orientation,* vertical or oblique

Subjects are required to detect the stripes against the background, leading to a *contrast threshold* C_L (minimum perceptible contrast) or its reciprocal the *contrast sensitivity* $1/C_L$. [The terms detectable modulation wave amplitude m or its inverse, sensitivity to amplitude modulation $1/m$, are also used.] Such experiments (e.g., Blakemore &

Campbell 1969; Campbell & Maffei 1970; Campbell et al. 1973) have been able to relate these functions very clearly to visual acuity and they are summarized here.

One of the functions most often studied has been the contrast sensitivity as a function of spatial frequency in cycles/degrees (figure 3.30) and at different retinal illuminations, that is, at the different mean luminance levels at which the experiments were carried out. The subject observes a grating (usually sinusoidal) and at each spatial frequency is required to adjust the contrast for the grating to be just perceptible (i.e., as soon as stripes are seen against the uniformly bright background). The experiment is repeated at different mean luminance levels (figures 3.30I and 3.31).

A family of curves with the following characteristics is obtained: At low luminance values, there is simply a progressive decrease in sensitivity with increasing grating spatial frequency until the curve cuts the abscissa (figure 3.31). For moderate and high luminance values, there appears a *maximal sensitivity* (at 4 cycles/degree in this case) beyond which the curve again falls until it cuts the abscissa. The point of intersection with the abscissa in fact indicates the perceptual limit for recognizing a grating pattern of maximal contrast ($C = m = 1$); here we are back to one of the methods for measuring acuity discussed above. But do not fail to notice that this whole family of curves gives much more information on the performance of the visual system than the single test of visual acuity. As an illustration, if the reader examines figure 3.32 and its legend, the existence of a maximum in the spatial resolution will be clearly apparent.

Finally, note that the curves are not exactly the same if the luminosity modulation is square wave rather than sinusoidal but basically their general shape is similar.

Figure 3.30   ▶
Studies of contrast and visual acuity and their interrelationships. *I*, Comparison of results in three cats (dots, triangles, and black squares) and in human (monocular) vision (open circles). Cat results are from evoked potential amplitudes, human from pyschophysics. *II*, Effect of adaptation at a given spatial frequency (7.1 cycles/deg). (*A*) Note the reduction in sensitivity for that spatial frequency but the lack of effect for other frequencies. (*B*) This curve, derived from (*A*), illustrates the relative elevation of the threshold as a function of spatial frequency. Note the tuning of adaptation in the spatial frequency channel, with the maximal threshold elevation (*arrow*) occurring at 7.1 cycles/deg. III. Similar results based on human (scalp) evoked potentials. Spatial frequencies (in cycles/degree) are: filled circles, 3.5; open circles, 9.0; squares, 18.0. Extrapolation of the curves yields the threshold detectable contrast (C_L). (From (I) Campbell et al. 1973, (II) Blakemore & Campbell 1969, III Campbell & Maffei 1970)

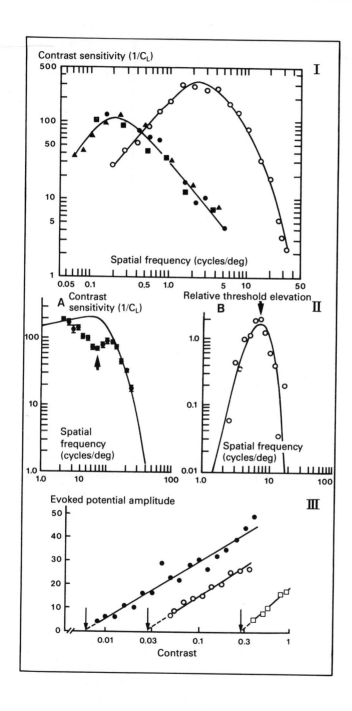

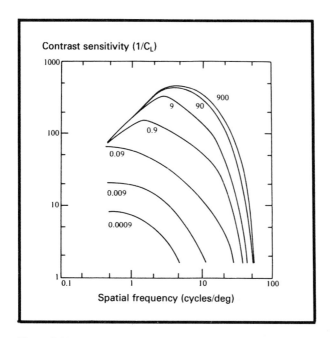

Figure 3.31
Family of spatial contrast-sensitivity curves for retinal illuminations between 0.0009 and 900 Td. Experimentation at 570 nm with subject observing grating through a 2-mm artificial pupil. (From Woodhouse & Barlow 1982)

Overall, it is possible to give some explanation of the negative slope of the curves at high spatial frequencies and the fact that the system is behaving as a low-pass optical filter. In every optical instrument (including the eye) that receives signals of increasing spatial frequency but of fixed contrast, the contrast of the image gets worse as the spatial frequency increases. A demodulation occurs, in particular one that is related to diffraction, such that a limit is reached to the resolving power of the system (Van Nes & Bouman 1967).

The optical modulation transfer function of the eye can be observed directly with an ophthalmoscope for different pupil apertures (e.g., Campbell & Gubisch 1966). Essentially it is similar to that of any optical instrument, although it does not correspond exactly to that of the ideal instrument (figure 3.33).

To be quite rigorous, the shape of the real perceptual curve as a function of spatial frequency does not correspond exactly with the transfer function of the eye that we have just described. There are obviously many possible reasons for the differences, such as influ-

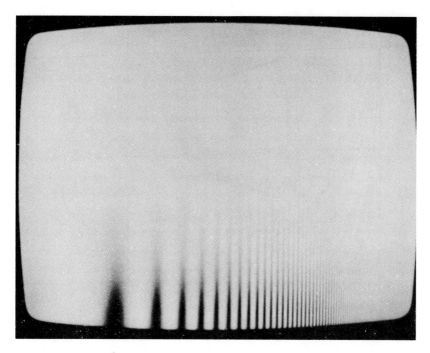

Figure 3.32
Variation of contrast sensitivity with spatial frequency for a grating. The contrast of
each bar with respect to the background decreases with increasing ordinate and the
spatial frequency of the grating increases with increasing abscissa. The implied contour
enclosing the limits of just-perceptible contrast approximates to the observer's visual
contrast sensitivity curve as a function of spatial frequency. (From Woodhouse &
Barlow 1982)

ences of the "retinal grain" or the operation of central neural mechanisms.

In contrast, the existence of a fall in sensitivity toward low spatial
frequencies does not apply to an optical system but implicates functional mechanisms throughout the collection of information channels
in the afferent pathways. We can suspect effects from the process of
surround inhibition that already exists in the periphery at the optic
nerve output from the retina to the next higher nucleus: stripes of
low spatial frequency (i.e., that are broad) can effectively excite a
central receptive field and its antagonistic surround at the same time
(see chapter 4, section 5) and a minimal response will ensue. We will
see later how it is possible to predict the shape of the spatial frequency curve from neuronal receptive fields by exploiting Fourier

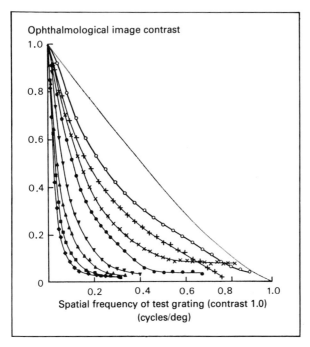

Figure 3.33
Spatial modulation transfer function for the human eye. Mean results for six subjects. The results are normalized to the highest spatial frequency transmitted by an ideal optical system for 570 nm light. Test grating contrast, 1.0. Dotted curve, performance of ideal optical system; different curves obtained for different pupil diameters (mm): open circles, 1.5; plus signs 2.0; crosses, 2.4; filled circles, 3.0; inverted triangles, 3.8; triangles, 4.9; squares, 5.8; diamonds, 6.6. (From Campbell and Gubisch 1966)

transforms. We will also see how, in more general terms, neurophysiological observations support these present results.

One important factor in contrast sensitivity is the retinal illumination. We have just seen that as this is reduced so is the spatial sensitivity, in such a way that below a certain illumination the maximum becomes degenerated and then eventually disappears, resulting in a monotonically decreasing function. Starting from such transfer functions, several others can be developed such as how spatial resolution (in cycles/degree) changes, at a given contrast, as a function of retinal illumination (figure 3.34). Notice that resolution improves up to 500 Td, then reaches a plateau. Certainly it is better the higher the contrast (Woodhouse & Barlow 1982).

Another experiment consists in adapting a subject to a grating of a given spatial frequency (i.e., the subject views this grating for some

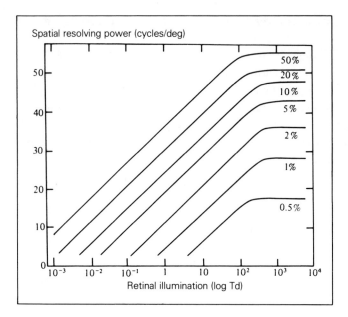

Figure 3.34
Relationship between spatial resolving power and average retinal illumination (parameter, grating contrast). Note that performance improves with increasing retinal illumination up to about 500 Td. Beyond that the performance stays constant. (From Woodhouse & Barlow 1982)

time). If the researcher then turns off the adapting field and immediately substitutes a test grating of the same spatial frequency as the first, the subject's contrast sensitivity is found to be diminished for some seconds thereafter. In contrast, after the same time of adaptation, the sensitivity for detecting gratings of another spatial frequency is little or not at all affected (see figure 3.30, IIA). [The grating is stationary in the subject's field of view during these experiments, unlike other more complicated ones that will be considered later with respect to temporal factors.] Quantitatively, starting from the curve of normal spatial frequency sensitivity and then by constructing a curve of the sensitivity loss after adaptation, again as a function of spatial frequency (see figure 3.30, IIB), the *spatial frequency specificity* of adaptation is seen to be the order of one octave bandwidth centered on the adapting spatial frequency. Campbell and his collaborators were thus able to conclude that in the visual system (of the human, the species in question) there exists *spatial frequency channels*, linear in operation, each one being sensitive to a limited range of spatial frequencies. The reader might be amused to use figure 3.35 to experience these adaptation effects.

More quantitatively, it is worthwhile considering the problem of the detectability of nonsinusoidal spatial patterns, such as square wave or triangular gratings (Blakemore & Campbell 1969; Campbell & Robson 1968). Having discovered that such a grating becomes detectable when one of its Fourier series components itself reaches threshold, they deduced that the visual system performs a linear analysis of spatial frequency, at least at threshold. The question that remained to be solved was whether such a harmonic analysis is effected by independent, separate, channels or by a single channel.

In modeling a channel, its output becomes the result of a filtering determined by its transfer function. In the multiple channel case, each narrow frequency band is treated by a particular channel, and detection operates independently in the channels.

[Some ideas developed by Campbell and Robson leaned in the direction of separate channels; when separate, scarcely adequate harmonic components are exploited, for example, they will not sum in the same way as would be predicted when they are within a single channel. Or again, the observation of a square wave grating of a given spatial frequency can be distinguished at a certain viewing distance from a sinusoidal one of the same spatial frequency on the condition that, at the same distance, the viewer can begin to perceive the contrast of a sinusoidal grating of adequate contrast and of three times the spatial frequency, in other words, perceive the third harmonic, that is prominent in the Fourier decomposition of a square wave.

Synthesizing the following Fourier series generates a square wave of amplitude $\pi/4$: $\sin\omega t + 1/3 \sin3\omega t + 1/5 \sin5\omega t + \ldots, 1/(2n + 1) \sin(2n + 1)\omega t$. In other words, following the authors' approach, if the constrast of a square wave grating is 50%, then the valid comparison is that the fundamental Fourier component will have a contrast $50 \times 4/\pi$ (63.7%) and the third harmonic of frequency $3f$ must have a contrast $(50 \times 4/\pi)/3 = 21.2\%$.

The arguments of Campbell and Robson were not devoid of critics, for the same type of response could have occurred in a model assuming that it was a question of one channel that then shared the analysis with several distinct analyzers. But many other more concrete tests, however, lent support to the idea of multiplicity, as, for example, that of Graham and Nachmias who in 1971 by adding two gratings

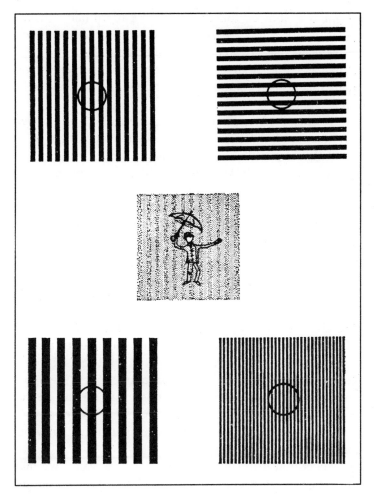

Figure 3.35
Demonstration of the selectivity of adaptation of a given spatial frequency channel. First, view the central figure from a distance of about 3 m and notice the person holding an umbrella. The superimposed grating of poor spatial contrast represents "rain." Next, look at the high-contrast vertical grating of the same spatial frequency (*upper left*), fixating on the interior of the circle for 60 s. After this adaptation, fixate on the central image once again and notice that the poor contrast central image ("rain") disappears for a few seconds and then is seen again. This effect does not occur if the high-contrast images with a different spatial frequency or a different orientation from the test grating are first fixated on and used as possible adaptors. (From Blakemore & Campbell 1969 and Barlow & Mollon 1982)

of frequency f and $3f$ showed that the complex pattern had a detectability that was *independent of the relative phase between the fundamental and the third harmonic* (see Graham 1977, Shapley & Lennie 1985—Trans.). In the case of a single channel such an independence was mathematically inconceivable, and this was therefore evidence in favor of multiple channels.]

Other experiments used stripes of varying orientation and showed that in the human subject the sensitivity is better for horizontal or vertical stripes than for oblique. With oblique stripes the optimal spatial frequency corresponds to increasing the relative separation of the stripes by 20%.

These experiments have been taken up once more using, not the subjective judgment of threshold by the subject but instead the global visual evoked potential recorded on the occipital region of the scalp by alternated spatial frequency gratings of a given spatial frequency, the contrast C of which is varied. In these experiments the dependent variable is not a threshold contrast but the amplitude A of the electrophysiological response.

Plotting the characteristic $A = f(C)$ for a given illumination reveals a linear relationship $A = k \log C$. Extrapolating this line, to zero A, gives contrast values that agree reasonably well with the subjective threshold contrast reported for the same spatial frequency (see figure 3.30III). It is permissible therefore to use this value for the liminal contrast sensitivity C_L. The characteristic, that can now clearly be written as $A = \log C/C_L$, will clearly vary with spatial frequency but its slope does not change very much.

We might expect that if this extrapolation for C_L is valid, we may redraw from this sort of data a curve of the variation of contrast sensitivity with spatial frequency that is identical with that obtained from psychophysically estimated thresholds. In essence this is what happens and is used as the justification for using evoked potentials as a valid measure of contrast sensitivity.

Similarly, plots of $A = \log C/C_L$ have been made (monocularly) for horizontal stripes to one eye and for vertical stripes to the other and are found to be almost identical. But if both gratings are exposed simultaneously (binocularly), each eye seeing both gratings, then the resulting curves behave like the sum of the individual responses for the different orientations. This is what would be expected if the system consisted of separate channels "tuned" to various orientations. Animal experiments, as we shall see, confirm this.

An analogous study was carried out in the cat, similarly exploiting the evoked potential amplitude A (this time measured on the occipital cortex itself) as evidence of contrast detection. As in humans, a linear relationship between A and log C was obtained, the slopes of the straight lines in this case being slightly different.

Profiting from results in human subjects, studies in the cat proceeded similarly by extrapolating the straight lines $A = f(C)$ to the abscissa, taking the point at which the abscissa is cut by the line as the value C_L (the contrast threshold) and plotting $1/C_L$ (contrast sensitivity) as a function of spatial frequency. A maximum was seen once more (i.e., a maximal contrast sensitivity), at least at adequate luminance values (see also Westheimer 1972).

However, the cat results differ from the human results in two ways: (1) there is no orientation preference (horizontal or vertical, rather than oblique), and (2) the point of maximal sensitivity has moved to lower spatial frequencies by a factor of about ten. Thus visual acuity of the cat is reduced similarly (0.2 cycles/degree maximum). Some investigations in the cat made by single unit measurements in the visual pathways will be described later.

The perception of contrast thresholds of simple or repetitive patterns has generated a variety of theoretical hypotheses that will be considered below during a discussion of data concerning the types of retinal receptors.

4 TEMPORAL EFFECTS: TEMPORAL RESOLUTION

Here we discuss how well the visual system detects short-duration stimuli, or successive stimuli following each other in given temporal patterns. There are a variety of observations to discuss but their common theme is the response to suprathreshold stimuli.

4.1 LUMINANCE OF BRIEF STIMULI

Consider a source delivering flashes of short duration ($d < 10$ ms). If the luminance, B, is low but suprathreshold (retinal illumination of the order of 1 Td), the perception depends on the product $B \cdot d$. In other words, the laws enunciated with respect to absolute thresholds (e.g., Bloch's law, Blondel and Rey's law) remain essentially the same in this case (figure 3.36, curve A).

In contrast, when the luminance is raised, a brief flash appears to be relatively brighter than a field of the same appearance but continuously illuminated. Proceeding by comparison and matching, it can

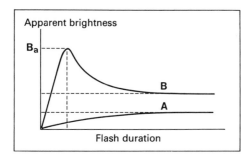

Figure 3.36
Variation of the apparent luminance of a brief flash as a function of the duration and intensity of the stimulus expressed as retinal illumination. The curve is constructed by comparing the apparent luminance with that of an adjustable luminance constant field. Retinal illumination: (A) 1 Td; (B) 200 Td. (The effect is known in France as "the pre-equilibrium waveform of Broca and Sulzer.") (From Le Grand 1964)

thus be shown that beyond duration of about 1 s a flash develops an apparent luminance curve of the shape shown in figure 3.36 (curve B), showing a maximum then a progressive return toward the real luminance. This *Broca and Sulzer effect* is sometimes referred to as a *pre-equilibrium wave* (see Piéron 1945).

4.2 PERCEPTUAL PERSISTENCE OF FLASHES

A light flash, however brief it might be, is perceived with an appreciable duration on the order of 150 ms. This persistence increases a little with increasing luminosity from 150 to 180 ms. We shall briefly examine the questions arising in the perception of consecutive images.

4.3 SENSITIVITY TO TEMPORAL CHANGES IN CONTRAST

The subject viewing a source whose luminosity fluctuates sinusoidally at a given frequency is required to adjust the contrast to perceptual threshold (once more the Michelson contrast is used: $C = (L_{max} - L_{min}) / 2L_m$. The frequency of the temporal modulation is then changed, and the subject adjusts to the liminal contrast again (see, e.g., Kelly 1961). In this way, plots of liminal contrast as a function of temporal frequency are obtained as above, usually taking the reciprocal S_c of the contrast as the dependent variable. An interesting parameter to investigate is the effect of the luminance or the retinal illumination. Adding this factor yields a family of curves (figure 3.37) from which the following facts can be deduced:

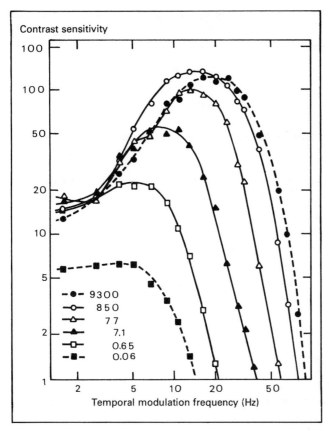

Figure 3.37
Temporal contrast sensitivity curves as a function of the stimulus' flicker frequency.
Large area stimulus: mean luminance (or more exactly, the corresponding retinal illumination) is specified as parameter (in Trolands, indicated to the left). Contrast sensitivity is expressed as reciprocal of the detectable amplitude modulation m, the luminance of the stimulus being given by $f(t) = L(1 + m\sin\omega t)$ where L is the mean amplitude and m ($0 < m < 1$) the sinusoidal modulation amplitude. Between 2 and 5 Hz modulation frequency the luminance only affects the sensitivity at very low values. Above 5 Hz the contrast sensitivity increases to a maximum that becomes larger with increasing luminance and then decreases. (From Kelly 1961 and Jameson & Hurvitch 1972)

• For moderate or high retinal illumination the contrast sensitivity passes through a maximum near frequencies between 10 and 25 Hz depending on the illumination.
• At each illumination there is a maximal frequency at which the subject no longer perceives any flicker in the stimulus even if the contrast change is 100%. This frequency is where the curve cuts the abscissa.
• This frequency intercept for no flicker perception varies with illumination.

Other studies have particularly concerned themselves with this rate for *critical flicker fusion frequency* (cff), which never exceeds 60 Hz even at the highest light intensities.

Evidence of "tuned channels" for different modulation rates of temporal contrast might be expected, as for spatial contrast. The results prove to be much less clear in the former than in the latter case. However, we shall see later that neurophysiology does reveal two types of receptor system, X cells with a tonic response and Y cells with a phasic response that are quite different in their temporal response characteristics.

4.4 CRITICAL FLICKER FUSION FREQUENCY: A DETAILED DISCUSSION

The cff, the frequency at which even for 100% contrast the subject sees no fluctuation, has been the object of much research concerned with variations as a function of differing stimulus parameters such as luminance, subtended angle, eccentricity, wavelength (refer to Pirenne 1962).

VARIATION WITH THE RETINAL REGION STIMULATED

In these experiments a 2° diameter white light field is projected to a variety of retinal eccentricities, 2°, 5°, and 15°. The independent variable is the retinal illumination, or the source luminance, and the dependent variable is the cff in hertz, with the eccentricity of the stimulus as parameter. [The Talbot-Plateau law states that when the subject sees a steady source beyond the frequency at which flicker is perceived, i.e., when fusion has occurred, the resulting luminance L_m is equal to that which would have been obtained if the light emitted during each period of its oscillation had been uniformly shared throughout the whole period. In other words, the apparent luminance L_m is equal to the physical luminance of the source L_i multiplied

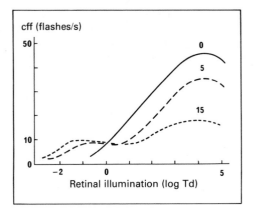

Figure 3.38
Relationship between critical flicker fusion frequency (cff) and retinal illumination for different eccentricities. Stimulus field 2°, white, projected on the retina at the fovea and 5° and 15° above it. The stimulus was applied in a background of constant luminance, equalized to that attained by applying the stimulus at rates above the flicker fusion frequency and maintained at that value throughout the test; 1.8 mm artificial pupil used. (From Pirenne and Marriott 1962)

by a certain coefficient. This coefficient equals $t_l/(t_l + t_o)$ where t_l is the time that the light is on during each period and t_o is for the light switched off, $(t_l + t_o)$ being the total duration of the period: $L_m = L_i \times t_l/(t_l + t_o)]$.

For a central retinal stimulation, the curve is uncomplicated, with the cff rising with illumination to a single maximum at about 10,000 Td, then decreasing once more (figure 3.38). At 5° where there is a considerable rod population, the curve has two parts: at high luminance it resembles the central retinal curve (presumably therefore is governed by cone outputs), whereas at low luminance a distinctly new regimen is apparent, presumably due to rods. At 15° where the cones are more rare and the rods more dense, the part of the curve corresponding to the cones is even more attenuated.

The above conclusion is confirmed by an experiment in which the test stimulus is always central but of greater and greater diameter (figure 3.39). For 0.3° and 2° the curve is purely foveal, and the change due to rods is apparent at 6° and even more so at 19°. In summary, at low luminances, flicker of the source is better detected in the periphery than in the fovea.

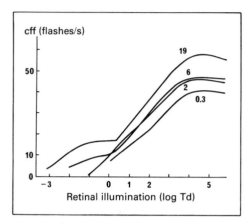

Figure 3.39
Relationship between cff and retinal illumination for stimuli fixated centrally but of different diameter (0.3°, 2°, 6°, 19°). Surrounding field, 35° diameter: luminance adjusted as in figure 3.38. (From Pirenne and Marriott 1962)

WAVELENGTH

Wavelength effects have been investigated, the subject fixating on a centrally situated spot, the wavelengths of the whole visual field being variable (figure 3.40). The results show two parts of the plots of cff. At high retinal illumination the points for all wavelengths sit practically on the same curve (attributed to cones), whereas at low illumination (attributed to rods) this curve extends more and more toward low luminance as the wavelength is diminished. However, it is not entirely proved that the whole of this lower part of the curves is entirely due to rods.

Notice, in this figure and earlier ones, that in the photopic range where the cones are in operation, the cff is essentially proportional to the log of the retinal illumination and is of the form: cff = a log L + b, where a is a constant between 10 and 15, over a range of retinal illumination of about 4 log units. [This is the *Ferry-Porter law*, originally proposed in 1892 by Ferry, who showed that "retinal persistence" varied proportionally with the inverse Log of the luminance. In 1902, Porter added some refinements; however, these measurements were rather approximate.]

CRITICAL FLICKER FUSION FREQUENCY IN MONOCHROMATS

Corresponding studies have been made in those monochromats in whom no indication of cone function has been found by other experiments. Essentially, the curves are like those found in normal subjects that have been attributed to rods, but it is also clear that for different colors or stimulus dimensions, such curves show singularities (at

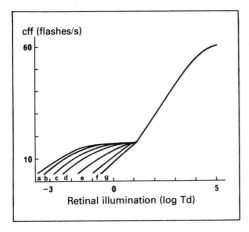

Figure 3.40
Relationship between cff and retinal illumination for different λ, between 450 and 670 nm. Test stimulus diameter 19°, surrounding field 35° (cf. figure 3.38) Wavelengths (in nm): *a*, 450; *b*, 490; *c*, 535; *d*, 575; *e*, 605; *f*, 625; *g*, 670. (From Pirenne and Marriott 1962)

least in some subjects) that suggest the existence of *two* types of mechanisms related to rods (figure 3.41.)

5 MOVEMENT PERCEPTION

The discussion of movement discrimination must go beyond the limits of pure detection to consider more complex aspects of the perception. We venture into this domain, which some consider especially complex, because the neurophysiology of the retina and pathways has demonstrated that the movement of a visual stimulus constitutes a fundamental visual characteristic that the nervous system treats selectively, as it does with many others.

In principle, two mechanisms are needed to underpin movement vision depending whether the eye is fixed and the image moves over the retina or whether the eye can follow the displacement of the object. The first strategy seems to have by far the greater precision. In any case, that is what we are going to discuss: experiments in which the subject is required to keep the gaze constant by fixating on a given point.

An essential distinction must be made at the outset between a real movement (MR) and an apparent one (MA), which we shall examine in turn (see Graham 1965; Anstis 1978; Burr & Ross 1986).

5.1 REAL MOVEMENT

To understand real movements, two more distinctions are needed; one concerns movement of a single target (single movement domain), and the other is the passage of a grating image (spatial frequency domain).

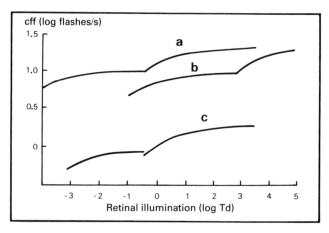

Figure 3.41
Critical flicker fusion frequency for a (rod) monochromat as a function of retinal illumination for two wavelengths (450 and 670 nm) and two spot diameters (3° and 19°). *a*, blue 19°; *b*, red 19°; *c*, blue 3°. The curves show two branches but the extent of the portion corresponding to low illumination is not changed by changing color (wavelength) in passing from blue to red (unlike in the normal). Similarly, the curves do not change shape when the stimulus diameter is changed. (From Pirenne and Marriott 1962)

SINGLE MOVEMENT DOMAIN

Suppose a target moves for d seconds with amplitude a (in minutes of arc) at a speed $v = da/dt$ (in minutes of arc per second). Then the variables are clearly not independent ($a = v \cdot d$) and one or the other threshold can be determined, the just perceptible a_{lim}, v_{lim}, or d_{lim}, as a function of one of the other variables. Thus v_{lim} can be measured as a function of d or a, d_{lim} as a function of v or a, a_{lim} as a function of d or v. In each case the movement threshold is specified as the limit of detecting the direction of a translation of the moving target, expressed in the appropriate dimensions.

Consider the case of the liminal velocity of movement v_{lim}. This quantity can be specified in a variety of ways (Leibowitz 1955). First, it is clear that at constant luminance the *just-perceptible speed* decreases as the duration of the exposure to the stimulus increases, up to relatively large values of d of about 16 s (figure 3.42). At constant duration, v_{lim} becomes smaller and smaller as the source luminance increases: Movement is best distinguished at very high luminances (figure 3.43). v_{lim} also varies as a function of retinal eccentricity of the image. The fovea appears to be more sensitive to movement than the

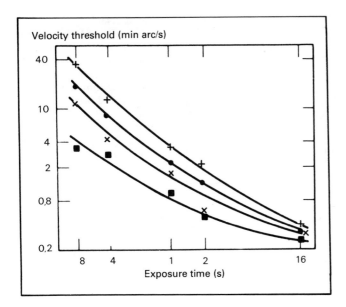

Figure 3.42
Threshold detectable velocities as a function of the duration of exposure in seconds at different luminance levels. Luminances: squares, 500 mL; crosses, 0.5 mL; circles, 0.05 mL; plus signs, 0.005 mL. (From Graham 1965)

periphery, values being the order of 1 min arc/s for foveal vision, 3 min arc/s at 5° eccentricity, 14 min arc/s at 10°, 34 min arc/s at 20° for constant d (of order several seconds) and fixed luminance. The smallest thresholds are attained when the movement takes place with respect to a visible fixed mark, at least in the case of long exposures, values being around 1 to 2 min arc/s with a fixed reference and 10 to 20 min arc/s without one, other things being equal.

Brown (1955) analyzed the influence of luminance and exposure time in discriminating the *direction of movement* (figure 3.44). More precisely, his hypothesis was that the movement discrimination for moderate velocities might depend on a relationship between luminance and duration, as mentioned above, according to a constant product $L \cdot d$. Measuring the threshold for detecting movement direction in terms of liminal luminance L_l for durations of exposure between 1 ms and 3.2 s, he clearly showed that for short durations it is not the luminance needed (L_l) that remains constant but the product of luminance and duration $L_l \cdot d$ for durations up to about 300 ms. Beyond that duration the liminal luminance does become constant. Here, once more, we see a reciprocity between light duration and light intensity for short durations.

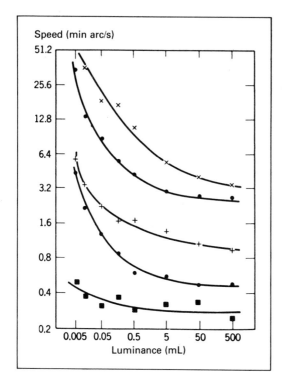

Speed (min arc/s)

Luminance (mL)

Figure 3.43
Minimal speed of a source for movement to be just perceived, as a function of luminance. Parameter: different exposure times, from the top downward, 1/8, 1/4, 1, 2, 16 s. (From Graham 1965)

Measurements of the *liminal duration of exposure* d_{lim} have also been made as a function of velocity. This variation has also been shown to be a reciprocal one, d_{lim} decreasing with increasing velocity.

Finally, a variety of observations have been made on the minimal absolute displacement a_{lim} (liminal displacement amplitude of a single movement that can be detected). Since 1906 a value of 20 sec arc has been agreed for this threshold in photopic conditions. The threshold rises as the periphery is approached, being 3 min arc at 20° and 5 min arc at 40°. [Notice, however, that this sensitivity decrease to movement is more gradual than the decrease in visual acuity for fixed stimuli. Notice also that in optimal conditions, i.e., at the fovea, the threshold in photopic conditions is less than the threshold for spatial discrimination. These factors pose some interesting problems.]

Studies of the *differential threshold for speed changes* have been made particularly using a cathode ray tube spot moving at a velocity v as the test object: The observer is required to detect a change dv (as acceleration or deceleration). The differential sensitivity, given by dv/v, is found to pass through a minimum situated at $v = 1$ to 2 deg/s

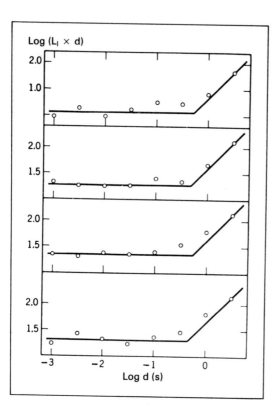

Log (L$_l$ × d)

Log d (s)

Figure 3.44
Relationship betweem liminal luminance L_l and the stimulus duration needed to discriminate the direction of movement of a target exposed for a time d. The horizontal straight line corresponds to a constant product $L_l × d$, the rising straight line to a constant L_l (four different subjects). (From Graham 1965)

and the variation detectable in this range is the order of 0.1 deg/s ($dv/v = 0.10$) (see Hick 1950; Notterman & Page 1957; figure 3.45).

As for the maximal velocity detectable, very high magnitudes of order 10,000 deg/s are reported in particular cases. Clearly, the range of detectable speeds is very wide.

DETECTION IN THE SPATIAL FREQUENCY DOMAIN

Measurements made in the temporal domain using grating images have much extended the study of the visual system's performance. Experiments are made with gratings of a given spatial frequency f in cycles per degree that are presented either with a periodic luminance variation, in principle sinusoidal, at η cycles/s or with a drift in the frontoparallel plane at a speed of v deg/s. In the latter case the three quantities are related by $η = f · v$. In many such experiments the dependent variable is the contrast or spatial luminance modulation specified as above $(L_{max} - L_{min})/(L_{max} + L_{min})$. It is difficult to describe

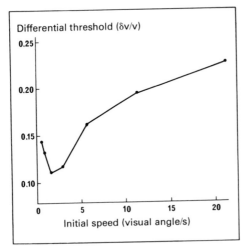

Figure 3.45
Differential threshold for detecting a change in target speed as a function of the speed. (From Sekuler et al. 1978)

all these experiments that are, it must be said, quite complicated. We will only discuss a few of them.

Mechanisms for Detecting the Direction of Movement:
Specificity of Adaptation
We saw earlier, after experiments on fixed gratings, the evidence for different detecting channels "tuned" for different spatial frequencies, that is, spatial frequency is detected in a "metathetic" way. What happens with drifting gratings? The use of drifting gratings has similarly given signs of the existence of channels for the detection of movements.

The experiment consists in measuring the contrast threshold before and after prolonged exposure to a grating moving in a given direction. Measuring the contrast threshold necessary for detecting that a grating of spatial frequency f is moving in a given direction, after having observed it drifting either in the same direction or in the opposite direction for some time, shows the existence of a *specific adaptation:*

• The contrast threshold for detecting a drifting grating increases after prolonged exposure to the same grating, of supraliminal contrast, drifting in the same direction.
• The detection contrast threshold for a grating drifting in the opposite direction is unchanged.
• The adaptation is greater and lasts longer the greater the contrast of the adapting grating, until the effect saturates.

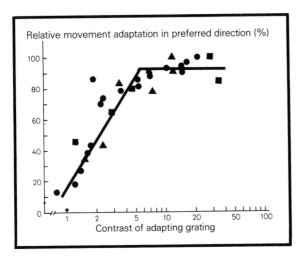

Figure 3.46
Psychophysical measures of adaptation to the movement of a grating in a given direction. Squares, squarewave adapting grating (0.38 cycles/deg liminal contrast 2.4%); triangles, sinusoidal adapting grating (3.4 cycles/deg liminal contrast 0.33%); circles, *relative duration* of the movement aftereffect (same ordinate scale) as a function of contrast of the adapting grating (4 cycles/deg liminal contrast 0.5%). (From Sekuler et al. 1978)

[In fact, these three observations are the result of a series of experiments (Pantle & Sekuler 1969; Sekuler et al. 1978) in which a subject is adapted by a grating drifting in a given direction with its velocity kept constant, the luminance contrast being the independent variable. After adaptation, the threshold contrast for detecting the same grating drifting in the same direction is increased, whereas the threshold for detecting movement in the opposite direction is hardly modified. The log of the differences between threshold elevation for movement in one direction and in the other is taken as a measure of the adaptation. The adaptation relationship is found to be linearly increasing with the adapting contrast, between log/log axes, up to a certain maximum plateau (contrast elevation 5 to 6 times) when the effect saturates (figure 3.46).]

The well-known postadaptation effect experienced after observing a drifting grating can be introduced naturally here. This is the illusion of movement in the opposite direction after the drifting is stopped (the "waterfall effect" described by Addams in 1834). The duration of this postadaptation effect is found to last longer the higher the contrast of the adapting grating. The effect's duration in fact closely follows the shape of the selective adaptation curve (see figure 3.46); therefore it is tempting to explain the effect as a disequilibrium between the two directionally selective mechanisms for opposed directions of movement that established itself at the stopping of the grating's drift. One mechanism will have been adapted and the other not; the latter might instead become temporarily excited for the time the adaptation lasts and in that way give an illusion of movement in the opposite direction.

Sekuler et al. (1978) have reported that the detecting mechanisms for movement direction operate independently, more or less, in the low luminance range also. This was shown by using a stationary grating of the same spatial frequency as moving gratings, alternating at the same temporal frequency and with the same contrast as one or other of the test drifting gratings. It can be shown mathematically that a stationary grating is equivalent to two gratings of half the contrast drifting in opposite directions.

[A drifting grating has a luminance profile that can be described by:

$$L_u(x, t) = L_0\{1 + m \cos(fx \pm \omega t)\},$$

where L_0 is the mean luminance, m the contrast, $f/2\pi$ the spatial frequency, x a point in the visual field, $\omega/2\pi$ the temporal frequency or rate of drift in hertz, and t the time. This is for the case of grating drifting at a rate ω. The sign $\pm \omega t$ shows that we are concerned with gratings drifting in one and the other direction.

The fixed, alternating grating has a luminance profile:

$$L_c(x, t) = L_0\{1 + m \cos(\omega t) \cdot \cos(fx)\}.$$

In spite of its stable appearance it can be analyzed trigonometrically into the sum of two functions representing two gratings each of half the contrast drifting in opposite directions:

$$L_c(x, t) = L_0\{1 + \tfrac{1}{2}m \cos(fx - \omega t) + \tfrac{1}{2}m(fx + \omega t)\}.]$$

If, therefore, the detectors are two independent direction-specific channels, the necessary contrast threshold of a stationary grating ought to be half that of one of the test gratings. And that is what they found.

Conversely, it is found that at high contrast there are signs of an inhibitory effect of one selective detector system on that dedicated for movement in the opposite direction.

The Influence of Temporal Frequency in the Detection of Moving Gratings
A certain number of observations suggest that at low spatial frequencies it is the *temporal frequency* in a drifting grating that is probably the determining feature in the response of the human observer's detection system.

When the contrast sensitivity as a function of velocity is measured for gratings of different spatial frequencies (<3 cycles/deg) a U-shaped function is found. It is notable that in all cases the optimal v obtained is an inverse function of the spatial frequency f, and this fixes the temporal frequency ($\eta = f \times v$) at a practically constant value of order 5 Hz (Watanabe et al. 1968).

Another supporting observation arises from the postdrift adaptation mentioned above. This effect also depends not on the spatial frequency but on the temporal frequency that the drift creates. To keep the latter constant, either f or v can be manipulated to keep the posteffect constant (Sekuler et al. 1978).

A whole series of other observations, from which we will only point out the main lines, lead to the same conclusion, namely, that the detection of a moving grating or, if you wish, its contrast sensitivity, is determined not by the velocity of displacement but rather by the *temporal frequency* of the contrast variations that the movement brings with it.

[When two gratings f and $3f$ move in phase, if the velocity were the important criterion the two gratings would be optimally visible at the same velocity. This is not so. The optimal speeds are different: It is the temporal frequency that is critical. In a new experiment Pantle (1970) used a square wave grating of low spatial frequency (0.38 cycles/deg) as the test stimulus after adaptation by gratings of spatial frequency between 0 and 23 cycles/deg. When the test grating moved at high rates (9 to 22/s) its threshold was only elevated by adapting graftings with spatial frequencies between 0.3 and 0.7 cycle/deg, which suggests that in this experiment it is the frequency of the fundamental component that dictates the threshold visibility of the moving grating, given that in this range of speeds the temporal frequency determined by that fundamental will be situated in the optimal band between 3.6 and 3.8 Hz (for any harmonics the temporal frequency would be >10). On the other hand, when the test grating is displaced slowly it is sensitive to adaptation by a grating of 1.4 cycles/deg, suggesting that it is now the third harmonic of the test grating (1.2 cycles/deg) that most contributes to its detection at low speeds. At these speeds the temporal frequency associated with the movement lies between 0.6 and 3.0 Hz (which is not optimal but is better than that created by the fundamental). In any case, the experiment shows that in a moving complex pattern it is those spatial components that, because of the velocity of movement, generate a temporal frequency of stimulation in the optimal frequency band that are most effective.

In the range of suprathreshold contrasts it seems that, here again, the temporal frequency determines the perception of complex spatial patterns that move at different speeds. Breitmeyer (1973) adapted subjects to random drifting patterns, then evaluated their power of adaptation by comparing the contrast thresholds for stationary gratings, between 0.4 and 10.5 cycles/deg before and after selective adaptation. Two speeds were used, 2.5 deg/s or 6.5 deg/s. After adaptation at 2.5 deg/s the threshold for the grating of 4 cycles/deg was most elevated, whereas after adaptation at 6.5 deg/s the spatial frequency of 1.5 cycles/deg was most affected. Note that in each case it is the product of the velocity by the spatial frequency that matters, that is, the temporal frequency, which in each case is around 10 Hz and is the common constant factor. It is thus tempting to conclude, as did the author, that the visual system contains analytical mechanisms in which the optimal velocity and the spatial frequency analyzed are in an inverse ratio and that the temporal frequency is the invariant quantity to be optimized.]

Movement Detection Mechanisms and Pattern Detection Mechanisms
Campbell's hypothesis of the existence of separate channels for the analysis of different spatial frequencies rested principally, as we have seen above, on the spatial frequency "tuned" nature of the sensitivity reduction after adaptation by different spatial frequencies. Yet it is notable that these experiments, exploiting stationary gratings only, generated no adaptation at frequencies less than 3 cycles/deg. Attempted adaptation at less than 3 cycles/deg merely produced an adaptation characteristic like one at 3 cycles/deg. There is thus an interpretive problem at low spatial frequencies.

In contrast, it was shown that the sensitivity to these same low spatial frequencies is notably increased if a temporal modulation is also added to the grating image (cf. Tolhurst 1973). The hypothesis was suggested that at very low spatial frequencies another sort of channel operates that has a high sensitivity to temporal frequency modulation.

One principal demonstration of this, which in addition allowed a separation between the treatment of spatial information from that of temporal information, concerned the existence of *two different thresholds* when the contrast of an observed grating is increased, depending on whether the grating was moved in the subject's field of view or presented with a simultaneous temporal modulation. One threshold measures the perception of the target's spatial organization without clearly recognizing any movement or flicker; the other threshold corresponds to movement or flicker perception with no clear perception of its spatial pattern (Van Nes & Bauman 1967; cf. Tolhurst 1973).

When a grating of low spatial frequency (<1 cycle/deg) drifts with some mean temporal frequency, say 4 Hz, the first contrast threshold found corresponds to the detection of the temporal modulation in the field without the spatial structure of the grating being discerned: The subject sees a flicker but no precise form. The contrast needs to be increased for any pattern to be detected.

Unlike this, at a higher grating spatial frequency (>3 cycles/deg) the first perception with increasing contrast in these gratings is the spatial structure, without flicker or movement being seen. These need a higher contrast to be perceived.

From all of this arises the hypothesis, now well supported, that there are two parallel processing channels in the visual system with different detectability thresholds for the two characteristics of a moving or flickering grating image, (1) one process detecting temporal modulation in the stimulus whether that variation is related to flicker or to drift and (2) another detecting spatial modulation of contrast or, extrapolating a little, the structure or form of the stimulus (Tolhurst 1973; see Sekuler et al. 1978; Bonnet 1984)

Contrast sensitivities as a function of both spatial frequency and temporal frequency can concurrently be specified for each of the two different systems (in the temporal detectors of movement or flicker and in the spatial detectors of form); see the schematic curves of figure 3.47.

Throughout the data collection during the last two decades concerning the existence of two retinal mechanisms, the one tonic (T) represented by the X ganglion cells and the other phasic (P) represented by the Y cells, it was natural to suggest that the T systems might well underpin form vision and the P system movement vision. But the truth is probably more complicated. We will return below to some of the pitfalls in these ideas, but it is appropriate to point out

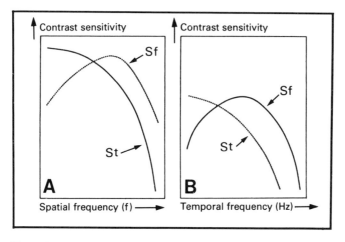

Figure 3.47
Theoretical characteristics of the contrast sensitivity of the form detector and of the movement detector in humans (based on studies by Kulikowski and Tolhurst 1973). Solid curves, sensitivity to flicker and movement (time domain) for a grating; dotted curves, sensitivity to spatial contrast (spatial domain); curves in (*A*), fixed temporal frequency; curves in (*B*), fixed spatial frequency. The curve with the maximum (Sf) is for the form detector in (*A*) and for the frequency detector in (*B*). (From Graham 1965)

here some observations that are based precisely on the duality of tonic and phasic systems. Research has been conducted on how the constrast sensitivity of the different systems of spatial frequency analysis change with stimulus exposure time (Legge 1978). The results show that for low spatial frequencies the *two systems* are involved, whereas only the tonic detectors remain in play at higher spatial frequencies.

5.2 APPARENT MOVEMENT (Φ PHENOMENON)

It is well known that if two spatially separated point sources are successively switched on after a small time interval the nervous system can interpret these two discrete stimuli, separated in time and space, in two quite disparate ways, either as a single continuous movement at a certain speed or as the switching on of two different spatially and temporally separated stimuli (see Anstis 1978).

Note first of all that several variables are concerned, not necessarily independent of one another: time difference t between the two stimuli; duration d_1 and d_2 of each of the two stimuli; distance between the stimuli; their intensities i_1 and i_2; shape and color, etc., whence arises the complexitiy of these studies (Wertheimer 1912; Korte 1915).

[The fact that there is a movement perception without real movement considerably engaged the attention of a certain school of psychologists. The gestalt movement, the "psychology of shape and form," arose partly from the recognition of this phenomenon.]

Assuming brief stimuli, one very important parameter is the time interval t. For an increasing t the subject experiences:

• For $t < 30$ ms, a simultaneous perception of the stimuli.
• Then a perception of (apparent) movement of a single stimulus from one place to the other, this perception being optimal for $t = 60$ ms approximately (sometimes designated as "movement β").
• For $t > 200$ ms, a successive presentation of different stimuli at different places is perceived; see Wertheimer (1912) and Korte (1915).

Under certain conditions, for certain combinations of the times of switching on the stimuli, of the interval t, and of the amplitude of translation, there is a special perception of a *phantom movement*, the perception of movement without the perception of displacement. The target is perceived as stationary at each point of its trajectory yet the impression of movement exists. This type of *stroboscopic perception* is important for cinematography.

Other researches illustrate the nature of continuing work in this field, notably the establishment of different subclasses of movement, following which Le Grand was moved to remark that "practically all the Greek alphabet has been exploited." Apart from the β movement, above, there are also an "α movement" concerned with the apparent size change in successive presentations; a "γ movement" concerned with an apparent growth or shrinkage of the object when successive presentations are accompanied by an increase or decrease in luminance; finally, a "δ movement," which is no doubt the most interesting. This concerns the case when the second stimulus is considerably brighter than the first, when the impression becomes one of a movement in the *opposite* direction (Korte 1915; Neuhaus 1930) from the second stimulus to the first.

Arising from these descriptive aspects, the apparent perception of movement has inspired many discussions in which both the visual pyschologist and visual physiologist become strongly engaged. One sensitive aspect of these discussions is whether apparent and real movement perception share the same neuronal mechanisms or exploit separate ones. Experimental psychologists tend to argue in some instances for the former and in other instances for the latter, whereas (as we shall see in chapter 5, section 3.35), physiologists tend to favor a single mechanism.

Arguments in experimental psychology for a *single mechanism* include:

• Apparent movements are not distinguished from real movements (the success of cinematography suggests that this is so but does not prove it).
• Apparent (stroboscopic) movement can, like a real movement, generate posteffects of apparent movement following direction-selective adaptation techniques.

The argument for *separate mechanisms* points out that for very rapid movements, the detector system for apparent movement appears to be much more sensitive than that for real movement, an apparent movement being perceived for speeds at which real movement is not perceived.

In fact, in a more eclectic view, Braddick (1974) suggests that apparent movement is linked with two distinct mechanisms that become involved in two different conditions:

• One operates for small displacement (≤15 min arc) and/or for short time intervals (<100 ms), with this one serving both real and apparent movements.
• A second operates for greater displacements (20 min to 20 deg arc or even more) that is only concerned with apparent movement.

An interesting extension to this idea of duality of movement mechanisms has been suggested by Anstis (1978), which relates to another question posed by experimental psychology: whether form recognition is a necessary condition for movement perception. In other words, must the subject perceive form to be able to perceive apparent movement or, in contrast, can the perception of movement precede any recognition of the object?

[The following has been established: (1) The random stereograms of Julesz (1978) (see figure 3.67 below) observed monocularly can generate sensations of movement for small displacements, without there being any perception of form (remembering the nature of the objects used). The detecting system seems to operate entirely as if it made a point-to-point comparison of the position at every instant. This sensation of apparent movement is obtained by alternately presenting an image to one eye then to the other. It is only obtained for separations <15 min arc. The hypothesis in this case is that the detectors of movement have operated before any detection of form. (2) For other apparent movement perceptions, point-by-point comparison is not possible, particularly when the perception concerns two configurations that *do not necessarily* have any point-by-point correlation between them. Here it becomes necessary to suggest that a global perception of the object's form must have preceded the perception of movement.]

These observations complement the preceding ones. Detection of movement before detection of form arises in systems for small movements that operate either for real or apparent movement. Detection of form before movement relies on a wide displacement system that is only used for apparent movements. It thus seems to be an economical arrangement for the nervous system to use two separate mechanisms, one for small amplitude displacements (which is always the case for real movements and can be the case for apparent ones), the other for the more global perception of apparent movements of large amplitude. This second system, "a comparator of discrete targets," has the difficult task of deciding whether there is a point-to-point correlation following two successive presentations, with all the possibilities of perceptual illusions that can accompany them. The interested reader is advised to consult specialized texts such as Rock (1975).

6 REAL COLOR VISION

We have already examined some aspects of color vision that assumed a model subject operating in very specific conditions, such as a restricted visual field of 2° to 3° solid angle, using foveal vision at high luminance (100 Td) against a neutral, low-luminance background. In the second stage of our study, we will consider certain questions arising in real color vision from a psychophysical and an experimental psychology viewpoint as well as reviewing some further theoretical proposals concerning the general perception of colors.

The last stage, which will be discussion in chapters 4 and 5, concerns the physiological and neurochemical aspects of color vision in which we will examine retinal and supraretinal mechanisms of color vision in the physiological sections proper of this book.

6.1 ASPECTS OF REAL COLOR VISION

Let us first consider some of the details of color vision as an actual observer experiences it in the real world (see, e.g., Marriott 1962, Le Grand 1964).

VISIBILITY OF THE SHORT WAVELENGTHS

It is probable that all the visibility coefficients V calculated for the violet (<420 nm) for the mean CIE observer have been underestimated for most groups of real observers. From this arise differences in the distribution coefficients in this region of the spectrum for real observers. Such disagreements have been shown, for example, by the fact that certain pigments based on oxides of Ti that have identical trichromatic coordinates for a given illumination C (and should therefore appear to have the same color) are easily distinguished by real observers. The explanation of this is probably that the diffuse reflection of the different pigments differs below 430 nm, whereas that difference is not taken into account for the (mythical) standard CIE mean observer and thus the relative weight of the violet in color vision seems to be underestimated for real observers.

COLORIMETRY FOR LATERAL VISION

Essentially, the colorimetric equation for central vision is also valid for slightly eccentric vision (2° to 6°). At most, a researcher would notice that the color chart is slightly deformed in eccentric vision; one of the reasons for this is, apparently, the diminution in the yellow macular pigment, which gives rise to a relatively lesser absorption of the blue in this pericentral region.

COLORIMETRY AT LOW LIGHT LEVELS

When the light levels exceed 100 Td the colorimetric laws remain valid, provided there is no dazzle. But in the scotopic region where the Purkinje effect changes luminosities, it is necessary to discover how chromaticity changes also. Essentially, low luminance color vision still obeys the diurnal visibility functions but superimposes on that color vision a supplementary luminance due to scotopic mechanisms which slowly and progressively "drown" color vision. As dark adaptation proceeds and scotopic vision predominates more and more, color vision is progressively lost. Scotopic univariance overcomes photopic trivariance: In twilight vision the system passes through a state of quadrivariance needing two lur

and two chromatic variables. In night vision, color

SUBJECTIVE ATTRIBUTES OF COLOR

Let us examine some color attributes that psychumᵤᵧ ᵣₑₑₒ
apart from those straightforward quantities of luminance and wavelength that we have already discussed with respect to color vision
(summarized in table 2.2).

Saturation

This term refers to the extent to which a color is "strong" or is relatively "washed out" in comparison with white. The objective coefficient of chromatic purity p that we defined above in discussing objective colorimetry certainly affects the passage from saturated to
washed out. But for a purity $p = 1$, not all colors have the same
subjective saturation. Thus violet appears to be maximally saturated,
whereas yellow (even for $p = 1$) seems quite close to white.

The Betzold-Brücke Phenomenon

Von Betzold (in 1873) and Brücke (in 1878) independently discovered
that variations in light level change the sensation of color. Practically,
an increase in luminance causes (1) a yellowing of red and of yellow-
green and (2) a movement toward blue of violet and blue-green.
There seem to be places in the spectrum that are invariable: the yellow of 571 nm and the blue of 476 nm, toward which other colors
tend to move with increasing luminance. Situated between these two
is a third invariant color (a bluish-green of 508 nm). Colors near to it
approach its color more closely with increasing luminance (see Walraven 1961). As a concrete example, two colors, one matching 525 nm
and the other 660 nm at 1000 Td, appear to have matches respectively
with the color of 545 and 636 nm at 100 Td. The change is thus far
from negligible. Experimentally investigating this slippage of color
with luminance has shown that the colors that remain stable are in
the yellow 571, the green 508, and the blue 476 nm.

Chromatic Hue

Experiments have shown that if white is added to a spectral light
the dominant color tends to change with the saturation change. By
introducing the concept of *hue*, it is then possible to make subjective
estimates of equal hue (from several subjects) and use these to draw
contours of equal hue on the XYZ color chart (figure 3.48). These are

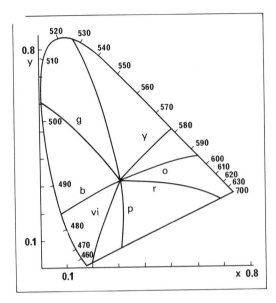

Figure 3.48
Lines of equal hue, for samples of 1% reflectance. *r, o, y, g, b,* and *vi* represent the colors of the spectrum; *p* represents purple (see text). (From Le Grand 1964)

clearly quite different from the theoretical straight lines that join white to the same dominant wavelength (compare figure 2.17).

Luminosity
Consider under this generalized term the factors that determine the visual luminance of a colored source, apart from affecting its color. With *primary sources* [primary and secondary light sources are defined in chapter 2, section 1.2], their subjective luminosity is usually described as the *brightness* of the source. *Secondary sources* are objects that are perceived as lighter or darker according to their reflectance. This is specified by the relative *lightness*.

Other things being equal, the *lightness* (Λ) increases with the reflectance (ρ). The way this occurs has been studied in detail and it is far from linear. Among the many discussions concerning such suprathreshold perception, some have proposed a Fechner type of log law:

$$\Lambda = a \log(1 + b\rho).$$

Others, among them Plateau (1872) preferred a power law:

$$\Lambda = a \cdot \rho^b.$$

In practice the experiments are well enough represented by the latter function with $a = 1.44$ and $b = 0.42$, with the convention that $\Lambda = 10$ when $\rho = 100\%$.

Objects of low lightness (which are very common in the natural world) generate an apparently new sort of tint in the range of orange, yellow, yellow-green, producing the *dull colors* (chestnut, olive, brown, etc.). These dull colors can, in a surprising way, have trichromatic coordinates that do not differ from those of a much lighter color. For example, a piece of chocolate and an orange peel have the same trichromatic coordinates. If the chocolate is lit 10 to 20 times more strongly than the orange peel, the visual stimuli are equivalent *on the condition that* the fragments are observed through a hole in a screen or any other device that only allows a restricted view and prevents any comparison or recognition of the objects. In the following sections we will briefly discuss the importance that lightness can assume in the perception of real colors.

DIFFERENTIAL THRESHOLDS FOR COLOR
The question here is to determine, at a fixed luminance and a given wavelength (λ), how the quantity $\delta\lambda$ varies for detecting a just-perceptible color change, also taking into account the spectral purity p (see chapter 2, sections 3.1, 3.2).

Variation of the Threshold Throughout the Spectrum
In these experiments the purity factor p is kept constant at $p = 1$ (i.e., the colors are all saturated) and $\delta\lambda$ is measured for all monochromatic λ. Practically, the subject observes two homogeneous fields A and B illuminated by monochromatic (narrow-waveband) light. The wavelength is fixed in A and is slowly changed in B until the subject signals a change in color perception of B with respect to A. An essential condition in these experiments is that there be no luminance difference between the two fields (and this can demand very strict experimental care).

Figure 3.49 illustrates the results expressed as the curve of $\delta\lambda$ as a function of λ. Notice that for the "normal" subject, there are two minima in sensitivity with practically the same $\delta\lambda$ value of around 1 nm. The first minimum is near 490 nm (moving from blue to green) and the second at 590 nm (moving from yellow to orange). In addition, another relative minimum is sometimes recorded at 440 nm. The field of observation in these experiments is about 2° solid angle (Wright 1946).

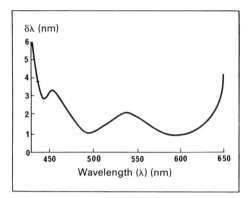

Figure 3.49
Differential sensitivity to wavelength change throughout the spectrum. (From Le Grand 1964)

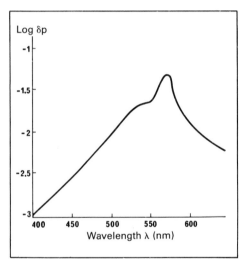

Figure 3.50
Differential sensitivity to color in the neighborhood of white (change δp) as a function of λ (see text). (From Le Grand 1964)

Threshold for the Perception of Colors Close to White
In this case experiments are concerned with keeping λ fixed and varying the colorimetric purity p (as defined in chapter 2, section 3.1), studying how easily the resulting color can be distinguished from white. In practice, the subject is asked to compare a white field of a given luminance B with a field in which δB has been subtracted from the white and replaced by δB of monochromatic light of wavelength λ. The subject signals the $\delta B_{o\lambda}$ at which the quality "colored" becomes just perceptible. Since, by definition $\delta p_{o\lambda} = (\delta B_{o\lambda})\,/B$, we can construct curves of the form $\log \delta p_{o\lambda} = f(\lambda)$ (figure 3.50).

Examining such curves shows that δp is maximal between 550 and 600 nm, this being where the subject is least sensitive to the colored nature of the source. In this region he or she perceives a luminance well before noticing that it is yellow.

Color Thesholds on the Color Chart
Following Wright and, notably, MacAdam we need to extend the representation of these differential thresholds to color onto the various regions of a color chart, such as the XYZ system. Tracing thresholds onto the plane of a color chart and not only between x-y coordinates implies measuring δλ not only in one direction at one point but in a variety of directions around it with respect to the chart's axes. In this way, MacAdam was able to plot values of the root mean square distinguishable thresholds for a variety of points on the chart in a variety of directions, at constant luminance (200 Td). The resultant ellipses (which bear his name) express the color differential thresholds for each point in the XYZ space. The shape of these areas shows that the thresholds are not identical, independent of the direction in which the wavelength of the monochromatic light is changed (figure 3.51).

The practical interest of such quantitative measures of color change is, for example, to evaluate a number of different gradations that separate two colors, or to establish the necessary tolerances between color samples that one wishes to use for matching, or in the limit even to establish what is the total number of distinct chromaticities. The latter, at the luminances used by MacAdam, numbers around 2000.

6.2 ANOMALIES OF COLOR VISION

The only way to approach so vast a topic here is by selecting some general themes of study (see Judd 1951, Marriott 1962, Le Grand 1964, Pokorny et al. 1979, Mollon 1982).

THE DYSCHROMATOPSIAS

For more than a century anomalies of color vision have been classified into a variety of essentially distinct groups, even though they are all described as dyschromatopsias. For some subjects with trivariant color vision (see chapter 2, section 3.1) the colorimetric equations show anomalies. Such subjects are referred to as *anomalous trichromats*. They used to be detected by asking the subject to match two fields, one being yellow and the other a mixture of red and green light. This showed up people who needed significantly higher proportions of red light than usual (even after taking into account normal

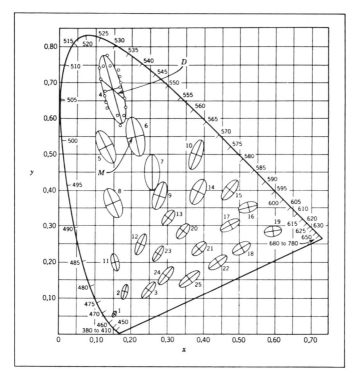

Figure 3.51
MacAdam ellipses. Each ellipse is drawn from points specifying 10 times the standard error in estimates of equal chromaticity, obtained by mean error methods. Retinal illumination held constant at 200 Td (see text). (From Le Grand 1964)

variability in this respect) and similarly those who needed much more green. (We do not have the space to enter into the details of the spectroscopes, Wright colorimeters, etc., actually used.) These subjects were characterized as *protanomalous* and *deuteranomalous*, respectively.

The visibility curve for the deuteranomalous subject differs rather little from the average ($V\lambda_{max}$ = 560 nm instead of 555 nm), whereas the maximum for the protanomalous individual is around 545 nm and is somewhat foreshortened at the red end (figure 3.52)

It is above all in the poor *differential* sensitivities throughout the spectrum (figure 3.53) that anomalous trichromats show their deficiencies. Thus protanomalous subjects (for saturated monochromatic lights) show, as in the normal, two minima at 490 and 590 nm, but these have larger than usual magnitudes and can also be more steeply

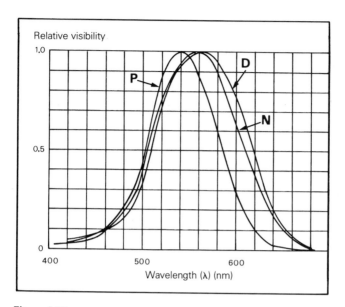

Figure 3.52
Relative visibility curves (equal spectral energies) for (*P*) 6 protanomalous subjects, (*D*) 6 deuteranomalous subjects, and (*N*) a normal subject. (From Graham 1965)

accentuated (figure 3.53, left). In deuteranomalous subjects the curves are less separated from those for the normal subject.

The curves of detection thresholds for colorimetric purity δp in the neighborhood of white are also abnormal, but whereas the deuteranomalous curves only deteriorate in the red, the protanomalous thresholds are higher throughout (figure 3.53, right). Subjectively, it is probable that the deuteranomalous see the spectrum more or less normally except near the red, which might look like a poorly saturated orange color, whereas the protanomalous see the whole spectrum as poorly saturated but with the red appearing to them as very dark because of the poor magnitude of $V\lambda$ in that wavelength region.

Other subjects present a different sort of color vision anomaly. In them the variance is reduced to two. These are *dichromats*; sometimes referred to as daltonians (recalling Dalton's diagnosis of his own color anomaly). Dichromats can be further classified as *protanopes* (red blind), *deuteranopes* (green blind), and much more rarely *tritanopes* (blue/green blind).

Protanopia and deuteranopia are sex-linked, recessive, hereditary phenomena; pure congenital tritanopia is a very rare deficiency and

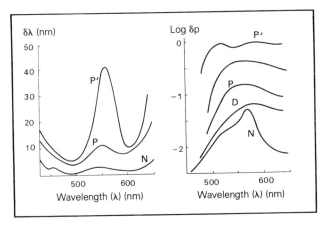

Figure 3.53
Differential sensitivity, throughout the spectrum, for saturated colors (*left*) and near white (*right*) in anomalous trichromats. In the two graphs several protanomalous subjects have been researched. *Left*, Note that the differential sensitivity to saturated colors shows two minima in normal subjects (N). Their contrast is more marked in protanomalous subjects (P) and there is also an abnormal reduction in sensitivity between the two minima. The deuteranomalous subjects show similar results but with lesser differences from normality, except a displacement of the second maximum towards 620 nm. *Right*, The colorimetric thresholds for hues near white for deuteranomalous subjects (D) are near the normal at short wavelengths but deteriorate in the red. In contrast, the protanomalous thresholds are higher throughout the spectrum. (From Le Grand 1964)

is not a sex-linked condition as are the other two dyschromatopsias. In contrast, the mechanisms concerned in the perception of blue are disproportionately sensitive to diseases such as retinitis pigmentosa or diabetes mellitus.

The dyschromatopsias, protanopia, deuteranopia, and tritanopia are considered to be linked to a deficit of long, medium, and short wavelength cones respectively (L, M, and S cones; chapter 4, section 1.3.3).

The visibility curve for dichromats differs from the normal. For protanopes the curve is truncated in the long wavelength region. In contrast, the differences are much less for deuteranopes. These effects are similar to those in the corresponding anomalous trichromats, namely the protanomalous and the deuteranomalous, respectively.

By definition, the colorimetric equations for these subjects only need two chromatic fluxes and not three to reproduce all perceived colors—for example, a primary blue and a primary red. The dichro-

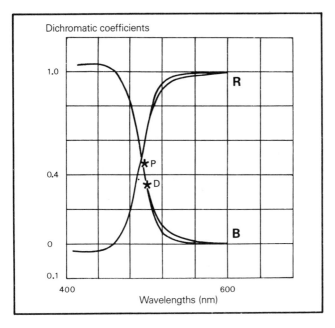

Figure 3.54
Mean dichromatic coefficients as a function of λ obtained from 8 protanopes and 7 deuteranopes for the red (R) and blue (B). P and D are the corresponding neutral points. Compare with figure 2.12. (From Graham 1965)

matic coefficients are similar in the two main populations of dichromats (figure 3.54). Because of this characteristic, the dichromat can find a certain color in the spectrum which to him appears white but cannot be matched with white by a normal subject or by an anomalous trichromat. The locating "point" for this anomalous white is in fact a narrow zone that is different for protanopes (490 to 498 nm, average 494 nm) and for deuteranopes (495 to 510 nm, average 502 nm); see figure 3.54. The case for tritanopia is harder to specify, because of its rarity. The neutral point seems to be around 570 nm.

The color sensation of a dichromat, in summary, seems to be reduced to a selection of two hues that are called yellow or blue with the color saturations being maximal at one and the other extremity of the spectrum.

Finally, dichromats show another notable characteristic. The values for the differential threshold throughout the spectrum [$\delta\lambda = f(\lambda)$] for distinguishing maximally saturated colors demonstrate that $\delta\lambda$ is higher than normal and the curve has a different shape: There is only

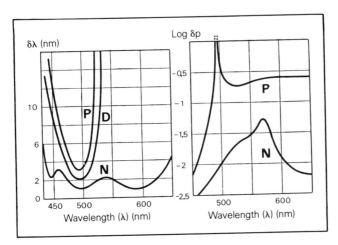

Figure 3.55
Differential sensitivities δλ throughout the spectrum for saturated colors (*left*) and
in the region of white (*right*) for dichromats. N, normal; D, deuteranopes; P, protanopes. (From Le Grand 1964)

one maximum, near the neutral point (i.e., around 490 to 500 nm;
figure 3.55). The curve of $\delta p = f(\lambda)$ is notably very different from the
normal in the region of white, where it shows a singularity where
$\delta p \to \infty$ at the neutral point which the subject confuses with a "true"
white.

Dichromats characteristically confuse colors. This phenomenon has
been subjected to many investigations. Referring to either the XYZ
or RGB color charts, the trichromat needs three coordinates to represent a color (as already illustrated in figure 2.14). In contrast, for a
dichromat one of the primaries will be lacking (say B) so that all the
colors $c1$, $c2$, and $c3$ situated on the straight line (GR) will not be
separable from a color $c4$ also situated on the line GR (550 to R) (figure
3.56). Such a straight line is called a *line of confusion*. There is a whole
family of them and for a given dichromat, experiment shows that all
the straight lines of confusion converge on a point called the *center
of confusion* (O in figure 3.56). One of the lines of confusion common
to a variety of dichromats is the practically rectilinear section between
R and 550 nm (G) (called a single color zone); another such line is
one for white that passes through the point W (of "true white") and
the neutral point N. From these facts it is possible to calculate the
coordinates for the points of confusion for protanopes ($x_p = 0.747$,
$y_p = 0.253$) and for deuteranopes ($x_d = 1.08$, $y_d = 0.08$); see figure

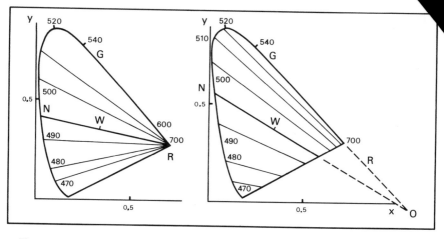

Figure 3.56
Diagrams illustrating color confusion in protanopes (*left*) and deuteranopes (*right*).
N, "neutral point"; W, white light. Point of confusion for deuteranope is O and for
the protanope R (see text). (From Le Grand 1964)

3.56. It seems that the point of confusion for tritanopes is in the violet
($x_t = 0.170$, $y_t = 0.000$); see figures 3.48 and 3.49.

Finally there are the subjects called *monochromats*. These cannot
discriminate colors in any way. Each color can be matched with another simply by making appropriate luminance changes. Most
monochromats—sometimes called "true achromats" or phota-
nopes—behave as though their retina were entirely deprived of cones
and only had rods ("rod monochromats"). In fact, their visibility
curve is like the normal subject's scotopic curve (maximum at about
500 nm). They are also photophobic and have a diminished visual
acuity.

Other rare monochromats, in contrast, seem to have a fovea with
cones but of only one sort. Their visibility curve has its maximum at
545 nm and the foveal visual acuity is normal. These cones seem to
be "green receptor" types. Some cone monochromats have been
found with only "blue cones" and a visibility maximum at 440 nm.
We will return later to some explanations of these anomalies.

ANOMALIES IN THE EUCHROMAT

Some deviations from trichromatic color mechanisms can be found
in normal subjects.

ıall Sources

ıs are found in color vision for small sources (on the
of arc), compared with that for larger fields (on the
ᴜ₁ ∠⁻). Not only is the differential threshold δλ higher, but
the *minimal differential threshold* is situated near 570 to 580 nm, just
like the characteristic of a tritanopic dichromat with the minimal
threshold in the yellow/orange. In fact, the experiments are very
difficult to perform because an absolutely immobile fixation of such
a small point is only possible for very small exposure times. This
central tritanopia,, demonstrable when the field is very small, is linked
to the *relative rarity of blue cone receptors.* (See the work of Mollon
referred to in the next section.)

Mollon and Polden (1977) have investigated this tritanopia. One
result establishes that after adapting the eye with yellow or red lights,
the sensitivity return in the short wavelengths is much slower than
it is, for example, after adaptation to white light and results in a
"transient tritanopia." Whatever might be the whole story, it is clear
that in general the blue receptors are significantly more scarce than
the other types of color receptors.

Peripheral Dichromatism

The phenomenon of defective color perception at increased eccentricity is not well understood and the data are controversial. Some claim
that the color sensations vanish unequally: green first of all, near 30°,
then red, yellow, and finally blue, near 45°. But in fact this "perimetry
of color sensation" seems to give imprecise and variable results at
present.

THEORIES OF COLOR VISION

We can now consider the attempts that have been made to specify
the true parameters of color vision without yet assuming a knowledge
of any of the physiological researches that have in some cases weak-
ened and in others strengthened the different hypotheses. To select
an appropriate theory, extensive data must be taken into account
such as the photopic visibility curve, Abney's law, the laws of colorimetry (visual trivariance, Grassman's laws, trichromatic coordinates,
luminosity of the primaries, etc.) as well as the data related to dyschromatopsias and certain psychological aspects of the perception of
color (saturation, brightness, Betzold-Brücke's phenomenon, etc.).
Traditionally color vision theory has been divided into two distinct
families. These, moreover, have very unequal importance.

The Young-Helmholtz Theory
In 1801 Young, after some preliminary references to it, fully launched the idea of three types of retinal receptors that are sensitive to three primary colors. The idea was adopted and amplified in 1852 by Helmholtz, who emphasized the fundamental fact that the choice of primary colors was essentially arbitrary. What later became known as the Young-Helmholtz theory comprised the following propositions:

• The visual organ contains three types of receptor R1, R2, R3, with three corresponding response *fundamentals* G1, G2, G3.
• Each receptor's spectral response G_i to an illumination energy distribution E_λ can be characterized by means of a wavelength-sensitive function $\bar{g}_i$ as follows:

$$G_i = f\bar{g}_i \cdot E_\lambda d_\lambda.$$

Color sensation is a function of the relative values of the three responses G_i.
• Perceived luminosity is a function of a linear combination of the three responses, therefore a function of the quantity $\Sigma L_i G_i$ where L_i is a constant: $L_1 G_1 + L_2 G_2 + L_3 G_3$. From this it can be seen that the expressions in G_i represent the primary colorimetric tristimulus coefficients, the $\bar{g}_i$ values are distribution coefficients, and the L_i terms are luminosity magnitudes. For this system to coincide with experimental systems (e.g., the XYZ system), the necessary and sufficient conditions are that there exist linear transformations between the tristimulus coefficients (or, what comes to the same thing, between the distribution coefficients).

Without going into great detail, let us point out that provided one adds a further condition (that white has uniform energy content) six magnitudes are needed (instead of nine) to specify the fundamentals.
Over the years, all variations have been determined by the choice of different types of fundamental; the choice sometimes being on the basis of theory, sometimes for practical purposes and even in certain cases inspired by experiment.
[Thus, one of the principles exploited was based on the study of dichromats, it being agreed that deficits are due to the *suppression* of one fundamental. In fact only two types of dichromat were known, protanopes and deuteranopes, so there remained some degree of uncertainty. This difficulty was resolved in various ways that we will not pursue in detail here. We might mention in this respect "König's

fundamentals," incorporating various solutions depending on the choice of the fundamental blue.

Another solution was suggested, also founded on dyschromatopsias but attributed this time to a *diminution*, not an abolition of a fundamental and on the *combination* of the red fundamental and the green fundamental in one and the same receptor to generate the sensation of yellow (Fick's fundamentals).

A third set of solutions consisted in taking note not of dyschromatopsias but of the effects of adaptation by colored lights. This was particularly exploited by Wright (1946).

A fourth approach consisted in *experimentally* determining the spectral absorptions of the three types of cones by using an original method concerned with investigating the discrimination of color on an adapting field (Stiles 1939).]

Consider, for the moment, Stile's approach (Boynton 1979, Marriott 1962, Barlow & Mollon 1982, Mollon 1982). This consisted in adapting chosen classes of cone with appropriate monochromatic lights in such a way that only one class of cone was left free from adaptation and available for study (figure 3.57).

A monochromatic flash of light of wavelength λ (for 200 ms, 1° field, foveal projection) is presented in the center of a wide concentric adapting field of a differnt wavelength μ. The detection threshold for the test flash U_λ is measured as a function of the luminance of the adapting field W_μ. The working hypotheses are that (1) each cone is only sensitive to one band of wavelengths and (2) the state of adaptation of other cones does not affect the sensitivity of the class being studied. For Stiles and those who adopted his methods this second hypothesis became a sort of essential role, the existence of which entirely determines the validity of the results ("principle of independent adaptation").

The key determination is how the detection threshold for a flash of wavelength λ (U_λ) varies as a function of the luminance W_μ of the adapting field of wavelength μ (from this can be plotted a detection/threshold curve of log U_λ as a function of log W_μ).

Then μ is varied, keeping λ constant. The result is that the curve moves along the abscissa. This slippage can be used as a measure of the *spectral sensitivity* of the receptors under study. To achieve this one measures for each value of μ the magnitude of W_μ needed to increase the threshold U_λ by a certain amount, always the same, fixed at, say, 10 times the absolute threshold U_λ in the absence of any

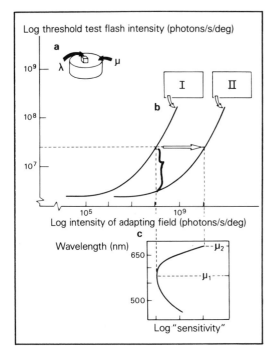

Figure 3.57
Studies of color sensitivities by Stiles's two-color method. (*a*) Spatial arrangement of
the test flash (λ) on the adapting field (μ). (*b*) Threshold/intensity curves for the same
test colors λ but for two different adapting colors μ_1 and μ_2. The horizontal dashed
line indicates the threshold elevation (1 log unit) chosen by Stiles as criterion. (*c*)
"Sensitivity" to the field. When μ_2 is used instead of μ_1, the threshold/intensity curve
is displaced along the abscissa by 2 log units. This corresponds in (*c*) to a threshold
elevation of 100. (From Mollon 1982)

adapting field whatsoever (figure 3.58A). From these measurements
the sensitivity of the receptors studied to the colored light of wavelength μ can be plotted.

Another strong point of interpretation in these experiments is that
when, for certain combinations of μ and λ values, abrupt changes
arise in the slopes of the experimentally determined curve at particular points (figure 3.58B), this is accepted as a sign that one spectrally
specific mechanism has been exchanged for another; in other words,
the effect has *changed from being mediated by one receptor class and is
taken over by another.*

Using such methods, Stiles identified certain distinct mechanisms
of color perception that he called "π mechanisms," three of which

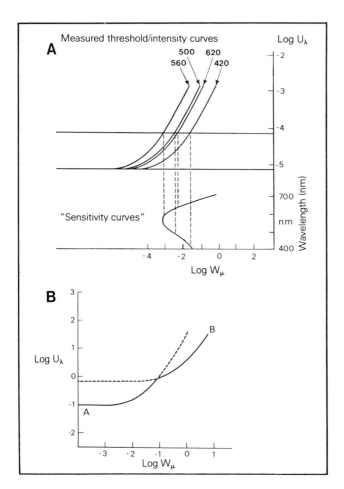

Figure 3.58
Characteristics of the "primary" color mechanisms determined by Stiles's method.
A, Threshold is determined for a small-area foveal flash in the presence of a wide
concentric field of luminance W and color (wavelength μ marked beside each curve in
nm). Four threshold/intensity curves are plotted, from which it is calculated how much
W_μ must be increased to raise the threshold (U_λ) by 1 log unit (cf. figure 3.57), obtaining
thereby a *sensitivity curve* for the system as a function of μ. This curve is shown in the
lower part of A with threshold along the horizontal axis and wavelengths on the
vertical axis. U_λ and W_μ are each expressed in erg · s · deg^{-2}. B, When a break is found
in the global sensitivity curve, the singular point is considered to indicate a transition
between two distinct color mechanisms. (From Marriott 1962)

had maximal sensitivities at wavelengths remarkably close to the maxima that were later measured by more direct methods of retinal receptor densitometry and spectrophotometry (described later). These mechanisms were maximally effective at 440 nm (π_3), 540 nm (π_4), and 570 nm (π_5). Stiles also described other mechanisms π_1 and π_2 at short wavelengths. The interpretation and discussion of these mechanisms in the blue would take us far from the present topic.

[Mechanisms linked with receptors for blue light pose a series of problems that are very different from any encountered in the other two color mechanisms. Many of the anomalies observed in this frequency band can be explained by the sparse population of short wavelength receptors, by their poor absolute sensitivity, by their high differential threshold ($\delta I / I > 9\%$), by their spatial integration (i,e., validity of Ricco's law) over a much more extensive area than for other colors, and by their temporal integration (Bloch's law) across a larger duration range. Added to all these difficulties is Stiles's evidence for a multiplicity of π mechanisms at that extremity of the spectrum. We will not develop these points further, but see Mollon (1982).]

The problem of luminosity detection, a question also posed by Young, relies for its resolution on very precise quantitative factors. This concerns the question of the *white receptor*. In this theory the perception of "photopic white" should occur by a summation of the outputs from several cones that results in this entirely novel visual sensation. However, summations of this sort do not necessarily obey Abney's law. To retain this law's validity, a supplementary receptor was suggested that only produced a sense of luminance. Among these suggestions must be counted that of Piéron (1945) of a *receptor tetrad* which comprised three cones, each containing one of the three visual pigments, with a fourth cone containing a mixture of them. The light would appear white after processing in this receptive unit when the inputs from the three cones were equivalent. Thus by mutual inhibition they annul each other's effects and leave only the white receptor active. In fact the existence of such cones ("à pigments mélangés") has not been shown by modern microspectrophotometric receptor measurements. Thus the problem of white sensation still remain largely undecided, and the reader interested in modern psychological studies of color vision is advised to consult specialized reviews, such as Mollon (1982).

Hering's Theory
In 1872 Hering introduced a second and quite different theory, this time from a viewpoint that was more radically related to psychological data. His explanation relied on the existence of six distinct sensations divided into three antagonistic couplings: white/black, yellow/blue, and red/green. These pairings correspond to the dual, opposed actions of light on three retinal substances, one *catabolic* action producing, depending on the substance, a sensation of white, or yellow, or red ("hot colors") and one *anabolic* action generating black, or blue, or green ("cold colors"). The first substance was destroyed by white and regenerated by black, an equilibrium between the two resulting in a shade of "retinal grey" that is quite distinct from the black, which can be created by simultaneous or successive contrast. The second substance was destroyed by yellow and regenerated by blue, responding neither to green nor to white nor to purple. The third substance was catabolized by red and regenerated by green, yellow, blue, and white light having no effect on it.

   This theory is clearly unacceptable on several grounds that need not be detailed here, apart from its obvious reliance on an obscure and unscientific reasoning that contrasts sharply with the trichromacy theory based on the quantitative laws of colorimetry. However, this has not prevented the discovery of a certain amount of physiological data, limited in their extent, that have fortuitously revived it, not at the level of retinal mechanisms but in some of the color antagonistic activity in the central visual pathways (see chapter 4). [A Hering type action in the supraretinal pathways had already been suggested in the "theory of zones" of early researchers (by Donders in 1881 and others) to justify the single nature of the perception of yellow, a characteristic that is not emphasized by the Young-Helmholtz theory.]

Color Constancy and Theories of Color Vision
Theories of color vision have assumed that the pathways and visual centers contain analyzers that are sensitive to particular wavelengths, and physiology has, as we shall see, largely confirmed this expectation. The color of a given object is directly linked with the dominant light frequency that it reflects from its surface, and there are a collection of cells in the visual cortex that respond preferentially to that color. However, this correlation arose largely from experiments in a laboratory situation (thus in danger of being very artificial) in which *separate isolated* colored fields were presented to the eye.

This is not normally the situation in real life, in which the color of objects seems to be *constant* for many and varied compositions of the incident light. Thus, for example, the leaf of a tree remains green even if the spatial composition of the light illuminating it varies over a considerable range. The observation of this "color constancy" is not new. Hering had demonstrated it in one of his classic experiments: Two cards of different color (one brown, the other blue) are examined in isolation, each lit by a different source. The illumination of the blue card can be adjusted so that it appears to be brown (this is always possible). If now the two cards are placed side by side under the illumination that made the blue card appear to be brown in isolation, it immediately appears to be its normal color, so long as it is seen with the brown card. Land's systematic observations (1974) have elaborated this sort of experiment by using matte-surfaced cards of different colors arranged in a mosaic of squares and rectangles that are observed under different intensities and different selected light wavelengths (long wavelengths or short wavelengths). Without going into detail (for which see Zeki 1990) it can be concluded that under a *global* viewing of a complex scene such as this mosaic, the fact that one or another band of wavelengths predominates in the reflected light from a given card in the mosaic does not modify its color. In summary, even if the color of a surface in isolation depends on the wavelength composition of the reflected light, there is not nearly so simple a relationship between the compositon of the wavelengths in the reflected light and the color perceived when the card is examined in its environmental context. This is to say that the perception of hue comprises color conservation, in a way that disobeys the laws of colorimetry, only when the visual pathways and centers are provided with *comparative elements* of information from various parts of the visual field.

These results have led to the hypothesis that a certain number of operations are effected from information on the *brightness* of a surface and this is linked with its *reflectance*, yielding a constant measure for a given object (Land 1974, 1983). It is assumed that in the neuronal centers some weighting operations are carried out from the whole gamut of individual local inputs based not on their absolute intensities but on the various brightnesses extant in the perceptual field.

It is interesting to recall in this respect an assertion that is apparently quite different but in fact is an essential function in color perception (Naka & Rushton 1966). Rushton effectively emphasized an inevitable confusion between light intensity and color signals at the level of a single photoreceptor. Each class of cone ("color receptor") cannot alone carry pure color information since the cell's response can be changed in the same way by appropriately changing either the color or the intensity of the light [or even both of them—Trans.] that stimulates it. The information carried by a cone is thus not unequivocal. This *principle of univariance* makes it essential that a comparison must be made beyond these receptors in the central nervous system, intraretinal and postretinal. Thus, from this aspect too, the perception of color may be regarded as the result of a central operation comparing the information received from each class of cone.

7 AFTERIMAGES

A subject who has been exposed to a very bright source and is suddenly plunged into darkness experiences, from that moment in time, sensations of luminosity and color called *afterimages* that follow one another in a complex series of events sometimes lasting for several seconds. These sensations, which recall the phenomena of successive contrast, have been studied seriously for some time and have gathered to themselves a very elaborate terminology (Brown 1965).

7.1 TERMINOLOGY

Primary stimulus: a stimulus that is the cause of afterimage (AI)
Positive afterimage: an AI that has the same arrangement of relative brightnesses as the primary stimulus
Negative afterimage: an AI with the arrangements of relative brightnesses reversed compared with the primary stimulus
Homochromatic afterimage: an AI with color distributions similar to the primary stimulus
Complementary afterimage: an AI in which the colors are throughout complementary to those in the primary stimulus
Original afterimage: an AI seen in darkness after exposure to the primary stimulus
Secondary stimulus: an extended field of uniform light upon which background an AI is perceived
Afterimage on a secondary stimulus: an AI perceived on the background of the secondary stimulus

7.2 CLASSES OF AFTERIMAGES

Descriptions of the exact temporal sequencing of afterimages are far from unanimous, presumably because these depend not only on the primary stimuli but also on the observer. Apparently a very favorable method of generating afterimages is to expose the subject to a short, intense flash, followed immediately by darkness. The subject then sees in succession:

1. A first positive AI, called a Hering AI (latency 50 ms, duration 50 ms).
2. A first negative AI.
3. A second positive AI, called a Purkinje AI or a Bidwell AI (latency 200 ms, duration 200 ms). The most constant phenomenon, this comprises, depending on the case, (a) a succession of different colors if the primary stimulus was white: blue–green–red–blue or green, or (b) colors complementary to the primary stimulus if it was colored.
4. A second negative AI.
5. A third positive AI, called a Hess AI (latency about 500 ms, slow disappearance up to about 900 ms, duration). It is less bright than the Purkinje AI and, depending on the case, it is likely to be homochromatic with the primary stimulus.
6. A third negative AI, often long lasting.
7. A fourth positive AI, very weak and inconstant, is sometimes reported.

Note: Negative AIs appear dark with respect to "retinal grey," which is the perception of the background visual field seen at rest in total darkness, a perception which itself is not totally black. This retinal phenomenon intrinsic to the eye (entoptic) has been variously called retinal chaos or noise, intrinsic retinal light, Eigengrau.

Conditions become complicated when an AI is viewed against a lit homogeneous field. The luminances, color, particular temporal exposures, and position of the retina all need to be considered. Essentially, if the eye is exposed to a white primary stimulus and the AIs are observed on a neutral homogeneous uniform field, the AIs follow the same sort of sequences as in darkness. Things are, not surprisingly, more complicated for (a) a colored primary stimulus on a neutral ground, (b) a white primary stimulus on a colored ground, and (c) a primary stimulus and a secondary colored ground. In case (a) one sees successively and briefly an AI of the same color, then predominantly an AI of grossly the complementary color (red → green, blue → yellow, for example). In cases (b) and (c) the result is approximately what would be obtained by mixing lights of the colors of the AI and the secondary field.

We will not pursue this analysis further. Researchers have studied the effects of a whole range of primary stimulus variables that determine the nature of AIs (area, duration, luminance, spectral content, homogeneity, etc.) as well as the retinal region stimulated, state of adaptation of the eye, and so on, but while their investigations have been meticulous, they do not lead to any great advance in understanding retinal mechanisms. Later, however, we will discuss some interesting physiological observations on the general ways in which afterimages arise.

[Certain other effects should be distinguished from afterimages proper. These include the effects, often very late, of dazzling light exposure. They can last for several minutes, in the course of which complementary brilliance and color changes are both clearly perceived (white → black, red → green, yellow → blue).]

8 VISUAL SPACE

We must now consider problems concerned with the visual perception of external space. Even though this perception is usually considered to be primarily a matter of binocular vision with coordinated eye movements, a certain importance for monocular visual mechanisms must also be taken into account. Our discussion will mostly concern the first aspect, followed by a less extensive look at the second. (For reviews, see Ogle 1962, Le Grand 1964, Graham 1965).

8.1 BINOCULAR SPATIAL VISION

Before considering the nature of the visual field, we need to consider the methodology for specification of a point in the visual field with respect to the point *F* that represents the fixation point of the gaze. Essentially, two methods of specification have been and continue to be used, depending on the researcher (see Bishop et al. 1962).

In traditional perimetry (figure 3.59A), rectangular axes are constructed with *F* as the origin. One is the *horizontal meridian* (HM), the other the *vertical meridian* (VM). The point under consideration (*P*) is specified by polar coordinates. Its vector radius **FP** is read from a series of parallel circles drawn for every degree between 0 at the origin and 90° (with + signs for *P* above *HM* and − for below). Its vector angle is usually specified clockwise with, for the upper half of the visual field, 0° at the left on *HM*, 90° above, 180° to the right on *HM* and continuing through the lower part of the field via 270°, below, to 360° (≡ 0° on *HM*). Note, however, that other conventions are sometimes used to specify longitude.

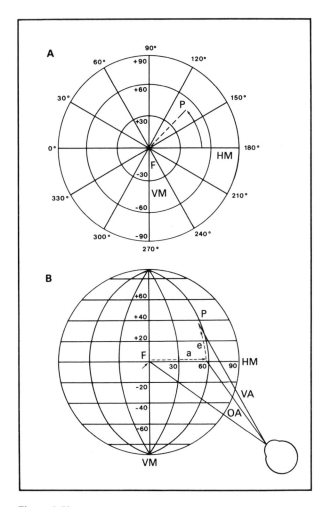

Figure 3.59
Ways of specifying a point *P* in visual space with respect to the fixation point *F*. HM,
(zero) horizontal meridian; VM, (zero) vertical meridian. *A*, Classic perimetry with
specifications in polar coordinates. Angular distance from *F* is shown in degrees, at
an angle (with respect to the HM). Conventionally 0° is at the left. The marking of the
parallels 210 to 330 is in fact redundant, since the same parallel is specified as positive
or negative depending on whether the point is above or below the HM. *B*, Method
more often used by experimentalists for defining two angular distances with respect
to the two principal axes HM and VM: azimuth (*a*) with respect to the VM and elevation
(*e*) with respect to the HM. OA, optic axis; VA, line of vision of *P*. In this method,
angles to the right of VM are positive and angles to the left are negative. (From Bishop
et al. 1962)

Another, more hybrid, specification is often used by experimentalists (but not, it seems, by ophthalmologists). This also uses the horizontal and vertical meridians *HM* and *VM* (figure 3.59B) but then a mixed system of straight lines parallel to *HM* numbered to +90° above HM and to −90° below together with arcs of circles, *meridians*, specified as angular distances from *VM*, 0° to +90° to the right and 0° to −90° to the left. The point *P* is specified in quasi-cartesian coordinates with an *azimuth*, positive or negative, with respect to *VM* and an *elevation*, positive or negative, with respect to *HM*.

Two principal operations are linked to binocular vision: convergence and stereoscopic vision (stereopsis). We shall discuss these in turn, but first we need to consider briefly a problem related to the visual field.

THE BINOCULAR VISUAL FIELD

We emphasized when discussing phylogenetic aspects in chapter 1 that the visual field may be divided into monocular and binocular fields, and we gave quantitative specifications of the visual fields of some vertebrate species. Let us now discuss some points concerning the human visual field, which is the concern of this chapter.

Perimetry shows that the contour of the monocular field is not circular because obstruction by the nose (and eyebrows and cheekbones) particularly restricts vision in the nasal direction (figure 3.60A). If binocular vision is measured instead, that is, the region of overlap between the two monocular fields, it is clear that the overlap is not total; to either side of the binocular field there is added a crescent of temporal monocular vision (figure 3.60B). The horizontal extension of vision by this crescent-shaped field along the horizontal meridian is about 25°.

CONVERGENCE

Convergence is defined as the fixation by the two eyes on a point *A* in the visual field, with the assumption that the two principal lines of gaze intersect at *A* and that corresponding images are formed on the two foveas, leading to a fusion of the two punctate retinal images. If the image of *A* were to fall on the fovea of one eye and outside the fovea of the other, the impression would be of two separate images (i.e., a subjective *diplopia*).

The simplest case is that of *symmetrical convergence*, when the two principal directions of gaze cut in the median plane of the interpupil-

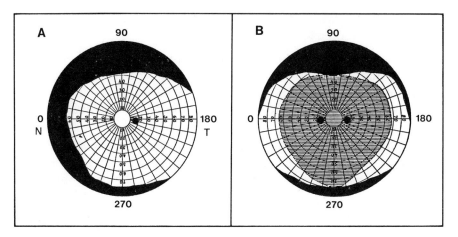

Figure 3.60
Monocular (*A*) and binocular (*B*) fields of human vision (plotted by conventional perimetry). *A*, Right monocular field; the black boundary marks the true limit of this field. Note its greater extension temporally (T) than nasally (N). The black circle marks the external projection of the blind spot. *B*, The cyclopean field; both sides of the binocular field are hatched (lateral extent in the HM ±60°) and the crescents of monocular vision are unshaded. The two blind spots are shown with respect to the central fixation point. Invisible regions are in black. (From Le Grand 1964)

lary line (or more rigorously, of the baseline joining the centers of rotation of the eyes w_1 and w_2). If λ is the angle of convergence, we may write (see figure 3.65A):

$$\tan (\lambda/2) = a/2d$$

where a is the interpupillary distance (not distinguished here from the baseline distance w_1w_2 which in humans = 61 mm) and d is the distance of point A from the straight line w_1w_2. For small angles the convergence in radians can be approximated by $\lambda = a/d$ and in degrees $\lambda = 57.3\ a/d$. Sometimes λ is expressed (Nagel 1861) as the reciprocal of the distance in meters from the fixation point A to the middle of the baseline. This *metric angle* has dimensions m^{-1}.

A more complex case is *asymmetrical convergence*, which arises when the fixation point A is to one side of the line w_1w_2. However, it can be shown without much difficulty that here also, accepting some approximations, the expression $\lambda = a/d$ in radians still holds.

In a subject with normal vision (emmetrope), as the fixation point gets closer, there is an accommodation (in focus) that keeps the foveal image sharp, in addition to the convergence of the gaze.

CORRESPONDING POINTS ON THE RETINA

Definitions
One might think that if the two eyes fixate on the same point in space
there should be an impression of *two different directions*. Pursuing this
line further, one might also imagine that if the two eyes examine the
same object there could result an impression of two different objects
in two different directions ("we see two images because we have to
eyes"). The facts are clearly quite otherwise, since the two images on
the two retinas normally give rise to a single percept in a single
direction (*principal direction*). These considerations, which may appear
to be trivial, in fact led to the classical notion of *corresponding points* on
the retina: pairs of points, one on each retina, for which simultaneous
stimulation leads to the sensation of a single external source. By
definition also, noncorresponding, disparate points give rise to two
distinct sensations (i.e., to a diplopia).

Vision in the Principal Directions
Suppose an upright subject with head held straight looks front to the
horizon. Geometrically, a line parallel to the baseline is defined as
horizontal and one perpendicular to it, and thus parallel to the vertical
meridian, is *vertical*. Under these conditions we can determine for
monocular vision (one eye being closed) the horizontal meridian h,
which is the retinal image of HM and the vertical meridian v, which
is the image of VM. Comparing the results so obtained for each eye,
we find that the vertical meridians are not parallel but converge toward the base of the visual field at an angle of about 2° in an emmetrope. From this we conclude that the eye generates, in the opposite
sense, a rotation of about 1° around the visual axis when it changes
from viewing HM, presented alone, to viewing VM, presented alone.
It is thus in a system of oblique axes h_1, v_1, h_2, and v_2, that we should,
to be completely rigorous, define the corresponding points on the
retina (but h_1 and h_2 are normally not so distinguished).

Definition of the Theoretical Horopter
Consider the definition of the *horopter*, namely, the locus of point
objects in visual space which, for a given position of the eyes (thus
of the direction of gaze), project on corresponding points in the retina. The simplest solution relies on the hypothesis that corresponding
points on the two retinas, assumed identical, comprise images of
pairs of points (E, F in figure 3.61) that are angularly equidistant.

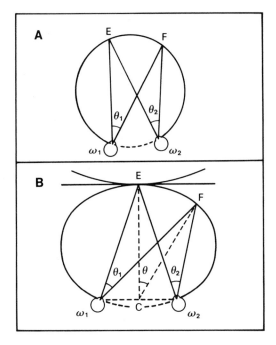

Figure 3.61
Theoretical and real horopters. *A,* Theoretical longitudinal (horizontal) horopter (Vieth-Müller circle). *B,* Example of a real, symmetrical horopter. θ_1 and θ_2, visual angles to points E and F; w_1 and w_2, optical centers of the eyes. For the elliptical, real horopter θ is the mean angle $(\theta_1 + \theta_2)/2$.

Under these conditions the horizontal *theoretical horopter,* which passes through both the baseline w_1w_2 (in practice through the entry pupils P_1P_2) and the fixation point, will clearly be the locus of points that are seen by the two eyes at the same angular separations θ from a given position ($\theta_1 = \theta_2$) or, what is geometrically the same thing, see two points P_1 and P_2 under the same angle of convergence. This must be a circle: It is called the Vieth-Müller circle (see figure 3.61A).

The Real Horizontal Horopter
The real situation is quite otherwise: In practice the horopter is not a circle (Ogle 1962, Le Grand 1964).

Experimental determination of the horopter. First consider the problems in experimentally determining corresponding points of the retina. A typical experiment consists of fixating on a point F marked on a vertical rod. To the side there is a second rod (T) that can be brought closer or farther away by the subject but only along the same line of sight of one eye (e.g., the left; figure 3.62). All precautions are taken to avoid extra clues being exploitable (e.g., the height of the rods). According to the position of the movable rod T (closer or farther away), the subject may have the following impressions:

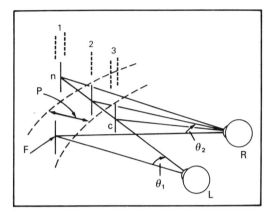

Figure 3.62
Perspective sketch of the principles of an apparatus for determining the human horizontal horopter. The eyes fixate on the point F. A movable rod can be displaced along the visual axis of the left eye (c to n). Depending on its position, the perception may be of two rods (diplopia) such as the dashed rods at (1) and (3), or of a single rod as dashed rod (2). The limits of the region for seeing P without diplopia are indicated by the double-ended arrow (see text; 1 illustrates uncrossed diplopia and 3 crossed diplopia. (From Ogle 1962)

- At a certain position the observer will perceive a single rod.
- When rod T is moved farther away, the observer will eventually perceive two rods seen subjectively in two directions that become more separated as the distance away from the observer becomes greater (*physiological diplopia*).
- Moving T closer to the observer from the position of a single fused image also generates a physiological diplopia.
- The "near" diplopia and the "far" diplopia are, however, distinguishable. If, for example, the subject closes the right eye the image to the right disappears in far diplopia, whereas the image to the left disappears in near diplopia. The first case is referred to as *direct* or *homonymous diplopia* and the second case as *crossed diplopia*.
- By definition, the intermediate region within which the two eyes see only a single object is the real horopter.

[Such experiments are simple in theory but difficult to achieve practically, and it pays to use trained subjects.]

This method is, however, not very accurate. A preferred procedure is one exploiting a *binocular vernier* technique (sometimes referred to as *of Nonius* after the name Nunez, a Portuguese mathematician of

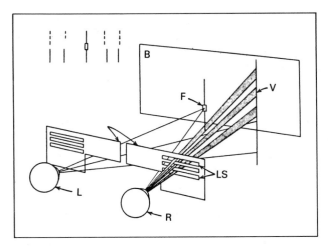

Figure 3.63
Sketch of apparatus to determine the horopter by the "binocular vernier" method.
The two eyes fixate on F and view the test image rod V in more peripheral vision.
This is seen by both eyes on a bright background (B) but as a continuous line by the
left eye (L) and as an interrupted line by the right eye (R) thanks to screens (arrows)
provided with appropriate longitudinal slits (LS). *Inset,* Two cases of images displaced
and two of images aligned with the rod V, the lower half being seen directly and the
upper half as interrupted. (From Ogle 1962)

the 16th century). This consists (figure 3.63) of asking a subject to
observe two different graphic patterns simultaneously with each eye.
The two eyes fixate on a point F on a horizontal line H (binocular
fixation point). But they can also see a vertical line V in lateral vision.
However, because of a system of gratings, one eye can only see the
half of line V that is above the horizontal and the other eye only the
half that is below. The subject fixating on F thus sees in lateral vision
one continuous and one interrupted line. The subject signals when
their *alignment* is achieved by changing the frontal distance of V.
Good in conception, this experiment remains difficult in application
for eccentricities exceeding about 10°.

Plotting the longitudinal horopter. Experimental measurements of the
horizontal horopter like the above have shown (1) that they are relatively imprecise, there being an appreciable range *in depth,* and (2)
that the mean position of this horopter is sited somewhere between
the theoretical Vieth-Müller circle and the "frontoparallel" plane
passing through F (see figure 3.61).

Given this situation and recognizing that most measurements are made in the horizontal plane or its immediate vicinity ($\pm 5°$), Ogle (1962) was able to demonstrate that the horopter is not a circle but a conic section reasonably well specified by the function

$$\cot \theta_2 - r_0 \cot \theta_1 = K$$

where θ_2 and θ_1 are the angles subtended at one and the other eye by the same segment EF, and K and r_0 are constants.

Assuming to begin with that $r_0 = 1$ and that the angles θ are small, then

$$\theta_1 - \theta_2 = h\theta_m^2$$

where θ_m is the mean $(\theta_1 + \theta_2)/2$ and the angles are expressed in radians. This curve (with the so-called Hering-Hildebrand deviation) is symmetrical with respect to the median plane and is more or less an ellipse (see figure 3.61B). In the right half of the visual field the visual angle of the right eye θ_2 is greater than the visual angle θ_1 of the left eye, the difference increasing with eccentricity. If, for example, $K = 0.12$ and $\theta_m = 10°$ eccentricity, the difference $\theta_2 - \theta_2$ is of the order 0.2° (12 min arc).

If, in contrast, $r_0 \neq 1$, the horopter ceases to be symmetrical with respect to the median plane. Vision is then in a state called *aniseikonia,* which we shall discuss further a little later.

There are a variety of considerations, that we will not detail here, which essentially justify the above description of the horopter as a conic section.

The Problem of "Panum's Area"
As we saw above, attempts to determine the real horopter experimentally lead to the delineation in depth of a certain *zone* within which fusion occurs, while diplopia occurs farther away and closer than that zone. This zone for fusion, called *Panum's area,* is measured by the minimal angle between the extreme positions for which the subject can attain fusion. Note in particular that this angle (and correlated to it the area) increases with increasing eccentricity. As an indication, Panum's area at eccentricity 0 has a depth of about 10 mm and at 20° about 15 mm, each for a viewing distance of 40 cm. The real horopter (figure 3.64) is clearly the mean curve.

The existence of Panum's area has been argued about and even denied. Effectively, the problem is to imagine how two images that

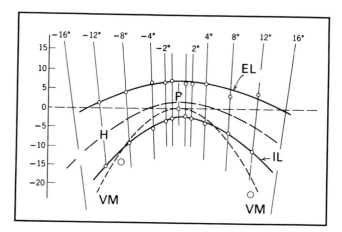

Figure 3.64
Panum's area. Data for the real horizontal horopter, illustrating the region of binocular fusion (Panum's area) and its external (EL) and internal (IL) limits. H, the horopter; VM, the Vieth-Müller circle (here transformed into an ellipse since the ordinates [in mm] are relatively doubled). The distance of vision was 40 cm. (From Ogle 1962)

are not strictly on corresponding points can fuse. Some authors have invoked explanations that to some extent avoid the issue and make the problem somewhat banal; an alternation between one eye and the other has been suggested. Another suggestion is that a minimal and irreducible difference arises when the subject directs his attention first to the fixation point then to the lateral object; this lowers the acuity ("fixation disparity"). We shall see later what the explanation is from neurophysiological experimentation.

STEREOPSIS

Our next step is to study *vision in depth,* that is, the translation into three dimensions of two-dimensional images, thanks to central nervous mechanisms. Its origin has been known since Wheatstone's demonstration in 1833, by a mirror arrangement, that an illusion of depth can be obtained by presenting a different image to each eye. Because the two retinal images of the same object are usually received from two different angles, there normally results a small retinal disparity between them of a few seconds of arc. It is this *binocular disparity* (sometimes called stereoscopic parallax), principally horizontal, that is the basis of depth perception.

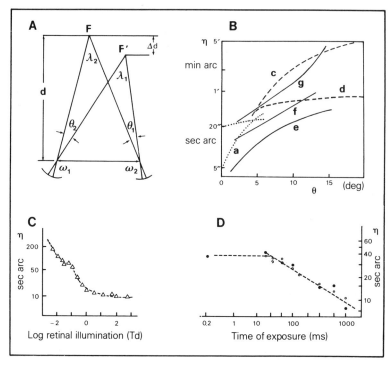

Figure 3.65
Studies of stereoscopic acuity. *A*, Sketch illustrating geometrical definitions (see text). *B*, Threshold stereoscopic acuity η as a function of the angle θ separating the objects compared. The different curves are for different experimenters and different experimental conditions. *C*, Stereoscopic acuity as a function of retinal illumination. *D*, Stereoscopic depth perception as a function of duration of exposure of the test objects. (*A* From Graham 1965; *B* from Le Grand 1964; *C*, *D* from Ogle 1962)

Stereoscopic Acuity

Suppose (figure 3.65A) that two adjacent points F and F' on the median plane are sited at slightly different distances d and $d + \delta d$ from the line $w_1 w_2$ between the entry pupils, that is, within the region of fusion of Panum's area. The segment FF' is seen at angles of gaze θ_1 and θ_2 and the angles of convergence are λ_1 and λ_2, respectively. Supposing θ_1 and θ_2 are slightly different, as are λ_1 and λ_2, we can arrive at the stereoscopic parallax, or binocular disparity, $\theta_2 - \theta_1$, its absolute value being equal to $\lambda_2 - \lambda_1$.

Defining the stereoscopic acuity η as the threshold, of a just-perceptible binocular disparity, we can also, knowing η, calculate the linear disparity δd that is just perceptible as a function of the distance

Table 3.1. The just-perceptible linear depth differences δd, both distal and proximal, as a function of depth d

d (m)	0.25	1	10	25	1,000
δd distal (mm)	0.05	0.9	91	580	∞
δd proximal (mm)	0.05	0.9	89	550	555,000

The threshold for a just-perceptible binocular disparity is taken as η = 12 sec arc.

d of the two targets from the observer. Making an approximate estimate (by putting tan η = η in radians, which is justified since the angles are small) we may write

$$\delta d = d^2 \cdot \eta / (w_1 w_2 - d \cdot \eta)$$

In this calculation it is supposed that the moving test target is farther away from the subject than the fixed target. For a proximal disparity (the test target closer to the subject with respect to the fixed target) it suffices to give η a negative sign.

This threshold η_t (determined by various methods we will not specify) can be remarkably small. Thus for η_t = 5 sec arc, a value found by several researchers, a depth change of 0.4 mm is perceived at a distance of 1 m if $w_1 w_2$ = 0.063 m. By the same argument, an object at 2.6 km is seen as in front of another sited at infinity. Clearly, the greater the distance the greater the just-perceptible separation in depth between the two objects. This difference becomes infinite—in other words, depth vision is lost—when d = $w_1 w_2 / \eta$. This, with the other values selected, happens at 3 km.

Under normal conditions the threshold is a little higher (12 sec arc). Using this value for η one can estimate the linear values δd (in millimeters) either distal (far) or proximal (near) as a function of d in meters (table 3.1). Note that as d increases, the distal difference increases more rapidly than the proximal difference such that it becomes infinite at about 1 km, where all vision in depth becomes negligible.

Factors Determining Stereoscopic Acuity
Stereoscopic acuity varies greatly between subjects but is uncorrelated with age or the level of accommodation. In contrast, there is a quite strong correlation between this and monocular acuity. Thus in a given individual the stereoscopic acuity decreases between the fovea and the periphery, as does monocular acuity. However, certain data show that stereoscopic acuity is not maximal at the central fovea itself but at several minutes of angle away (15' to 21').

Good retinal illumination is favorable to good stereoscopic acuity and so is good contrast. If either factor increases, then η decreases. Notice, however, that the curve (figure 3.65C) shows a point of discontinuity which recalls several others that give evidence of duality of retinal mechanisms. The same explanation is no doubt valid here: Cones and rods each play their part in binocular acuity but at different luminance levels, the one in photopic and the other in scotopic conditions. [In appreciation of depth differences of two opaque bars it is the illumination of the background that matters; in the same discrimination of two lit targets, it is their luminance that matters.]

Another factor is the horizontal distance between the two points that the observer is attempting to separate in depth in the visual field. Other things being equal, the best depth discrimination is attained for small angular separations. For small target separations (up to about 5°) the threshold increases approximately linearly as the separation increases. For wider separations, in contrast, this threshold seems to stabilize at a constant value (figure 3.65B).

When the refraction of the two eyes is not identical (e.g., as in anisometropia, or in an emmetrope when a special lens is placed in front of one eye that changes the size of the image but not the focus), one speaks of *aniseikonia*. In this case the horopter is no longer symmetrical with respect to the median plane, and complicated stereoscopic effects can result. However, this effect is essentially a curiosity because there is usually some compensation after a relatively short time (several days).

Mechanisms for Stereoscopic Acuity
Researchers investigating binocular vision in depth have posited two underlying mechanisms. The so-called *static* theory attributes depth perception to the small disparity between the two retinal images without any additional active involvement by the eye. In other words, this theory rests chiefly on the difference $\theta_1 - \theta_2$ in the expression above. A second (*dynamic*) theory exists which, in contrast, relies on a central role for changes in convergence (i.e., tiny movements by the eyes), this time emphasizing the difference $\lambda_1 - \lambda_2$. A compelling support for the first theory is that a tachystoscopic presentation (using a very brief flash), which excludes the possibility of any eye movement, allows depth discrimination as before. Studies by Ogle (1962) of visual stereoacuity as a function of exposure time of the targets give interesting evidence on this point:

• For very short stimulus durations (0.2 ms), stereoscopic vision occurs, therefore excluding eye movements as a *necessary* factor in stereoscopy.

• Stereoscopic acuity remains on a practically constant plateau up to a stimulus duration of around 6 ms.

• Between 6 and 100 ms acuity increases considerably (figure 3.65D). At this time fine eye movements must presumably be taken into consideration (Riggs et al. 1954) since the mean amplitude of eye movements have been shown to increase with exposure duration (from 5 to 180 sec arc as exposure times increase from 20 to 1000 ms, the relation being linear in log/log coordinates).

Illusions of depth produced by viewing two flat two-dimensional figures have been studied for some time. Two well-known methods used are the following.

1. *Stereoscopes.* After Wheatstone's first apparatus, based on the artificial distortion of the baseline (w_1w_2) for the two eyes by mirrors, another system invented more or less simultaneously by Wheatstone, Brewster, and Helmholtz came rapidly into vogue (figure 3.66). This is founded on the viewing of two adjacent images (stereograms) of the same object but taken from appropriately separated viewpoints. These are examined through lenses that place the images at infinity and thus prevents any convergence and accommodation but still very effectively generates depth perception (Rock 1975).

2. *Anaglyphs.* Depth illusions are created in this second method, not by spatially separating the two images by optic arrangements but instead by ensuring that when a pair of suitably displaced images is viewed, each eye can see only one of the pair. The classic method was to have the two images in different colors, which allowed different color filters before each eye to filter out one of the images. Alternatively (and this has been used in the cinema), the two stereoscopic images are projected in polarized light, the planes of polarization at the two projectors being at right angles. This viewer wears spectacles that carry transparent Polaroid disks also polarized at right angles in each eye. Once again, each eye can see only one image.

Problems Posed by Stereoscopic Vision
Experimental psychology continues to unearth a number of difficulties that underly the interpretation of mechanisms for depth vision. We will only examine a few examples here (see also Barlow & Mollon 1982).

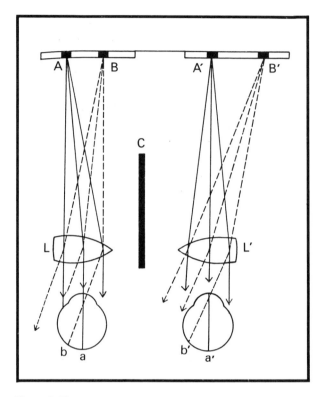

Figure 3.66
Stereoscopic apparatus (Wheatstone, Brewer, Helmholtz). Two adjacent images each comprise two lines (in which A is seen along rays A and A' and B along B and B') that are slightly differently displaced, ($AB \neq A'B'$), constituting a stereogram. The images are separated by the partition C and are each visible to one eye only through the half lenses L, L'. These lenses render the rays parallel so the images appear at infinity. There will be neither convergence nor accommodation, yet the two retinal images ab, $a'b'$, ($ab \neq a'b'$) give rise to relief and depth. (From Rock 1975)

One of the most important concerns the establishment of point-to-point comparisons between the two retinal images. When this is a matter of real, unambiguous figures with easily identifiable characteristics (comprising bars, angles, etc.) with visual binocular horizontal disparity, there seems to be no great problem, particularly if it can be shown that stereoscopy can be preceded by a cognitive stage involving form recognition in the two images.

However, this operation becomes much more difficult to conceive when the images concerned are each an apparently random constella-

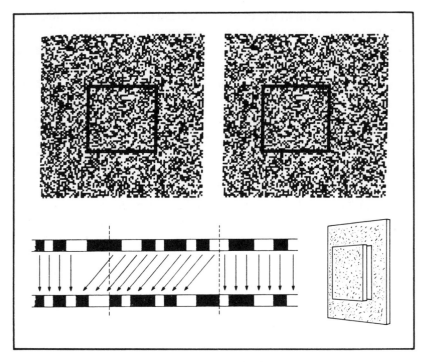

Figure 3.67
Random dot stereogram. The two halves are almost identical, except that a central region, which is a subassembly (shown here surrounded by the square boundary), has suffered a translation between the two stereograms. Observation of these in a stereoscope generates a sensation of relief (sketch, *lower right*). [Note: The square boundaries shown here do not appear in the viewed stereograms.] *Lower left*, Principle of translation of a segment of the random pattern which displaces the image seen by one eye with respect to that seen by the other, which gives rise to the sensation of relief. (From Barlow & Mollon 1982 and Rock 1975)

tion of spots (random-dot stereograms, RDS) of the type that Julesz (1978) in particular has studied using anaglyphs (figure 3.67).

How can the examination of such collections of points by an anaglyph method (e.g., viewed through different-colored spectacles) reveal a shape, whereas such a shape is invisible in a monocular view? What procedure can the visual system use to resolve the ambiguities and compare the many points two by two? This situation, and others raised by experimental psychology, suggest that the comparison mechanism must precede shape recognition rather than follow it. From this point of view, stereoscopic vision becomes a fundamental and early mechanism in the treatment of visual information, independent of perceptual processing and subsequent recognition.

A second aspect of the problem concerns the type of evidence used to establish correspondences. In this respect, it is absolutely necessary that local differences in intensity can be detected and exploited. Quite a series of observations involving the manipulation of images, in particular by spatial filtering and measurement of the second derivative of spatial intensity variations (*zero-crossings* in particular), seem to underline the importance of this as an essential part of the operating characteristics of stereoscopic mechanisms (Marr & Poggio 1976). (We will return to this later in chapter 5.)

Another basic problem to be resolved concerns the second stage of stereopsis, namely, how, following recognition and identification of corresponding points in the object, a representation of three-dimensional space is arrived at with perception of actual distances and directions. Theoreticians and experimentalists agree that extra data are needed to make this reconstruction and that the appreciation of horizontal parallax cannot alone be regarded as sufficient. Two sorts of solution have been suggested: (1) either the extra information is extraretinal in origin, exploiting a knowledge of eye convergence ("far" and "near") and the direction of gaze, or (2) *vertical disparity* between the two retinal images is introduced as supplementary information (Mayhew & Longuet-Higgins 1982). There is a particular observation by Ogle (1962) concerning the importance of vertical parallax. A cylindrical lens placed in front of one eye introduces a slight enlargement of that image in the vertical direction (without altering the horizontal disparity or the extraretinal information). This profoundly affects binocular vision.

In addition, studies based on either RDS or on simpler visual shapes where there is no risk of ambiguity have proposed distinctions between (1) *local stereopsis*, for which only a limited number of elements are needed to effect fusion of retinal images and perception of depth (because there is no ambiguity) and (2) a *global stereopsis*, which implies an operation that must review a number of possible correspondences before finally selecting the one most likely to generate a three-dimensional perception of form.

Another pair of opposing types of stereopsis has been proposed, both of which are in the *local* category. They concern two sorts of depth perception, *broad* (or *coarse*) and *fine*, the distinction being defined by the size of the object that generates the perception of

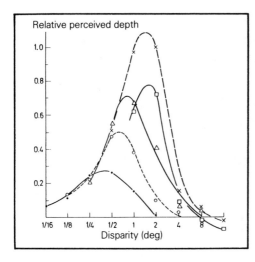

Figure 3.68
Relative depth perceived in local stereoscopy as a function of binocular disparity. The different curves relate to different bar widths: dots, 3 min arc; open circles, 6 min; triangles, 12 min; crosses, 24 min; squares, 48 min. The height of the bars is 30 min arc in each case. (From Richards & Kaye 1974)

depth. Fine stereopsis concerns the vision of objects or bars that have small dimensions and parallax values not exceeding 0.5°, whereas broad stereopsis concerns wide objects with considerably larger interocular disparities. In fact, the distinction between broad and fine stereopsis does not seem to have been experimentally proved. Thus it is possible to show by careful experiment that presenting a subject with bars of a given size but of increasing disparity, the sensation of depth passes through a maximum and then decreases. The experimental curves are different for various sizes of bars; their peak moves along the abscissa with the point of maximal depth perception increasing as the width of the bars increases (figure 3.68).

It is also clear, however, that as the size of the object increases, the curve changes without any sort of discontinuity or bimodality that might be expected to signal a change from one operational mechanism of depth perception to another (figure 3.68; Richards & Kaye 1974). Consequently, the idea of a continuum seems to be a better concept: not a division into two mechanisms but rather a multiplicity of spatial frequency detector mechanisms, tuned so that some are used for the lower spatial frequencies and others for the higher. Later we shall discuss the agreement between some of these proposals from experimental psychology and some of the results of experimental neurophysiology and also, in more general terms, the present neurobiological state of the problems of stereoscopy (Poggio & Poggio 1984).

8.2 MONOCULAR SPATIAL VISION

Despite the clear importance of binocular mechanisms in spatial vision, there remains the question of what part monocular mechanisms might play in depth perception. Depending on the situation, this topic might be divided into four different aspects of varying importance, as discussed below.

MONOCULAR PARALLAX

The most important factor in monocular parallax seems to be whether movement is of the target or of the head and eyes. The number of actual conditions is clearly very large and we will only discuss a few.

Target Movement
When a three-dimensional target moves in front of the eyes, all points on the object have the same linear velocity but their angular velocity with respect to the retina (or their angular displacement in a given time interval) depends on their distance from the eye. In the case of a simple circular movement with the eye as its center, or for a translation in the frontal plane, the angular speed of parallax ω can be calculated as the differential with respect to time of the angular parallax $\delta\theta$:

$$\omega = d(\delta\theta)/dt = (\delta r/r) \cdot d\theta/dt,$$

where r and $r + \delta r$ are respectively the distances from the eye of the two neighboring points for which monocular viewing can generate a depth perception. (The order of magnitude of ω is 40 sec arc/s.)

Head Movements with Stationary Object
While movements of the eyes within the orbit do not seem to be very effective for depth discrimination, movements of the head are, in contrast, very useful. It is clear that, for certain restricted ranges of head movement and with an immobile target, the type of quantitative expression used in the estimates given above remain valid.

OVERLAP

Another factor is overlap, in which a closer object partially obscures one that is farther away. In overlap, the preception of the continuous contours that exist in real objects and a detection of their *points of intersection* are exploited. It is the position of these points of intersection that, according to quite complicated laws, determines which figure is the closer. We will not elaborate this point any further here.

ACCOMMODATION

We quote this as a factor in depth perception because it is so often referred to. The idea is evidently that either the effort of contraction of the ciliary muscles themselves or even the effort of convergence (by the interplay of convergence and accommodation, which persists even if one eye is closed) can be consciously perceived and generates a depth perception. In fact, such speculations are overall disappointing: If any such factor does intervene it can only be at short distances on the order of 1 m.

ANGLES, SIZE AND SHAPE

These are in no way absolute parameters but rather help the appreciation of relative distances between one object and another based on all sorts of comparisons between objects that are visible at the same time as well as appealing to elements in the subject's cognitive repertoire (past experience, recognition of the object, etc.) which are consciously perceived and act as a depth cue. These factors are not uninteresting but they remain rather limited in our present purpose for establishing agreed physiological data. We will therefore not continue to discuss them nor will the equally diverting and rich collection of data to be found in the specialized literature on the multifarious other details of stereoscopic vision be discussed further here.

4

Genesis and Elaboration of Signals in the Retina

The global view of visual mechanisms as previously described in psychophysical terms is enriched by an underpinning of finer detail from investigations of individual functional mechanisms throughout the separate levels of the visual nervous system. As we consider these investigations, our study will be divided into two stages. The first is concerned with retinal processing, where it has been possible to push the analysis of detail toward the cellular and even the molecular level. The second stage, which is the focus of chapter 5, concerns the mechanisms determining responses of individual neuronal units at the various organizational levels beyond the retina, using appropriate analytical methods.

This chapter begins by discussing two aspects of retinal processing, (1) the biochemistry of the retinal photopigments and (2) the global nervous response of the retina as witnessed by the electroretinogram. Earlier experiments that generated essential data in these two areas have since been elaborated and extended by the single-unit study of receptor mechanisms.

Following these, we will discuss various electrophysiological researches and the complementary methods such as neurochemical examination (particularly by immunocytochemistry) and fine-structure investigations that together have yielded models concerned with the genesis of receptor signals by light inputs and their further transformation in retinal neuronal networks. Some of these are now quite well understood.

1 RETINAL PHOTOCHEMISTRY

Apart from the more detailed electrophysiological and neurochemical studies to be examined later, there is a collection of research work that, although carried out some time ago, firmly established the essential characteristics of the intermediate photochemical link in the causal chain light stimulus $\rightarrow$ neuronal output signals.

1.1 THE RETINAL PHOTOPIGMENTS: GENERAL

To be physiologically effective, a retinal pigment must absorb light according to certain photochemical laws. Although a wide variety of light receptors exist across the animal kingdom, it is likely that the individual receptor photopigments that can be recognized in different species are all related chromoproteins and are relatively few in number.

GENERAL METHODS OF STUDYING SPECTRAL ABSORPTION

Pigments in Solution
The oldest and still current method for studying pigments consists in first extracting them from the retina into solution. These pigments are not in fact directly water soluble but can be brought into aqueous solution by adding digitonin or bile salts. The study of these solutions has established their absorption characteristics as a function of wavelength as well as the stage-by-stage photochemistry of their decomposition by light (Dartnall 1962). In practice, several techniques are exploited to measure pigment absorption.

Absorption spectra. The pigment solution is crossed by a flux of incident monochromatic light I_i of wavelength λ. The light intensity I_t transmitted through the solution is measured and the amount absorbed I_a deduced from $I_a = I_i - I_t$.

In practice, the variation of I_a with wavelength is plotted as a function of λ, expressing I_a as a percentage of the incident intensity I_i, thus as the fraction $100 \times (I_a/I_i)$ or $100(I_i - I_t)/I_i$. Note that these plots depend on the pigment concentration (the greater this is, the wider the curves become) and also on the thickness of the layer traversed by the light. A first simplification is to normalize them by referring them all to their maximal magnitudes (figure 4.1, left).

Spectral optical density. The two difficulties above are obviated by using an expression that is independent of the thickness of the layer crossed by the light (l) and of the concentration of the solution (C). Consider an element of thickness dl of the absorbing layer. If I is the incident light intensity and dI the amount absorbed by the element then, from Lambert's and Beer's laws for absorbing fluids, we may write

$$dI/I = \alpha_\lambda \cdot C \cdot dl$$

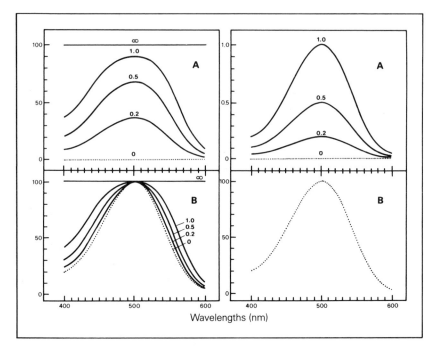

Wavelengths (nm)

Figure 4.1
Absorption spectra and optical density spectra. *Left*, Absorption spectra of solutions of frog visual pigment at different concentrations. (A) Curves are in percentage absorption (ordinate); (B) ordinate values of curves are normalized as percent of maximum. *Right*, Optical density spectra for the three concentrations on the left. (A) Ordinate is optical density; (B) curves are normalized as % of maximum optical density. Note that in this latter case they coincide, independently of concentration. (From Dartnall 1962)

where α_λ, the absorption coefficient (or absorption factor) depends on λ.

Integrating this equation between the limits I_i (incident intensity) and I_t (intensity transmitted) gives the *optical density* (O.D.) at the wavelength λ:

$$\text{Log}\,(I_i/I_t) = \alpha_\lambda \cdot C \cdot l.$$

In practice $\log_{10}$ units are preferred so that the optical density (D_λ) becomes:

$$D_\lambda = \log_{10}(I_i/I_t) = (1/2.3)\alpha_\lambda \cdot C \cdot l.$$

Following this, if D_λ is referred to the maximal value of D_λ (D_{max}) we end up with a way of expressing D_λ as a function of λ that involves neither the concentration nor the thickness of the sample:

$D_\lambda/D_{max} = (\alpha_\lambda \cdot C \cdot l)/(\alpha_{max} \cdot C \cdot l) = \alpha_\lambda/\alpha_{max}$.

This yields a curve of *spectral density* (figure 4.1, right). Since

$D_\lambda = \log_{10}(I_i/I_t)$,

then

$10^{D_\lambda} = I_i/I_t$

and the absorption is given by

$I_a/I_i = (I_i - I_t)/I_i = 1 - 10^{-D_\lambda}$.

Developing the series for $1 - 10^{-D_\lambda}$ and neglecting higher terms we finally obtain (figure 4.2a).

$I_a/I_t = 2.303 D_\lambda$.

The two characteristics, spectral density and spectral absorption, are important. In fact, intrinsically, a visual pigment is effectively specified by its spectral density distribution; nevertheless, when it is a matter of comparing the plots of one pigment's spectral sensitivities with those of other pigments or with related phenomena in the same pigment, it is more appropriate for a true comparison to use the absorption spectrum corresponding to the concentration of the pigment in the photoreceptors.

Difference spectra. One of the difficulties in measuring the spectral density of a pigment is the existence of impurities or of other substances that also absorb light in a wavelength-dependent way. For this reason it is often profitable to use *difference spectra.* These are obtained by measuring the spectrum of the colored pigment, then subtracting the corresponding spectrum measured after the pigment has been bleached by light, all other factors remaining the same. In this way extraneous sources of absorption can be eliminated.

Figure 4.2b concerns the pigment rhodopsin. It shows the relative changes in density produced by bleaching (ordinate: reduction in density upward, increase downward). Note that the difference spectrum remains the same whether there are impurities present or not. The decrease is zero around 425 nm, maximal around 500 nm, and becomes zero again near 600 nm. Below 425 nm the density has

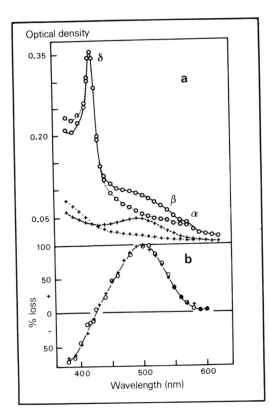

Figure 4.2
Density spectra and differ-
ence spectra. *a*, Density spectra before (solid lines) and
after (dotted lines) bleaching.
The two upper curves are for
a solution strongly contaminated with blood from the retina; the lower curves are for
a relatively pure solution. The
contaminated case shows the
three absorption peaks of oxy-
hemoglobin (α, β, and δ). *b*,
The difference spectra obtained by subtracting either
the upper two curves (impure
solution) or the lower two
(relatively pure solution), the
ordinates for each case in (*b*)
being the relative loss in optical density as a percentage of
the maximal loss. Notice how
these curves coincide for the
two cases of measurement on
pure or impure solutions.
(From Dartnall 1962)

increased because the product of decomposition is more absorbent
there than the original colored substance.

Action spectra. Some studies, particularly those carried out in vivo,
have been conducted in the opposite way, by determining what
quantity of light at each wavelength (e.g., expressed as quanta) is
needed to bleach a given quantity of rhodopsin, or matches a phenomenon that depends directly on such a photolysis. This method
yields an *action spectrum.*

Reflection Densitometry
Rushton and his group (Rushton & Campbell 1954 and also Weale
1959) were preeminent in devising and using a method that allows
the study of visual pigments in situ in the living eye, thanks to a
reflectometry technique normally referred to as *retinal densitometry.*
    A known luminous flux of monochromatic light is projected on the
retina, and the reflected luminous flux is measured at a variety of

selected wavelengths λ. In practice, this flux is only about 1% or less of the incident light flux and clearly is also an inverse function of the amount of light absorbed in the retinal tissue. From these data— following a whole series of very careful experimental precautions that we cannot elaborate upon here—it is possible to calculate the absorption spectrum of the pigment or pigments that have been (doubly) traversed by the incident pencil of light after reflection at the back of the retina. It is possible at the same time to compare the results with the psychophysically determined state of vision, before and after adaptation, for example.

This highly elegant method was specifically designed for human investigations by Rushton and his colleagues. In their first publication, Campbell and Rushton (1955) essentially validated the method by showing that with retinal densitometry they could quantify the amount and the principal functional characteristics of rhodopsin in the living extrafoveal peripheral retina. Rushton (as we shall see below) later used the method to research cone pigments, even though this latter problem presents considerable difficulties related to interfering parasitic absorptions and also to the resolving power and sensitivity of the system.

Microspectrophotometric Measurements
The introduction of microspectrophotometric methods to analyze the absorption in an isolated piece of retinal outer segment, by exploiting a microscopic bundle of monochromatic rays traversing the sample, also facilitated considerable progress. It has been applied to the receptors of various species, as we shall see below.

Essentially, the apparatus consists in a monochromatic light source plus associated devices arranged to apply micropulses of light to the preparation. Then a photomultiplier detector and associated electronic apparatus present the data in a two-dimensional XY display. Two light bundles are projected in parallel, one crossing part of the outer segment and the other the entire optical system except for the specimen, serving thereby as a reference beam. The whole spectrum is swept by monochromatic flashes that are as brief as possible (to minimize pigment bleaching) and are spatially well focused. The quantity of light actually absorbed by that part of the outer segment is measured at each wavelength λ. The curve of $A(\lambda)$ (percentage absorption) as a function of λ is plotted.

$A(\lambda) = 1 - (I_m/I_r)$

where I_m is the intensity of the emerging measuring beam and I_r the intensity of the reference beam.

One of the major difficulties in this technique arises from the orientation of the receptors with respect to the monochromatic microbeam. In fact, a large number of results, particularly from the first experiments, were taken with the monochromatic beam traversing the receptors along their long axis. Under these conditions, the danger of lateral diffusion and scattering of light is quite high, particularly by the retinal neuronal network, which inevitably was present, with light incident on it. More recently, researchers pressing the analyses further have been obliged to operate with laterally incident light beams, attacking the receptors in the outer segment from the side. The measurements have proved to be more reliable under these conditions.

KINETICS OF PIGMENT BLEACHING AND REGENERATION

Another indispensable set of data concerns the kinetics of the decomposition of the retinal photosensitive pigments by light and their resynthesis in the dark.

Decomposition in vitro

Let C_0 be the initial pigment concentration in solution and C_t be its concentration after exposure to light for a time t to an incident light flux of intensity I. For these, the simplest possible conditions, we may write:

$\text{Log } C_0/C_t = k \cdot I \cdot t$

or

$C_t = C_0 \exp(-k \cdot I \cdot t).$

The coefficient k needs explanation: It comprises two terms, the absorption coefficient α_λ of the pigment as a function of λ and a coefficient γ called the *quantum efficiency* of the stimulus, which is the number of pigment molecules decomposed per single quantum of light absorbed. Thus we may write:

$C_t = C_0 \exp(-\alpha_\lambda \cdot \gamma \cdot I \cdot t)$

In practice, γ is independent of temperature, concentration, solution pH, and the incident flux. Thus C_t is essentially a function of the two parameters I and α_λ, that is, of the incident light intensity and of the photosensitivity of the pigment throughout the spectrum. In this, the most simple in vitro condition, there is no resynthesis of the pigment in darkness.

Actual Events in Vivo

In fact, the problem is not quite so simple since the in vivo decomposition is reversible, as is experimentally demonstrable, and it is necessary for this reason to use formulas of the type: $S \rightleftharpoons P + A$, where S is the photosensitive pigment and P and A are the products of decomposition.

If (a) is the initial concentration of S and (x) is the concentration of the products of decomposition at time (t), then at time t the rate of decomposition dx/dt is proportional to the incident light intensity I and to some power m of the concentration.

At the same time t, a resynthesis of S is also occurring, and this is proportional to a power n of the concentration (x) of the decomposition products. We may write therefore:

$$dx/dt = k_1 \cdot I(a - x)^m - k_2 \cdot x^n$$

where k_1 and k_2 are two constants, and the exponents m and n, according to researchers, are 1 and 2, respectively.

If, in particular, we are interested in the resynthesis of the pigment in the dark, then $I = 0$ and the relationship becomes

$$dx/dt = -k_2 x^n$$

or in practice

$$dx/dt = -k_2 x^2.$$

What is the real significance of such estimates? In principle, the reasoning is simple: Insofar as a given retinal pigment is concerned in mechanisms of photoreception, some of the changes of visual sensitivity might well be expected to be correlated with the properties of this pigment, particularly (1) the variation of retinal sensitivity with wavelength, determined by the spectral variation of light absorption, and (2) the variation of the absolute threshold with dark and light adaptation, depending on the kinetics of pigment breakdown and regeneration. We will discuss the actual situation below.

1.2 RHODOPSIN

THE CHEMICAL COMPOSITION OF RHODOPSIN AND PORPHYROPSIN

Rhodopsin is the main pigment found in mammals, birds, and reptiles. Its absorption spectrum in the visible, from corrected in vitro measurements in solution, shows a maximal absorption at wavelengths (λ_{max}) between 470 nm and 525 nm according to species.

In freshwater fish, in contrast, the predominant pigment shows a λ_{max} displaced toward the longer wavelengths (510 to 540 nm). This pigment is called *porphyropsin (retinal violet)*.

Rhodopsin is formed by the association of a protein (opsin) with a chromophore. The latter is the aldehyde of vitamin A_1, which is an alcohol, *retinol*. The aldehyde is called retinaldehyde 1, retinal 1, or retinene.

Porphyropsin differs from rhodopsin in that the aldehyde is of vitamin A_2 (dehydroretinol), which is distinguished from vitamin A_1 by an extra conjugated bond in its structure (3-4 dehydroretinaldehyde, or retinal 2). In either case, retinal 1 or retinal 2, X ray and nuclear magnetic resonance studies have shown that it is the 11-*cis* isomer that links with opsin (figure 4.3).

If a detailed spectrum of rhodopsin is measured throughout the spectrum in both the visible and ultraviolet (figure 4.4, where bovine rhodopsin is shown as a typical example) three peaks are visible: one near 500 nm corresponds to the chromophore in the visible as does the peak at 350 nm in the ultraviolet. A third, very large peak in the far ultraviolet (280 nm) is linked with absorption by the acid amine groups of opsin.

The differences between rhodopsin (derived from vitamin A_1) and porphyropsin (derived from vitamin A_2) lead to some interesting ecological comparisons. The most marked contrasts are in fish, though there are some exceptions. Essentially, marine species have rhodopsin and freshwater fish have porphyropsin, while euryhaline fish can carry either type of pigment. Certain migratory fish (lamprey, eel, salmon, and trout) show a transformation from rhodopsin to porphyropsin according to their migratory phase. In the batrachians, the passage from aquatic to terrestrial life is accompanied by a change from porphyropsin in the tadpole to rhodopsin in the adult frog. [Note that the differences between rhodopsin and porphyropsin λ_{max} values can be quite small, e.g., gecko rhodopsin 524 nm, carp porphyropsin 523 nm.]

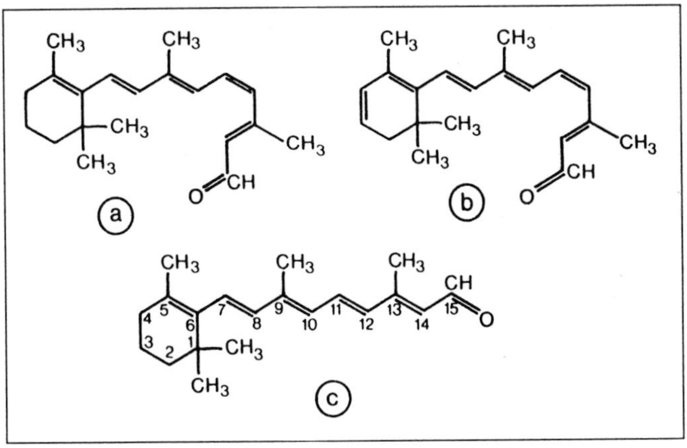

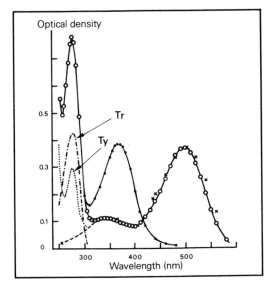

Figure 4.3
Structure of vitamin A aldehydes. *a*, 11-*cis* retinal of vitamin A_1; *b*, 11-*cis* retinal of vitamin A_2; *c*, all-*trans* retinal of vitamin A_1 (see text).

Figure 4.4
Density spectrum of rhodopsin. Typical density spectrum of a pure extract of bovine Rh with λ_{max} at 498 nm for pH 9.2 (curve passing through the open circles). The curve passing through the filled circles is the spectrum after bleaching. Note that the principal peak in the visible at 498 nm and the second less contrasting peak at 340 nm (*cis*-band) are replaced by a peak at 370 nm (alkaline indicator yellow; see section 1.2). The band at 278 nm, linked essentially with tryptophan (Tr) and tyrosine (Ty) is in contrast not affected by bleaching. The crosses represent the curve for frog rhodopsin (502 nm). (From Dartnall 1962)

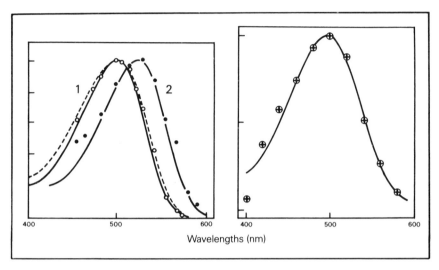

Wavelengths (nm)

Figure 4.5
Pigment spectra and spectral sensitivities. *Left,* Spectra of visual pigments and spectral sensitivities for frog (1) and tench (2). The continuous curves are absorption spectra; the open and filled circles refer to the appropriate visual sensitivities observed behaviorally. For the frog, the dashed curve refers to the percentage light absorption calculated from in vivo measurements. *Right,* Comparison of the spectral density curve of human rods and dark-adapted human spectral sensitivity (crosses). (From Dartnall 1962)

The absorption spectrum of rhodopsin (and similarly, in freshwater fish, of the porphyropsin) in the visible coincides well with the plot of the scotopic sensitivity curve for the species in question, provided the absorption spectra are corrected for any absorptions in the eye media (figure 4.5). This confirms the essential role that the pigments were judged to play in the functioning of the receptors in which they are localized. The relationships between pigment absorption and visual sensitivity can be analyzed in a variety of ways: in humans by psychophysical investigations with an additional spectrophotometric confirmation by reflection densitometry methods (Rushton 1956, 1965, 1972). In animals, the scotopic sensitivity curve can be derived from behavioral studies, although such studies are often very difficult.

PHOTOLYSIS IN VITRO

The literature contains an abundance of data on the intermediate processes in the breakdown of rhodopsin in vitro. Nowadays some of this information has probably only a residual historic interest, but its study, at least in summary, should not be completely neglected. These intermediate compounds unfortunately have only an extremely brief lifetime and for the most part can only be identified by low-temperature spectrophotometry. Not everything is fully understood in these stages of the bleaching process: Let us look at the essential milestones, best understood for bovine rhodopsin (figure 4.6; Abrahamson & Wiesenfeld 1972).

Hypsorhodopsin and Bathorhodopsin (Prelumirhodopsin)
At very low temperatures ($-250°C$) illumination of rhodopsin generates a first product, hypsorhodopsin ($\lambda_{max} = 430$ nm) and around $-195°C$ a second, bathorhodopsin, also known as *prelumirhodopsin* ($\lambda_{max} = 548$ nm). There is still disagreement concerning the conformation of these molecules. It seems that they might begin to show the torsion in 11-12 (see figure 4.3) moving towards the all-*trans* conformation but without having fully attained that.

Lumirhodopsin
In darkness and at a much higher temperature (not above $-40°C$), prelumirhodopsin gives rise to a compound lumirhodopsin which in the bovine case has $\lambda_{max} = 497$ nm. The compound is stable at that temperature (in practice the temperature of solid carbon dioxide, "CO_2 snow"). Its characteristics have been evaluated at $-25°C$, but it is extremely transient and remains poorly understood. It is, however, universally agreed that at this stage the structure is certainly all-*trans*.

Metarhodopsin
When lumirhodopsin is allowed to warm to $-20°C$ or $-15°C$ it is transformed into another compound called metarhodopsin I. Equally, illumination of rhodopsin at $-20°C$ in solution produces the same compound (stable to $-15°C$). In the vertebrates, warming to $0°C$ or changing the ionic conditions or pH causes metarhodopsin I to change, reversibly, to metarhodopsin II with the loss of a proton:

Metarhodopsin I + $H^+ \rightleftharpoons$ metarhodopsin II
($\lambda_{max} = 476$ nm)   ($\lambda_{max} = 380$ nm)

Pararhodopsin and N-Retinylidene-Opsin
Solutions of rhodopsin may, during exposure to light and at temperatures above $0°C$, contain a compound called *transient orange* or pararhodopsin ($\lambda_{max} = 465$ nm). The exact nature of this substance is

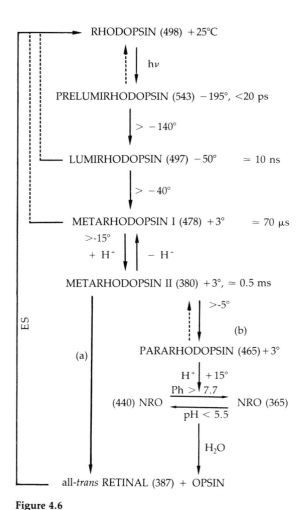

Figure 4.6
Reaction sequence for the photolysis of bovine rhodopsin in vitro. The λ_{max} is shown for each intermediary component and the temperature (in °C) at which it was measured. The approximate half-life of the first terms is indicated, being very brief for the prelumirhodopsin (<20 ps), 500 times longer for lumirhodopsin, $35 \cdot 10^5$ times more for metarhodopsin I, and $25 \cdot 10^6$ times more for meta-II NRO (N-retinylidene opsin). There is still discussion about the later stages. The direct path *a* is preferred by Matthews et al. (1963) and trajectory *b* is proposed by Ostroy et al. (1966). Para-Rh is also referred to as metarhodopsin III and is the same as the old "transient orange." NRO 440, the acid component, and NRO 365, the basic component, constitute the pH-sensitive system (called for some time "indicator yellow"). The dashed arrows indicate possible resyntheses caused by light (photoregeneration). The path ES shows the enzymatic synthesis starting from retinal and opsin. (After Abrahamson & Wiesenfeldt 1972 and modified according to Kropf 1972)

disputed but it has been established to be a derivative of metarhodopsin II.

Above 5°C in darkness, pararhodopsin is decomposed into the final products *trans*retinaldehyde and opsin (λ_{max} = 307 nm). The way in which these final components are generated remains controversial, as we shall see.

There exists another intermediate compound in this transformation, N-retinylidene-opsin, a compound derived from N-retinyl-opsin, that has already been mentioned above in discussing the structure of the pigment. It forms a Schiff base between (this time all-*trans*) retinaldehyde and the amino group of opsin. The sensitivity of N-retinylidene-opsin to pH gave it its older name *indicator yellow*. Depending on pH, the compound exists in two states (λ_{max} = 440 nm at pH 5.5 and λ_{max} = 365 nm at pH 7.7).

There is still much discussion about the final stages of this process. Some regard the final step as a direct passage from metarhodopsin II to the final stage of retinal and opsin (Matthews et al. 1963; see figure 4.6a.) with products like pararhodopsin (sometimes called *metarhodopsin III*) and indicator yellow being only by-products. Others regard these latter compounds as essential intermediates (figure 4.6b). For a detailed discussion of this already long-standing problem, see in particular Dartnall (1962) and Morton (1972).

PHOTOLYSIS OF RHODOPSIN IN VIVO

We need to ask what the functional importance of these transitory states is, taking into account that the structure of rhodopsin has been worked out (see below). Some points should be kept in mind which, in spite of considerable advances, still throw doubt on our full understanding of this phenomenon.

While considering, for instance, the arrangement of the molecules of rhodopsin in the outer segment of the rods (see below), one question is whether the above scheme for the breakdown of rhodopsin in vitro remains valid in vivo (e.g., studied in suspensions of rods).

Prelumirhodopsin and lumirhodopsin seem to have been properly identified in situ in spite of experimental difficulties and of certain differences in λ_{max} values in situ and in solution. The presence of metarhodopsin is also rather certain, with λ_{max} at 480 nm and 380 nm. Their breakdown kinetics also seem to be very similar to what is observed in vitro in solution. Pararhodopsin has also been identified in the rods of some species. An essential difference is that in the retina, apparently, breakdown can go as far as a final stage of retinol (vitamin A), which implies the presence at that level of an enzyme system to support the necessary dehydrogenation reaction:

$$\text{(retinal} \xrightarrow{+2H} \text{retinol)}$$

An order of magnitude for the lifetimes of these intermediate stages must also be established at physiological temperatures. The following seem to be probable: on the order of several microseconds to reach metarhodopsin I; about 1 ms for the transition metarhodopsin I → metarhodopsin II; finally, on the order of minutes for the final stage metarhodopsin II → free retinal + opsin.

If the transition from transient orange to indicator yellow (which is disputed, as we have seen) is ignored, we might agree that:

• Isomerization is over by the lumirhodopsin stage at the latest
• Bleaching occurs in the meta-I to meta-II stage, the meta-II stage corresponding to the Rh* (activated rhodopsin; see below).
• The final stage is the hydrolysis of meta-II into retinal and opsin.

REGENERATION OF RHODOPSIN

Just as the breakdown of rhodopsin is a necessary intermediate in the process of excitation in the retina, its regeneration is also a necessary condition to restore visual sensitivity to the rods after light exposure. We shall study some of the questions concerned with this resynthesis (cf. Bauman 1972).

Synthesis from Opsin plus Retinal or Opsin plus Retinol
In vitro.   Incubation in darkness of retinal and opsin (the two components present as a result of former bleaching) can generate some resynthesis of rhodopsin (figure 4.7; the numbers in parentheses in the following discussion correspond to the numbered syntheses in the diagram). It can be shown, however, that this synthesis only takes place if the retinal has already been isomerized to the 11-*cis* state (1). Another synthesis is possible (2), this time starting from opsin and from retinol, not retinal, provided an alcohol dehydrogenase, with NAD (nicotinamide adenine dinucleotide) as coenzyme, are acting. The retinol must equally be the isomer 11-*cis*. Up to the present no one has succeeded in effecting the isomerization *trans* → *cis* in vitro with a useful yield.

In vivo.   In excised retinas or in isolated visual receptors in suspension, results have been very variable. Essentially, the expected resyn-

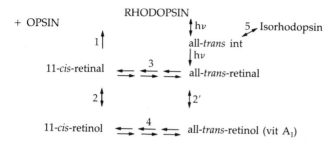

Figure 4.7
Diagram of the synthetic and breakdown processes for rhodopsin. Bleaching by light (hν) normally leads to all-trans retinal via pathway (5). Under certain conditions it can also lead to unstable all-*trans* intermediates (all-*trans* int). Under particular light-stimulations, either photoregeneration of Rh is possible (by a reversible reaction) but photoregeneration can also proceed (via 5) to form isorhodopsin (9-*cis* component). In vitro, regeneration of Rh in the dark can be effected from 11-*cis*-retinal (1) or in the presence of NAD and alcohol dehydrogenase from 11-*cis*-retinol (2). In vivo only, these syntheses can take place from all-*trans* retinal (vitamin A₁) catalysed by retinal-isomerase (3) or even from all-*trans*-retinol by pathways (2' then 3). The possibility of a synthesis through isomerization of all-*trans* retinal via (4) then (2) and (1) remains an open question. (After Dartnall 1972)

thesis is seen, even starting from retinol. In this case, the isomerase being present, synthesis can now take place starting from all-*trans* retinal (3) or even from all-*trans* retinol, given in this instance, the intervention of an oxidoreduction enzyme system (2'). The direct isomerization from all-*trans* retinal (pathway 4) remains hypothetical.

The respective roles of the pigmented epithelium and of the outer segments of the rods, where the enzyme systems are particularly located, remain disputed. [We should certainly reiterate the effect of vitamin A deficiency, known to carry with it a reduction in rhodopsin content and a corresponding rise in the absolute threshold in poor light (night blindness).]

Such analyses as these have been made in various species and the general idea that seems to emerge is that there is a complex exchange between the receptor level and the pigmented layer. Studies in the frog, in light adaptation when rhodopsin is decomposing, show that retinol migrates from the retina toward the pigmented layer by a slow process. The opposite migration occurs during resynthesis of Rh, which suggests the possibility of a constant interchange between these two levels. The mechanisms are not the same across species in all details, although the general principle of an interchange between these two levels might well remain valid.

Resynthesis from the Intermediate Products

So far we have considered the most interesting effects concerning the resynthesis of rhodopsin (Rh) from the products of complete breakdown (which probably corresponds with the events in the retina itself). Having done this, it is not irrelevant to discuss some of the observations concerned with rhodopsin resynthesis from the unstable intermediate products.

In this respect, the results are interesting but somewhat paradoxical to the extent that a certain amount of resynthesis has been observed (both in vitro and in vivo) during light exposure. It is true that this is chiefly of concern in very intense and very brief light exposures: A first stimulation (in practice, one quantum) acting on Rh will initiate an isomerization with the creation of an unstable product; but a second quantum, thereafter acting on this unstable product, can under certain conditions at least start the opposite process (i.e., a return toward a compound higher up in the decomposition's chain of events). This process, called *photoregeneration*, can initiate either a regeneration of rhodopsin from the first unstable breakdown products (prelumiRh, lumiRh, or metaRh I) or a return from the stage paraRh to the stage metaRh II (see figure 4.6). Photoregeneration leads to a parallel synthesis of a compound *isorhodopsin* containing the 9-*cis* isomer: This is an artefact not normally present in the retina (figure 4.7).

RHODOPSIN REGENERATION AND DARK ADAPTATION

In principle, the regeneration of rhodopsin ought to be related to the reduction in the absolute threshold that occurs during dark adaptation. Studies of relationships between the amount of rhodopsin regenerated and the threshold have led to very precise correlations, but they are not linear. It is quite clear that rather small changes in Rh suffice to modify the thresholds by proportionally much greater amounts.

In practice, experiments in animals and humans have shown a proportionality between *the amount of unregenerated Rh and the log of the threshold*, described by an expression of the form

$$s/s_0 = \exp[a(1 - p)]$$

where s is the present value of the threshold, s_0 the value after total dark adaptation, a is a constant, and $(1 - p)$ the quantity of pigment decomposed at this moment (or *free opsin*).

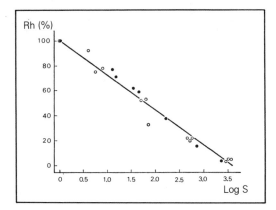

Figure 4.8
Rhodopsin and dark adaptation. Relationship between the retina's content of Rh and the threshold of vision in dark-adapted rats after exposure to a bright light (open circles) and in animals rendered "night blind" by deficiencies in vitamin A (filled circles). In each case the same relationship is observed: The log threshold (S) increases linearly with the reduction in the Rh concentration. (From Barlow 1972)

A good example of this sort of work is that by Dowling (1960) in the albino rat. The evidence used in this case was the amplitude of wave b of the animal's electroretinogram. A given level of dark adaptation was taken as parameter in this experiment and the curve of the amplitude of b was plotted as a function of log of the stimulus intensity. Extrapolating each curve so obtained to $b = 0$ determined what was taken to be the corresponding absolute threshold. In each case, the rhodopsin amount present was immediately measured after sacrifice. A linear relationship with a negative slope was found between this Rh and the log of the "absolute threshold"; see figure 4.8, where one point for each retina studied is shown and thus one point for each adaptation level explored.

Another interesting and exactly comparable correlation was made by the same author on rats rendered nyctaloptic by a prolonged deprivation of vitamin A. For each group of animals, for whatever length of vitamin A deprivation, the log of the threshold visibility (this time in darkness whatever might have been the level of adaptation) was seen once again to be linearly dependent on the final amount of Rh.

In humans, measurements in vivo by retinal densitometry combined with simultaneous measurement of the visual threshold at the same place on the retina were carried out by Rushton (1961). In normal subjects, these measurements verified that the time for total regeneration of Rh in dark adaptation corresponded well with the time taken for the absolute threshold sensitivity to reach its maximal value (40 minutes), with the rods beginning to show their adaptation after about 8 minutes in the dark. The regeneration of Rh, as measured by densitometry, was shown to have an exponential time course as

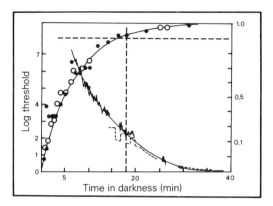

Figure 4.9
Human dark adaptation and the regeneration of rhodopsin. Rising curve: regeneration
of rhodopsin (right ordinate) for a normal subject (open circles) and for a "rod monochromat" with normal scotopic vision but very deficient photopic vision (filled circles).
Falling curves: dark adaptation curves (left ordinate) for a rod monochromat (irregular
trace) and for a normal subject (dotted curves). (From Rushton 1961)

a function of time in the dark. Another interesting illustration of the
nonlinearity of the relationship between Rh amount and absolute
threshold is that when 90% of the Rh is regenerated, the threshold
(measured in green light) is still 2 log units higher than the final value
obtained in adaptation (the total extent of the threshold change being
7 log units) (figure 4.9; see Rushton 1956). However, this experiment
can not be taken very far in the normal subject because of the intervention of cones with their more rapid adaptation, the existence of
which confuses the situation and does not allow the two changes
(absolute threshold and Rh) to be fully studied in isolation. The work
was repeated in rod monochromats, who have no foveal cone vision
(Rushton 1965). In this case, the Rh amount (more exactly, the
amount of Rh not regenerated) and the log threshold [now measur-
able over a 7 log unit range—Trans.] shows a linear correlation over
the whole time course and absorption range. According to Rushton's
measurements, the value of the constant (a) in the equation derived
above is around 20 (figure 4.10).

The correlation between Rh amount and threshold in animals and
humans is clearly more complicated than if the regeneration of Rh
had merely raised the sensitivity by the same percentage as the
amount of regeneration, that is, in proportion to the extra light absorbed by the extra pigment. A detailed explanation of this effect is
still to be found.

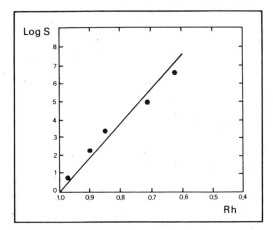

Figure 4.10
Relationship between log threshold (S) and the fraction of rhodopsin present (Rh) for a "rod monochromat"—a person lacking cones and thus color blind. (From Rushton 1965b)

RHODOPSIN IN SITU

We now arrive at the recent studies that have been fundamental as a basis for our knowledge of the structure of rhodopsin in situ. A stumbling block in research was removed by the effective application of biophysical techniques and above all by exploiting molecular biological approaches. These analyses have chiefly been conducted on bovine rhodopsin and more recently on other pigments such as those in drosophila that are less abundant but nevertheless have become accurately accessible with new techniques.

Arrangement of the Rhodopsin Molecules
We already know that the outer segments of the rods, which contain the rhodopsin, comprise a stack of disks (figure 4.11). The molecules of rhodopsin are confined to each disk. Some interesting data are concerned with the orientation of the rhodopsin molecules in the disks. This leads to a dichroism in the rods: When they are observed in polarized light they show different optical densities according to the plane of polarization with respect to the long axis of the receptor, the optical density being higher when the plane is perpendicular to that axis and very much less when it is parallel. These results, in spite of the arguments they have inspired, are nevertheless probably the first sensible indication in favor of a preferred common orientation in the population of molecules of the chromophore with respect to the long axis of the outer segment.

More recently x-ray studies and neutron diffraction imaging techniques have given rise to the scheme according to which an Rh mole-

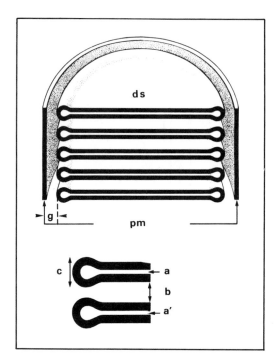

Figure 4.11
Morphology of the outer segment of a rod receptor. *Above*,
Note the arrangement of the
disks. *ds* is the disk surface
and the arrows *pm* indicate
the external plasma mem-
brane. The disk population
occupies most of the outer
segment except for a marginal
zone marked *g*. *Below*, A
sketch of the relative proportions of the disks, including
the thickness of the disk's
outer border, or "disk rim"
(*c*), the interdisk space (*b*),
and the intradisk spaces (a,
a'). Orders of magnitude according to EM observations
are: total radius of the outer
segment 3 μm: g = 0.01–0.02
μm; b = 0.015 μm; distance
between the centers of two
consecutive disks, 0.03 μm.
(From Steinberg et al. 1980)

cule constitutes a sort of transmembrane cylinder, with half of its
mass buried in the lipid bilayer of the disk and the rest spilling over
("like a head of a mushroom") at the two surfaces, the interdisk
(external) and the intradisk (cytoplasmic) (figure 4.12). According to
measurements of circular dichroism, each Rh molecule contains about
60% α-helical structure; from the infrared dichroism and diamagnetic
anisotropy of the membrane, it is also deduced that the helices are
essentially oriented perpendicularly to the plane of the membrane
(figure 4.13; see also Schwartz et al. 1975, Saibel et al. 1976, Dratz et
al. 1979, Chabre 1981, Dratz & Hargrave 1983).

Each rod contains about 600 to 2000 disks according to species, and
the disks repeat at about every 295Å. Taking into account the Rh
content of the receptor gives the image of a receptor surface liberally
sprinkled with quasi-cylindrical Rh molecules about 60 Å long,
spaced apart on the average by about 56 Å. The total number of Rh
molecules per disk is between $2 \cdot 10^4$ and $8 \cdot 10^5$ according to species.

The Structure of Rhodopsin

The use of recombinant DNA techniques allowed considerable advances in research, including the determination of the structure of

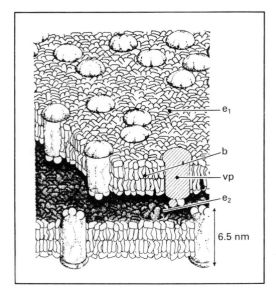

Figure 4.12
Model of a rod's outer segment disk membrane. Note the two membranes constituting the faces of a disk. Each is composed of a bilayer of lipid molecules within which are sited the pigment molecules (mushroom shapes). The three spheres at the base of the pigment molecule represent the sugar groups that maintain the orientation of the molecule. e_1, interdisk space; e_2, intradisk space; b, lipid bilayer; vp, visual pigment. (From Dratz & Hargrave 1983)

opsin (see Dratz & Hargrave 1983, Baehr & Appleburry 1986 for a detailed bibliography).

Bovine opsin is a polypeptide chain of 40 to 50 kD, with 348 amino acids for which the sequencing and the spatial configuration are well determined. It comprises seven transmembranal segments (I to VII) with each segment constituted by a helix of 21 to 28 essentially hydrophobic amino acids inserted into a lipid bilayer. The remainder of the amino acids are situated externally on the cytoplasmic interdisk and intradisk sides.

On the *cytoplasmic side* (figure 4.14, SCy) is sited the carboxylic terminal. At this level proceed the interactions that lead to the transduction cascade that we shall consider later (linked to the protein G). The hydrophilic residues of serine and of threonine are also found here. These can be phosphorylated under the influence of a rhodopsin-kinase.

On the *intradisk side,* where the amino terminal of the molecule is sited, the surface displays two oligosaccharide chains (in Asn_2 and Asn_{15}). The function of these sites for glycolysis is unknown.

Linkage with retinal. Segment VII contains the lysine (Lys 296) to which the 11-*cis* retinal is attached covalently as a Schiff base (retinyl-lysine). The retinal molecule is practically parallel to the plane of the membrane (inclination 16°) which the old measurements of dichroism had already predicted (see above). This Schiff base of retinal is pro-

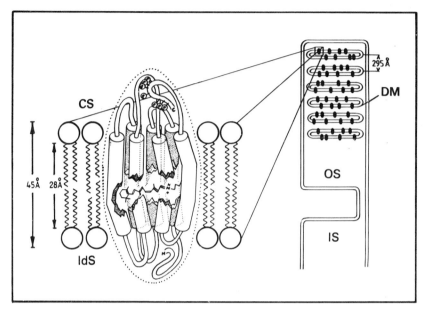

Figure 4.13
Rod outer segment. *Right,* Diagram of the outer segment (OS) of a rod as seen in
longitudinal section showing the disks and their disk membranes (DM). Inner segment
is marked IS. This diagram is not to scale since there are 600 to 2000 disks per rod and
$2 \cdot 10^4$ to $8 \cdot 10^5$ molecules of rhodopsin, depending on species (molecules represented
here by the black ovals). *Left,* Representation of the disk membrane showing the
cytoplasmic surface (CS) and the intradisk surface (IdS), the bilipid layer, and a molecule of rhodopsin. The latter is shown here as an elongated bundle of irregular helices.
The site of the junction with 11-*cis* retinal is represented as practically parallel to the
plane of the membrane. The small circles containing the letter P represent the sites for
phosphorylation. (From Dratz & Hargrave 1983)

teinated and buried in the membrane. There are assumed to be two
other possible anchorage points near the C_{11} – C_{12} junction with
retinal; these could be either an Asn (on chain 2) or a Glu (on chain 3).

Finally, the conformational change of the chromophore (isomerization of 11-*cis* retinal) will bring with it a conformational change of the
protein. Let us review what is known of the course of the isomerization under the effect of light.

The *cis* conformation shows an incurving chain. Under illumination
there is isomerization to the all-*trans* state. Because the retinal is not
free to move but is buried in the protein, the basal energy needed
for isomeration is on the order of 1 eV (whereas if the retinal were
free, without any torsional energy existing, the energy for isomerization would have only been 0.02 eV).

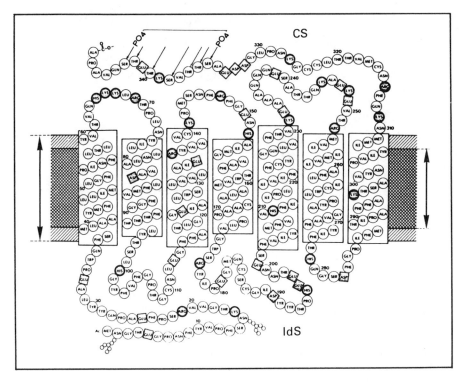

Figure 4.14
Model of the organization of the polypeptide chain of rhodopsin in its relationship
with the lipid bilayer and the disk membrane. The carboxyl terminal is situated at
the interdisk cytoplasm side of the cell (CS). The amino acids with positively charged
lateral chains are represented by shaded circles and those with negative lateral chains
by shaded squares. The sugar fragments are the small circles near the aminated terminals at the intradisk surface IdS. The helices I to VII are shown here from left to right.
In the lateral hatched areas, the central part with cross-hatching represents the distance
between the hydrophilic parts of the bilayer. (From Dratz & Hargrave 1983)

This isomerization has two time courses. The first stage lasts some
picoseconds, when complete isomerization is retarded by the conformation of the protein. In the second stage, the molecule changes to
its final form more slowly (10^{-4} ms), this change being effected in
the rest of the protein.

The second membrane of the external segment, the plasma membrane, is where, after isomerization, the ionic changes are generated
that eventually lead to the generation of neuronal discharges. This
will be discussed below.

It is worth noting also that bovine opsin and that from *Drosophila* enjoy very close homologies. The amino acid residues are identical within 35%. The two of them have seven hydrophobic transmembrane segments linked with hydrophilic chains that are either cytoplasmic or extracellular.

1.3 CONE PIGMENTS

The identification of cone pigments—the necessary mediators of color vision where it exists—was made in three stages, the results of which have had very unequal direct significance.

CONVENTIONAL BIOCHEMICAL STUDIES

This first method need not occupy us very long. Recognizing the small proportion of cones in mixed retinas, researchers have usually used all cone retinas, predominantly of birds, to make the pigment extraction less hazardous. Thus Wald and colleagues (1955) were able to extract a pigment *iodopsin* from the chicken. This pigment has been subjected to much study (perhaps not so intensively as rhodopsin) with the following main results:

• λ_{max} is at 562 nm, considerably displaced to the red compared with rhodopsin.
• Apparently it is likely that this pigment contains the same chromophore as rhodopsin but differs from Rh in its protein.
• Its photodecomposition gives rise to a series of intermediate compounds whose sequence seems very like that for rhodopsin (prelumi-Iodopsin, lumi, meta-I, meta-II-Iodopsin, and all-*trans*-retinal plus opsin). The details of λ_{max} and the temperature characteristics (Morton 1972) are very much like those for the homologous products of rhodopsin.
• The iodopsin absorption spectrum corresponds very closely to the photopic visibility curve for the species considered (in this case, chicken).

The fact that one is dealing with a single cone pigment, however, does not solve the problems encountered elsewhere, of separating out different pigments corresponding to different color receptors. These results have thus only a minor interest in this context. [In birds there are also colored lipid inclusions, the intervention of which is not excluded as a factor in their color vision].

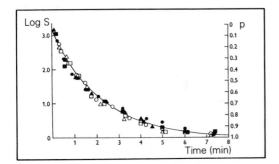

Figure 4.15
Kinetics of the regeneration of erythrolabe measured on three occasions for a dark-adapting deuteranope (filled symbols). The open symbols are for threshold(s) measurements (taken between those for erythrolabe concentration) during corresponding dark adaptation times. p, % regeneration of erythrolabe. (From Rushton 1965a)

REFLECTOMETRY (RETINAL DENSITOMETRY) STUDIES

Rushton's retinal densitometry method has certainly advanced our knowledge of the pigments responsible for human color vision (Rushton 1972). Two principal photolabile substances have been identified in the fovea of human subjects: *chlorolabe* and *erythrolabe*. However, this experimental analysis of pigment amounts is most easily done in dichromats, since in trichromats these pigments coexist in the same retinal region and in about the same general wavelength range.

In (red blind) protanopes, the pigment measured is chlorolabe and its absorption curve is like the photopic visibility curve for such subjects, with λ_{max} at 535 nm, in the green (Rushton 1963, 1972).

In deuteranopes, daltonian subjects who confuse red and greens and who are less sensitive in the green, it is the other pigment erythrolabe that can be measured alone with its λ_{max} at 570 nm in the bright red. Here again, the photopic visibility curve and the pigment absorption coincide well (figure 4.15; see Rushton 1965a, 1972).

In addition, Rushton (1965b, 1972) extended these studies for each type of subject into the kinetics of regeneration of the corresponding pigment during dark adaptation. In this way, he was able to establish in each case an excellent parallelism between pigment regeneration and the threshold. Once more, the measurements led to an expression of the form $s/s_0 = \exp[a(1 - p)]$—as above for rhodopsin and rod adaptation—with a lower value for the factor a of about 3.

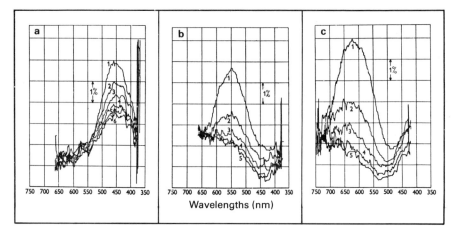

Wavelengths (nm)

Figure 4.16
Absorption spectra of three outer segments of cones isolated from the retina of the carp that show absorption maxima in three different spectral regions. (Ordinates: % absorption, scaled in 1% steps). The successive diminutions of absorption result from a progressive pigment bleaching after each spectral sweep needed to make the measurement. (From MacNichol 1964)

Unfortunately, such measurements could not be extended by Rushton to tritanopes (extremely rare subjects) to investigate the third pigment (called *cyanolabe*) postulated by the trichromacy theory [in part because of the very small concentration of "blue cones"—Trans.]. Neither did the technique have sufficient spatial selectivity to determine whether the pigments were located in the same or in different cones.

MICROSPECTROPHOTOMETRIC ANALYSIS

Microspectrophotometry, used to study difference spectra in single cones, has facilitated the most significant recent advances in studying color vision.

In *carp*, a species presumed to have color vision, MacNichol (1964) and Marks (1965) discovered that the maximum absorption in cones clustered around three values *but with only a single maximum per single cone:* 455 ± 15 nm, 530 ± 5 nm, 625 ± 5 nm. This showed for the first time that there are indeed three different categories of pigments in a species endowed with color vision, and that a given cone contains only one of those pigments (figure 4.16).

These three cone pigments are again different from that existing in

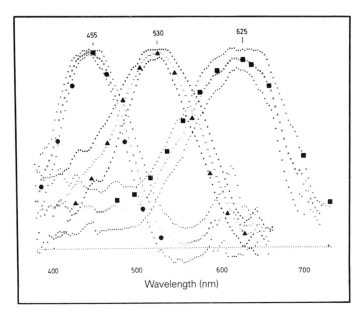

Figure 4.17
Mean difference spectra for three types of cone in the carp. Each mean curve is flanked by its standard deviation curves (for 8, 10, and 9 experiments, for the blue, green, and red cones, respectively). The symbols trace out the standard (Dartnall) absorption curves calculated for peaks at 455, 530, and 625 nm. Note that the differences between the actual and theoretical curves are rather small. (From Marks 1965)

the rods, which in this particular case contain a type A_2 rhodopsin (porphyropsin) since they are from freshwater species.

It was also demonstrated that the experimental points, obtained from a large number of receptors over the whole spectrum, show absorption curve shapes that are entirely comparable with the pigment curves for which Dartnall (1962) was able to devise a normalized shape, the "Dartnall monogram" (figure 4.17).

Recently, microspectrophotometry in another cyprinid revealed a fourth type of cone with a sensitivity maximum near 355 to 360 nm, that is, far into the violet (almost ultraviolet). This posed a problem (discussed by Bowmaker 1983) for postulating a universal trichromacy, since there is a possible tetrachromacy in these animals.

In *primates* (monkeys and humans), the same sort of detailed results have also been achieved. The maxima for isolated cones are in this case near 445 nm (blue), 5535 nm (green), and 570 nm (yellow), respectively. Thus the data for our own vision now enjoys a proof

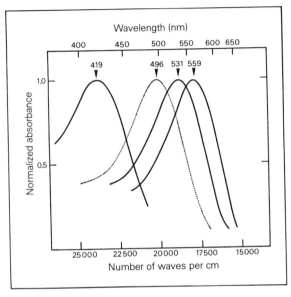

Figure 4.18
Absorption curves for the four pigments in the normal human retina. The solid curves
are for the three types of cone and the dotted curve for the rods. Absorbance is
normalized, i.e., expressed as a fraction of each maximal value. Results are based on
microspectrophotometric measurements on 137 receptors. (From Mollon 1982)

that its trichromatic system of color vision comprises three different
pigments that are carried separately in three types of cones (figure
4.18). The first results were due to Brown and Wald (1963) and Marks,
Dobelle, and MacNichol (1964); see also Bowmaker and Dartnall
(1980). Note that the λ_{max} values for two of the three pigments coincide with the retinal densitometry measurements in humans by Rushton, who specified 535 nm λ_{max} for chlorolabe and 570 nm for erythrolabe.

More recently, Bowmaker et al. (1980) have reexamined single primate cones on a large number of receptors, using *lateral*-beam penetration of the outer segment (see section 1.1). The values they report
are a little different from the above, as figure 4.18 and table 4.1 show
(notice that the so-called red cones and blue cones are in fact in
the yellow and the violet!). These authors prefer to talk of S (short
wavelength), M (mid wavelength), and L (long wavelength) cones.
They also compared their data with Stile's work relating to mechanisms π_4 and π_5; the agreement is essentially very satisfactory. Note

Table 4.1. Values of (primate) pigment λ_{max} determined by microspectrophotometry (nm)

Species	S cones	Rods	M cones	L cones
Human	419	496	531	559
Rhesus	*	503	535	566
Cynomolgus	419	500	535	567
Saimiri	429	499	535	568
Cebus	*	499	535	*

*Not measured.

that microspectrophotometry has also confirmed, as expected, that rhodopsin is well localized in rods (this being "true rhodopsin" [A_1]).

In *birds* the story of color vision is a long one. Before the multiple types of avian cones and pigments were recognized and only the existence of iodopsin had been proved (λ_{max} 560 to 565 nm), it was suggested that color vision in this group was entirely effected by light-filtering in the colored oil droplet inclusions of the receptors. This hypothesis fell when it was shown that abolition of the pigment in the inclusions by a suitably restricted dietary regimen did not abolish color vision.

Microspectrophotometry has recently discovered three types of cones in diverse bird species (notably in the pigeon) with λ_{max} values 560 to 570 nm, 495 to 515 nm, and 460 to 465 nm, respectively. However, the problem remains particularly complicated by the presence of different types of oil drops. Five sorts have been distinguished and, optically, they undeniably exert a filtering effect, cutting the transmission of shorter wavelengths by the cartenoids that the pigments contain. Each oily inclusion is characterized by its λ_{50}, the wavelength at which the transmission is only 50% (representing an absorbance of 0.3).

Values of λ_{50} found in the pigeon are: 473, 522, 554, 570, and 610 nm. It is possible to calculate the spectral sensitivity of each type of cone by combining the absorption spectra data for the pigment in the outer segment with the filtering action by one or the other type of oil droplet inclusion. It becomes clear that the sensitivity is modified in the red and yellow sectors of the retina (figure 4.19). For this reason, at least five types of cones exist in the red sector and at least five in the yellow sector (see chapter 1, section 5.1) but in different proportions. Correspondingly, the two sectors have different overall

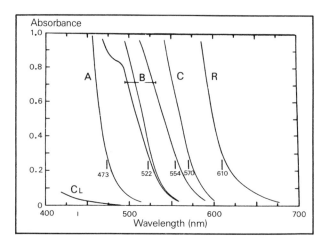

Figure 4.19
Absorption spectra of oil-drop inclusions in the red sector of the pigeon retina. The curves C_L ("clear"), A, C, and R ("red") concern the different inclusions in the simple cones; B is for the double cones. The absorption of the B inclusions varies between the limits indicated, according to the location of the cone within the red sector. The wavelengths marked in the diagram show the places for 50% transmission through the inclusions (absorbance 0.3). (From Bowmaker 1980)

spectral sensitivities. This had been separately confirmed by behavioral studies.

In spite of the presence of these inclusions, which limit the waveband transmitted toward the blue side, vision in the short wavelengths does exist in some diurnal birds like the pigeon. That they are sensitive in the region 360 to 400 nm (i.e., in the near ultraviolet) has once again been proved behaviorally.

To explain this sensitivity it seems that the eye media in these birds are optically transparent out to 350 nm, and there exist, at least in the red retinal region in the pigeon, cones that carry *colorless inclusions* also transmitting to 350 nm. Thus here is a fourth type of receptor; once more a tetrachromacy hypothesis arises, this time in birds.

Considering the wider question of the different ecological status in the birds, certain conclusions can be drawn relating this to the density and characteristics of the retinal inclusions. In nocturnal birds (owls) there are very few colored inclusions and few cones; swallows have only 5% to 15% of such inclusions, perhaps because they depend for their food predominantly on the perception of silhouettes against the short wavelength background of the sky; diurnal passeriformes have in contrast 50% to 80% of red and orange inclusions; among marine species, some (seagull) have almost as many, perhaps for good vision from the air, whereas others (cormorant) have few, perhaps for the better detection of underwater prey where vision in the shorter wavelengths is an advantage (Bowmaker 1980).

THE CONE PIGMENTS FOR COLOR VISION AND THEIR GENES

Studies based on a molecular biology approach have now brought essentially new data on the structure of the cone pigments. Nathans and colleagues (1986a,b) were able to isolate and sequence the genomic and complementary DNA clones that encode the proteins of three cone pigments. The first assumption was that the nucleotide sequence of the cone pigments presents a basic homology with that of the rod pigment rhodopsin. After isolating and characterizing the complementary DNA and genomic DNA clones encoding bovine rhodopsin, this DNA sequence was used to probe libraries of human genomic DNA. After screening, the hybridizing clones fell into three classes. The genomic DNA segments were finally compared to mRNA from retinas obtained at autopsy of normal subjects. From this comparison, the authors could conclude that, the first class being rhodopsin, the second class (only a very small part of the retinal cDNA, comparable to the very low ratio of blue cones vs. rods) was likely to be the blue pigment gene, and the third class (a higher proportion) included both green and red pigment genes. The results may be summarized as follows:

• The three human cone pigments thus identified and the rod pigment form a single family of homologous proteins encoded by the corresponding members of a family of genes.
• The amino acid sequence of the proteins of the three pigments show 41 ± 1% identity with Rh.
• The red and green pigment genes have a high degree of homology (96% mutual identity). They both show a lower (43%) degree of homology with the blue pigment gene.
• The red and green pigment genes are located on the X chromosome, whereas the blue pigment location is probably autosomic. Moreover, the data indicate that while the red gene is unique, the number of green pigment genes varies in normal individuals, from one to several.
• All pigments present, like Rh, have seven transmembrane seg-

ments that are similar, with no insertion or deletion needed when optimally aligned (figure 4.20).
• All pigments have a lysine corresponding to that at position 296 of Rh, for covalent attachment to the 11-*cis* retinal.
• The three cytoplasmic loops, likely points of contact with transducin (see below) are also conserved.
• The carboxyl terminal regions all contain serin and threonine residues, which in bovine rhodopsin are the site for light-dependent phosphorylation by rhodopsin kinase. By analogy with rhodopsin, it is supposed that such a kinase action also turns off cone pigments when light activation takes place.

The question remains of how the various opsins might modify the environment of the 11-*cis* retinal so that its absorption spectrum is appropriately shifted. Basically the same mechanism may exist as in rods with rhodopsin (attachment of retinal cavalently to the amino group of lysine by way of a protonated Schiff base; transfer of positive charges from the Schiff base nitrogen to retinal's conjugated π-electron system through photic excitation). From this basic Rh model, the authors speculated that the positively or negatively charged intramembrane amino acids near the Schiff base might facilitate either the excited state or the ground state and thus modify the absorption spectrum. These charges are actually different in the blue pigment, in Rh, and in the R and G pigments; these differences may partly account for spectral absorption differences. In sum, retinal tuning may be changed by interaction with neighboring amino acid charges. (See also Nathans 1987—Trans.)

DYSCHROMATOPSIAS AND RETINAL PIGMENTS

We shall not discuss here all the hypotheses that have been advanced to explain color vision anomalies in humans. Let us remember that Dalton postulated an anomaly in the absorption of the eye media, a hypothesis that was quickly denied. Young and Maxwell introduced the essentially correct idea that color vision deficits are due to functional deficits in the receptors. This work, taken up and developed by Helmholtz, led to the attribution of dyschromatopsia to the reduction of the number of degrees of freedom in the color mechanisms from 3 to 2, these being associated with deficits in the absorbing pigments. This interpretation arose at the time when other experimenters proposed that the reduction in the number of degrees of

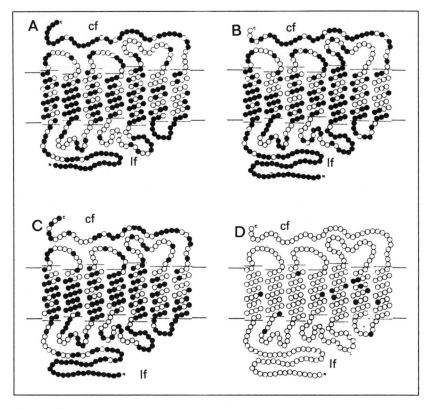

Figure 4.20
Pairwise comparisons of the four human visual pigments. Amino acid identities are white and differences are black. A, Blue vs. rhodopsin; B, green vs. rhodopsin; C, green vs. blue; D, red vs. green. Note that the red and green pigments are most alike. For each comparison, the amino acids were optimally aligned. This required no insertions or deletions except when comparing the carboxyl termini of the green (or red) with the blue pigment. When intramembrane regions are optimally aligned, the amino-proximal tails, on the intradiskal or luminal face (lf) of the red and green pigments are 16 amino acids longer than for rhodopsin; the carboxyl-proximal tails, on the cytoplasmic face (cf) are the same length. When optimally aligned, the amino- and carboxyl-proximal tails of the blue pigment are 3 amino acids shorter and longer, respectively, than for rhodopsin. (From Nathans et al. 1986a)

freedom was linked (a third possible *a priori* hypothesis) to an anomaly in the neuronal connections, an interpretation which is no longer considered.

Nearer our time, Rushton, as we have already emphasized, identified the two pigments erythrolabe and chlorolabe, absorbing in the red and green, respectively and also the probability of a third, cyanolabe, in the blue. Microspectrophotometry thereafter reinforced this experimental work and established that foveal trichromacy was linked with the existence of three pigments, with one pigment per cone. As a corollary, dichromatism is due to the absence of one of the pigments. Only one of the pigments, erythrolabe or chlorolabe, was found by Rushton in dichromats; protanopes only have chlorolabe, deuteranopes only erythrolabe.

However, the explanation is not without its snags. A difficulty arises with respect to anomalous trichromats, the protanomalous and the deuteranomalous because trichromacy only proposes three pigments. A variety of suggestions was made, for example, that in certain subjects some cones might contain a mixture of erythrolabe and chlorolabe. In its simplest form, this hypothesis does not hold if it is agreed that the pigment amounts rather than the receptor determine the amount of absorption at different wavelengths. Another suggestion was that there might be not three cone pigments but four or even five, one of these extra pigments being present in the protanomalous and the other in the deuteranomalous.

A recent systematic study of this problem leads to another explanation that can be summarized as follows: (i) Each pigment (erythrolabe, chlorolabe, and the less well defined one, cyanolabe) does not correspond to strictly identical and constant λ_{max} values in their absorption spectra. A detailed examination has shown a certain variability from subject to subject. The "standard C.I.E. observer" defined by the Commission Inernational de l'Éclairage is, after all, a mythical average individual, and differences from his characteristics and real subjects may be considerable if pains are taken to make careful and systematic measurements.

Such systematic investigations have, in summary, demonstrated that the three pigments comprise three subsets of pigments, the "red" group (Rushton's erythrolabe) having a λ_{max} spread between 565 and 575 nm, the "green" (chlorolabe) group between 525 and 540 nm, and the "blue" group between 420 and 440 nm.

Correspondingly, the following hypothesis is advanced:

• In the trichromat the three separate pigments are each from a different group of pigments.
• In the anomalous trichromat *and* the dichromat, two pigments belong to the same subset.
• If the pigments are different but all belong to the same subset, chlorolabe, the subject is protanomalous.
• If the pigments are different but all belong to the same subset, erythrolabe, the subject is deuteranomalous.
• If the pigments are *identical*, the subject will be protanope or deuteranope depending on whether the two pigments are both "green" or both "red" classes, respectively.

Further work is needed to test the hypothesis more fully. It has the merit of finding a certain unification for the various dyschromatopsias, dichromatism being a limiting case of the anomalous trichromatism that occupies an intermediate stage (Bowmaker 1983; see also the discussions in chapter 3 and in Mollon 1982).

Classic genetic data have long suggested that red and green color blindness is caused by alterations in the genes encoding red and green visual pigments. This hypothesis has been verified through a molecular genetics approach (Nathans et al. 1986b). Subjects with typical color vision defects (protanope and deuteranope dichromats, and anomalous red-green trichromats) were selected.

Genomic DNA from subjects with various red-green deficiencies were analyzed with the cloned red and green pigment genes as probes (see above). The observed genotypes appeared to result from unequal recombination or gene conversion or both. The loci responsible for variation in red cone sensitivity and those for variation in green sensitivity both map to the distal part of the q arm of the X chromosome. A very interesting and detailed study is provided by the authors to show how a dichromat's genetic structure may be (1) deuteranope with a single red pigment gene and no green pigment or one red-green hybrid gene; or (2) protanope with a more complex structure with one hybrid gene (red-green) and a variable number of intact green genes (zero, one or two). Different combinations may produce the same phenotype.

Anomalous trichromats were also considered in this investigation. The data have indicated that they correspond to a very complex, unequal intragenic recombination between R and G pigment genes; in *anomalous green sensitivity* (deuteranomalous), one red gene plus a variable number of hybrid and green genes; in *anomalous red sensitivity* (protanomalous), one hybrid red-green gene plus two or more green genes. Distinct unequal intragenic exchanges may, according to this view, lead to a variety of phenotypes, from anomalous trichromats to dichromats. As noted above, the two sets of anomalies may thus belong to a continuum of alterations with a common mechanism of unequal exchanges or gene conversions.

2 THE ELECTRORETINOGRAM

When the retina is illuminated, electric potential differences develop between the cornea and the posterior surface of the eye with a complex time course. These constitute the electroretinogram (ERG). In practice, the ERG is normally recorded between an electrode on the cornea and another ("indifferent electrode") on nonoptical tissue.

[In a resting state the eye presents a steady potential difference called the "corneoretinal potential," the cornea being positive with respect to the base of the eyeball. This dipole creates an electric field in the conducting media of the head. Any change in the position of the dipole, and thus any ocular movement, generates changes in this field and therefore in the potential differences detectable in the vicinity of the eyeball. These are exploited in electro-oculography (the recording of eye movements). We only cite this phenomenon for the reader to remember that it is instrumentally quite distinct from ERG recording.]

2.1 DESCRIPTION

The various ERG components have been inventoried according to the type of stimulus that evokes them. After short-duration stimuli (figure 4.20) of a predominantly rod retina (cat) there are three successive components (Brown 1968): *a*, cornea negative [meaning that the cornea is negative with respect to the back of the eye, though in practice with respect to an "indifferent" reference electrode. Conventionally, ERG records are arranged so that cornea positive deflections are represented upward.] There follows *b*, the principal component, cornea positive, followed by a return to negativity, with even a negative overshoot at the end of the stimulus (OFF effect). Finally, well after the end of the stimulus, there follows a positive *c* component that can last for more than a second (figure 4.21).

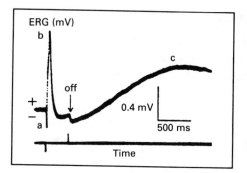

Figure 4.21
ERG following a brief stimulus
(cat). The ERG was measured between an electrode in the vitreous
humor and a reference electrode in
the orbit behind the eye. Positivity
of the active electrode is upward.
The signal marker (lower trace)
shows the onset and offset of the
stimulus. Voltage scale: 0.4 mV;
time scale: 500 ms. (From Brown
1968)

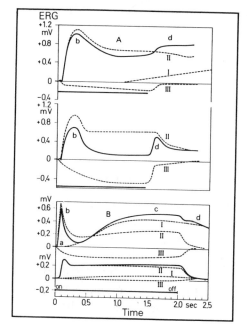

Figure 4.22
Standard analysis of the ERG into
three components. (PI, PII, PIII).
A (*upper*) ERG in frog retina, rich
in cones, when dark adapted and
(*lower*) when in the light. B, Cat
ERG, predominantly rods, at two
light intensities, 14 mL above and
0.14 mL below, for a sustained stimulus of 2.0-s duration (horizontal
bar). (From Granit 1947)

This *c* component can in no way be considered an OFF effect. In
fact, when the stimulus is a maintained step, the *c* wave develops
during the stimulus while the light is still on. The end of this stimulus
generates a new negative potential variation that can transiently in-
terrupt the development of the *c* wave (figure 4.22B).

In other retinas where cones predominate, the end of a long stimulus is signaled, mainly in the light-adapted state, by a second deflection like *b* (i.e., positive) that is called the *d* wave; in addition, the *c*
wave is feeble or absent (figure 4.22A).

2.2 A FORMAL MODEL FOR THE THREE COMPONENTS

Granit (1947) recognized that, given differences such as these, the ERG could be represented as the result of three fundamental "P" processes: two, PI and PII, being cornea positive and the other, PIII, cornea negative. This theory was based on extensive observations of ERG variation as a function of the most diverse conditions of stimulation (intensity, duration, color, etc.) and of the state of adaptation, even after certain pharmacological manipulations (which we have no space to detail here).

According to this scheme, the actual waves seen are the result of an algebraic interplay between these three components (figure 4.21). For example:

1. Initiation of PIII is responsible for the *a* wave.
2. Its suppression initiates the development of the *d* wave.
3. Initiation of PII generates the *b* wave.
4. Suppression of PII can generate a negative OFF wave (figure 4.21B).
5. When this suppression occurs during the development of a *d* wave, the latter is momentarily diminished.
6. Process PI is essentially responsible for the *c* wave.

Let us now enumerate some of the characteristic observations that led to localizing these ERG components and defining their substrate. Above all, this involves assertions of a certain independence between the *a*, *b*, *c*, *d*, and OFF components that is explained (with greater or lesser precision, it must be said) in terms of three separate hypothetical systems. At worst, these observations are just phenomenological; at best, they have sometimes permitted an attribution of the components to their own real substrate.

When the intensity of the stimulus is progressively decreased, (e.g., in the cat), the *a* and *c* components of the ERG disappear first and the only survivor is *b*. The suggestion according to the scheme described above is that the ERG is displaying only process PII.

In a retina rich in cones (frog) that is light adapted there is a large *d* wave, while the component *c*, seen in the dark-adapted state, disappears in the light. From this Granit made some estimates of the amplitudes of PII and PIII, as shown in figure 4.21A.

The effects of ether are a classic example of the separateness of the components. There is a rapid decrease in *c*, also of PI therefore; a progressive reduction of *b*, genrated by PII, and a prolonged persis-

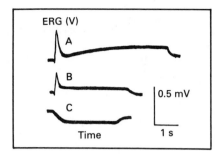

Figure 4.23
The progressive effects of ether on the cat ERG. (A) Control, (B) after 20 min and (C) after 31 min of ether administration. (From Rodieck 1972)

tence of a negativity, which signals the persistence of PIII (figure 4.23; see Rodieck 1972).

Lidocaine (Xylocaine) generates a perhaps more easily interpreted separation of the waves: It abolishes *b* without affecting *c* or *a*. Since this substance is known to act very rapidly on the responses of neuronal elements, we conclude that the *b* wave depends more strongly than *a* or *c* on retinal cellular mechanisms and thus involves either the receptors or some other neuronal elements.

The eye's vasculature comprises a retinal circulation proper and also a circulation called *choroidal*. The former essentially supplies the inner nuclear layer (bipolar cells) and the ganglion cell layer; the latter serves the receptor stages and the outer layers (pigmented epithelium). Thus, on interrupting the retinal circulation and that alone, wave *b* disappears (and therefore process PII) whereas the others remain, in particular component *a*. This sign of the survival of process PIII signals its outer layer origin.

In certain species (e.g., squirrel) separation by interrupting the circulation is not possible. But another method—injecting sodium *L*-aspartate into the vitreous humor (Furukawa & Hanawa 1955)— allows the isolation of PIII. Figure 4.24 clearly illustrates the progressive diminution of PII (*b*) and the progressive unmasking of PIII (*a*); see Raisanen and Dawis (1983).

Finally, another classic pharmacological separation of the effects is made possible by using different sodium compounds. Whereas sodium azide increases wave *c*, sodium iodate reduces this component (related to the PI system). The interesting point from these experiments arose from subsequent histology. The pigmented epithelium was shown to be effectively destroyed by the iodate, and it is highly probable that this is correlated with the disappearance of PI (wave *c*); thus the substrate for PI might well be the pigment epithelium.

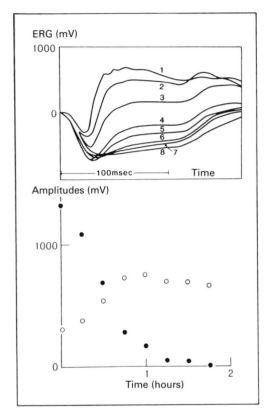

Figure 4.24
Effect of sodium aspartate on the squirrel ERG. *Above,* Mean ERG measured every 15 min during an infusion of sodium aspartate (100 nM of solution into the vitreous humor at the rate of 1.5 ml/h). ERG 1 is the normal standard ERG response. Note the disappearance of wave *b* that unmasks the single component PIII. *Below,* Amplitude of wave *b* in filled circles and of the negative wave PIII in open circles. (From Raisanen & Dawis 1983)

Detailed examination has shown that PII comprises two subcomponents, the first a short-lasting (*phasic*) wave *b* proper, which is the origin of the spike at the onset of the stimulus, and a second one lasting throughout the stimulus (*steady component*), *b*-DC. Interrupting the retinal circulation removes *b*-DC, like *b*. In contrast, lidocaine suppresses only *b*, leaving *b*-DC untouched, which must therefore be separate from *b* (Brown 1968).

Finally (and not the most negligible data), the ERG is not modified by retrograde degeneration of the ganglion cells following transection of the optic nerve. The ganglion cells and their axons do not therefore play any part in the generation of the ERG.

In terms of these "external" tests of the ERG the following observations summarize the situation:

• Wave *b* is the component most clearly associated with activity of the receptors and the retinal neuronal network.

• PI and PII find their origin in structures external to the retina, PI probably in the pigmentary layer, and PIII at a level that remains uncertain.

Further progress in this area depended on the more detailed analyses that follow.

2.3 RECENT ELECTROPHYSIOLOGICAL STUDIES: THE LOCAL ERG

Developments in microelectrode electrophysiology chiefly in the last decade have been applied to recording "local" ERG (LERG) potentials. These have notably advanced our knowledge of the ERG.

EXPERIMENTAL PRECAUTIONS

Successful microelectrode retinal recordings necessitate a variety of experimental precautions.

• To eliminate, when recording an LERG, those parts of the global ERG (summation of all the LERG) that originate far from the electrode tip while retaining the activity of cells that are immediately below the microelectrode. Experiment shows that, for geometrical reasons, an electrode placed in the vitreous humor is practically silent and can be used as a reference electrode.
• To exploit very restricted punctate light stimuli to excite only the region immediately situated below the microelectrode.
• To compare the LERG recorded in the fovea, where receptors dominate and the bipolar and ganglion cells are effectively lacking, with measurements made more peripherally.
• To arrange electrode penetrations that are normal to the retinal layers and to measure electrode depth as accurately as possible between the surface and the deep pigment epithelium.
• To block, if necessary, the retinal circulation without interrupting the choroidal system. As we have seen, this clamping affects the inner nuclear layer, whereas the receptors and the pigment epithelium retain a normal circulation.

RESULTS

The following discussion of such LERG measurements is based particularly on the detailed reports of Brown (1968) and his collaborators.

Laminar Analysis of the ERG

Brown and Wiesel (1961) first and others later carried out a serious "sectional" analysis of the ERG in which they paid particular atten-

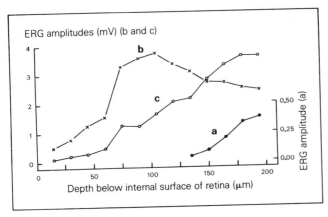

Figure 4.25
Amplitude of the components *a*, *b*, and *c* of the cat ERG as a function of the depth
of penetration of the microelectrode. At 200 μm the microelectrode reaches the receptor level. The indifferent electrode is in the vitreous humor. Stimulus: 3.0 mm diameter
bright spot centered on the region penetrated, 71 lumen/meter, 50-ms duration and
applied every 5 s. (From Brown & Wiesel 1961)

tion to the level at which the polarity of the different potentials reversed. They were thus able to make laminar explorations along the
radial dipole that represents the ERG generator. (The identification
of the reversal site of a potential is one of the most powerful means
of localizing its source.) Among other important results (figure 4.25),
they found that wave *c* reverses at the level of the pigment epithelium
(sometimes referred to as "membrane r" in ERG work. See p. 177,
Davson 1976), thus confirming its origin at that level. Juxtacellular
and intracellular measurements in the epithelial cells later confirmed
this result (Steinberg et al. 1983).

An equally important discovery is that wave *a* seemed to be localized at the level of the receptors themselves. This has been amply
confirmed by other measurements, as we shall see.

The origins of wave *b* and its DC component potential, judged by
their reversals, seem to be localized in a region delimited by the outer
boundary of the inner nuclear layer and the inner boundary of the
inner plexiform layer; this strongly suggests that the bipolar cells are
a likely source of these potentials. In fact, as we shall see later, the
case of wave *b* is much more complicated, and we cannot remain
satisfied with this conclusion for very long. Nevertheless, an electrode sited at the inner side of the pigmented layer records inverted
a and *b* waves, whereas wave *c* is not inverted there.

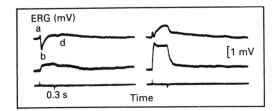

Figure 4.26
Local ERG (LERG) in cynomolgus. Comparison of LERG responses recorded in the periphery (*left*) and the fovea (*right*) by a deep electrode localized near membrane r (where responses are like normal ERG). Upper curve, normal retinal circulation; second curve, after clamping retinal circulation; lower curve, stimulus marker. Reference electrode in the vitreous humor. Stimulus diameter: 0.25 mm centered on the electrode. Stimulus duration: 0.3 s. (From Brown 1968)

The Late Receptor Potential (LRP)

In cynomolgus that has been light adapted to practically abolish wave *c*, clamping the retinal circulation removes wave *b*-DC, and nothing is left but a slow variation of the same polarity as wave *a*. This wave follows the time course postulated by Granit for mechanism PIII.

In addition, a local analysis with fine electrodes has demonstrated that PIII is particularly prominent in the fovea, where there are only receptors and no other nervous tissue, while it has less prominence in the periphery (figure 4.26), thus confirming that PIII is directly linked to receptor activity. Laminar investigation of the LRP during clamped retinal circulation essentially confirms, from the sign of the potentials recorded at different levels, that effectively the LRP has its origins in the receptors (figure 4.27).

Comparison of cone-dominant and rod-dominant retinas has shown that the recovery time for the rod LRP is much slower than for the cone. Moreover, the difference in amplitude and shape of the OFF response (which is slow and negative in rods but is the positive *d* wave in cones) is interpreted as being due to a complex interaction between the effects of interrupting the direct current component and interrupting the LRP. Fundamentally, the components are similar in the two types of retinas, but the LRP falls rapidly in the cones and slowly in the rods, leading to the differences seen (figure 4.28).

The Early Receptor Potential (ERP)

We will now discuss the early receptor potential, or ERP. The latency of potential PIII (in other words, of the LRP) posed problems since it was hard to imagine that, starting 1.7 ms after the stimulus, it could

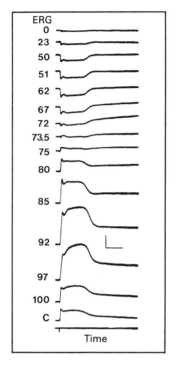

Figure 4.27
Variation of the late receptor potential (LRP) in cynomolgus, isolated by clamping the retinal circulation, as a function of depth of the recording microelectrode. Reference electrode is in the vitreous humor. The depth of the electrode is shown as percent of the maximal depth, which is near the choroid and is counted as 100%. Record C is touching the choroid. Stimulus: flash applied at the time indicated in the lowest trace, repeated every 10 s. Scale: 1 mV, 100 ms. (From Brown 1968)

give information about the earliest processes in the photoreceptors. It was thus judged to be important that after an intense stimulus a very early response can be observed (latency 60 μs)—initially negative, then positive—both in the fovea and in the periphery of monkey retina. A microelectrode sited near the receptors shows that this is larger in the fovea than in the periphery (Brown & Murakami 1964, Cone 1967; figure 4.29).

There is strong evidence that this ERP is linked with the visual pigments and their photolysis at the level of the outer segment of the receptors. In albino rats the action spectrum of the ERP coincides effectively with the absorption spectrum of rhodopsin, and its amplitude is proportional to the amount of rhodopsin activated by light: It disappears when all the rhodopsin has been bleached. In albino rabbits it has even been possible to uncover, by retinal densitometry, a parallelism between the ERP's generation and the appearance of the intermediate components of photolysis (meta- and pararhodopsin).

However, these suggestions concerning the origin of the ERP are not immune to attack from critics. There is no doubt that the potential has to do with the photochemistry of the pigments in the outer seg-

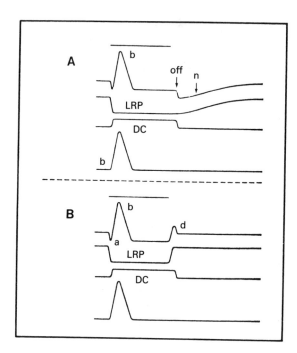

Figure 4.28
Schematic interpretation of the components *a*, *b*, and *d*, after taking account of the time course of the LRP and of the *b*-DC component (see text). ERG of light-adapted mammalian retina for (*A*) predominantly rod retina and (*B*) predominantly cone retina. Standard arrangement: active electrode in front of the eye and reference electrode behind. Wave *c* is not shown. Further explanation in the text. (From Brown 1968)

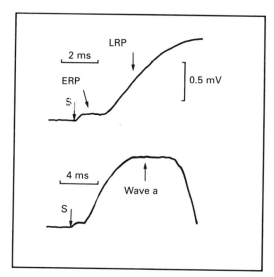

Figure 4.29
Time course of early (ERP) and late (LRP) receptor potentials in the albino rat and their relation to wave *a*. Recording at two different sweep speeds. Stimulus: a brief flash (vertical arrows) repeated every 10 s. The active electrode is deep in the retina at the level where wave *a* is maximal. (From Cone 1967)

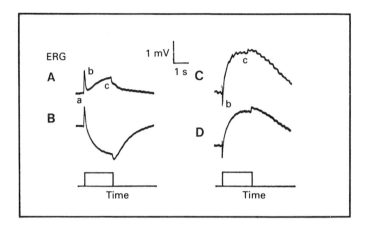

Figure 4.30
ERG and LERG recorded before (*above*) and after (*below*) intravenous infusion of
150 mg of sodium iodate. By normal conventions, deflection upward means positive
at the active electrode. The indifferent electrode is sited behind the eye for the ERG
and in the vitreous humor for the LERG. *A*, Normal ERG with components *a*, *b*, and
c. *C*, Identification of these components in the LERG where *a* and *b* are inverted
because of the deep electrode position. *B* and *D*, Same activities after treatment with
sodium iodate. Stimulus intensity: 140 lux. (From Rodieck 1972)

ment of the receptors, which necessarily implies that it is concerned
with the earliest stage of the physiological generation of retinal signals. But, taking into account the conditions under which the ERP is
generated (very powerful, brief, light flashes) it could well result from
a *photoregeneration* of pigment from one or other of the intermediate
unstable products of photodecomposition (see section 1.2).

The "r" Potential: A New Definition of Wave c
Rodiek (1972) emphasized that certain aspects of ERG component
generation were inexplicable by the then fashionable hypotheses. In
particular, there were problems with wave *c*, since the measured
deep LERG component does not seem to be suppressed by sodium
iodate, as it ought to be from arguments based solely on global ERG
measurements. On the contrary, it retains a very large amplitude
(figure 4.30).
    Rodiek proposed the existence of a new component, wave "r,"
positive, of large amplitude, and arising in the pigmented epithelium.
He also suggested that the LRP potential, linked with the receptors,
is larger than proposed by the hypothesis that links it only with
component PIII. In this scheme, wave *c*, classically identified with

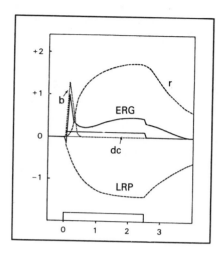

Figure 4.31
Modified scheme for the components of the ERG in cat (see text). (From Rodieck 1972)

PI, in fact results from an algebraic sum of two components, "r" and the LRP. As for wave b-DC, it remains the same as its original conception by Brown (figure 4.31). This new scheme allows a more subtle interpretation of the changes seen in wave c, for example, its presence in the pigmented rat but its absence in the albino rat under the same conditions, where it is replaced by an opposite, negative, wave (Weidner 1976).

2.4 IONIC MECHANISMS: GLIAL CELLS AND THE ERG COMPONENTS

At the same time as purely electrophysiological aspects of the ERG were being developed (and continue to develop), other approaches increased our understanding of its components, both in terms of ionic mechanisms and the role, which now seems to be a major one, of the glial cells and the pigment epithelium.

THE ORIGIN OF WAVE b

We saw above how, based on electrophysiological measurements, wave b was related to the activity of bipolar cells, the essential argument being its localization in the vicinity of the inner nuclear layer. However, the question seems now to be much more complicated than that suggests.

The interpretation of wave b is in fact much more firmly attributable to a participation of the glial Müller cells which extend throughout the thickness of the retina, practically from its inner to its outer boundaries (see chapter 1, section 8). Thus Miller and Dowling (1970) showed by intracellular recordings that the response to a light stimulus in these cells is a depolarization for which the latency of onset and the rise time are very much like those of wave *b*.

This hypothesis has a second aspect that is concerned with the effect of *extracellular potassium concentration* ($[K^+]_{out}$). The particular sensitivity of glial cells to $[K^+]_{out}$ having been known for some time (see Kuffler & Nichols 1966), Miller and Dowling (1970) then proposed the following chain of effects: A light stimulus increases intraretinal $[K^+]_{out}$ and this increase produces in its turn a depolarization of the Müller cells. This activity generates a transretinal current (which is radial because of the geometrical distribution of the cells) and this is seen as the *b* wave, the principal cornea positive component of the ERG.

In its major outlines, this scheme remains valid today, even though, naturally, it has been much refined in detail during the last few years. According to the initial hypothesis, the release of K^+ ions in the *distal* retinal region (i.e., near the receptors) was regarded as responsible for the depolarization of the Müller cells. More recent work based on the local measurement of $[K^+]_{out}$ by ion-selective electrodes has considerably elaborated the scheme. It has been recognized (Kline et al. 1978, Newman & Odette 1984) that there are in fact *two retinal levels* where stimulation causes a local increase in $[K^+]_{out}$: (1) a proximal zone in the vicinity of the amacrine cells (distal part of the inner plexiform layer) as well as (2) a separate distal zone, situated in the outer plexiform layer, no doubt in the vicinity of the bipolar cells (depolarizing Bi; see section 4.1). At these two levels, increases in K^+ have a time course that essentially justifies their involvement in the genesis of wave *b*.

However, there remain arguments to be considered concerning whether the distal source can be the only one that contributes to wave *b*: The kinetics of the K^+ release at this level vary like wave *b* under the influence of a variety of manipulations (stimulus size, pharmacological effects); and stimulation affects distal $[K^+]_{out}$ and the global ERG similarly, whereas the proximal $[K^+]_{out}$ is affected differently (see Dick & Miller 1978).

Examining the ionic exchanges as above has been accompanied by fine-scale electrophysiological measurements aimed at comparing level by level how the two phenomena, ionic and electrophysiological, develop in the different retinal layers. The traditional method of recording the local electroretinogram (LERG) was used first (figure 4.32). However, a more recently developed approach, the measure-

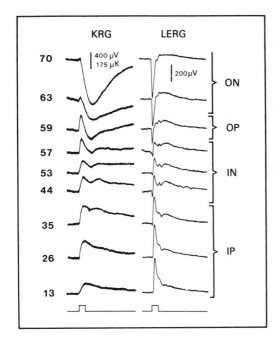

Figure 4.32
Variation of the "potassium retinogram," or KRG (measured by ion selective electrode, see text) and of the LERG as a function of depth in the retina. Responses to stimuli (of duration 1 s, intensity log $I = -5$) measured with respect to a reference electrode at the sclera. Moving from the outer distal to the inner proximal regions of the retina, responses are indicated for: ON, outer nuclear layer; OP, outer plexiform layer; IN, inner nuclear layer; IP, inner plexiform layer. (From Kline et al. 1978)

ment of "current source density" (Newmann 1980), has a better spatial resolution. The method of measuring the density of current sources has been much used in investigating central nervous responses electrophysiologically. It is based on measuring the second derivative of the vector current density (laplacian ∇^2). [Mathematically, this procedure is in principle the same as the one we derive briefly later in the addendum to chapter 5, section 3.3 concerning the quite different problem of spatial discrimination of vision.]

This technique showed the existence of two localized "sinks" of lines of current, that is, two precise retinal levels where there is an ingoing current from the extracellular medium to the Müller cells. An important adjunct is that these two sinks of maximal ingoing current to the glial cells coincide spatially with the two regions of $[K^+]_{out}$ increase, the outer (OPL) and inner (IPL) plexiform layers (figure 4.33).

This strict parallelism between ingoing currents and increases $[K^+]_{out}$ resolves one problem but introduces another. It is fully agreed that these entering currents flow into the Müller cells, but at what level do they exit? At present there are two hypotheses between which it is not yet possible to decide: the existence of a current

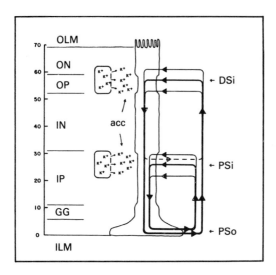

Figure 4.33
Illustrating the "potassium hypothesis" for the generation of wave *b*. Increase of
[K$^+$]$_{out}$ in the distal inner plexiform layer and at the outer plexiform layer causes two
inward currents in the Müller cell. Essentially, the corresponding site for the return of
these lines of currents is via the foot of the glial cell near the surface of the retina. The
current returns in extracellular space from this latter source to the two "sinks," thus
generating wave *b*. Ordinate: scale of depth (nm) in the retina. OLM, outer limiting
membrane; ON, outer nuclear layer; OP, outer plexiform layer; IN, inner nuclear layer;
IP, inner plexiform layer; GG, ganglion layer; ILM, inner limiting membrane; DSi and
PSi, distal and proximal current sinks; PSo, proximal current source. (From Newmann
1980)

"source" at a point in the Müller cell that is halfway between the two
sinks (Kline et al. 1978) or, in contrast, a current exit from the single
foot of the glial cell (i.e., by its proximal extremity). The arguments
are inconclusive, with perhaps a preference for those proposing a
particularly high permeability for K$^+$ at the level of the glial foot, the
proximal region of the cell situated at the inner limiting membrane.

An objection to these proposals is the difference between the time
course of the depolarizing response of the Müller cell and that of
wave *b*, which is much shorter. In fact, a simulation based on a
quantitative model in which quite a range of variables interact (including current densities and Müller cell K$^+$ permeabilities) has provided an answer to this objection (Newmann & Odette 1984). [The
"potassium hypothesis" has also been criticized because it is not always experimentally observed. In fact, the maintenance of this sort
of mechanism is dependent on the metabolic integrity of the retinal

tissue: The most detailed measurements have been made on isolated retinas].

In summary, it seems likely from this sort of investigation that wave b is a secondary consequence of the depolarizing activity in the bipolar cells in some way channeled and amplified by the Müller cells.

THE ORIGIN OF WAVE c

Other researchers have been more concerned with the very slow wave c of the ERG, sometimes identified with mechanism PI, sometimes, to the contrary, seen as a more complicated interaction between an amplified PIII and a component linked with membrane "r" (at the level of the layer of the pigmented epithelium). Quite a series of tests show, as we have already pointed out, a location for the generators of this component in the most distal part of the retina, the pigmented layer (retinal pigmented epithelium, P) because (1) destruction of this layer by sodium iodate abolishes c without affecting the discharge of axons in the optic nerve nor altering the components a, b, and d of the ERG; and (2) intracellular measurements in the cells of the pigment epithelium show a hyperpolarization on the order of 20 mV in response to light stimulation, and this has a time course identical with that of wave c.

This wave is not necessarily the result of synaptic action but could be the consequence of an extracellular change in the concentration of some ion species. Once again, potassium is discovered to be involved. Measurements of the concentration $[K^+]_{out}$ following a light stimulus show a slow, late lowering of this concentration in the extracellular medium surrounding the outer segments of the receptors (rods in particular), and therefore affecting the subretinal space. A series of experiments have confirmed this hypothesis (Oakley 1979; Oakley et al. 1976, 1979). The lowering of $[K^+]_{out}$ has the same onset time course as wave c, and the two phenomena vary in parallel if the light stimulus intensity or color is changed (figure 4.34). Finally, a linear relationship has been found between the wave c amplitude and log $[K^+]_{out}$.

Three stages need to be considered concerning the mechanisms involved. First, why, following a light stimulus, does the external potassium concentration decrease in the subretinal region and near the receptors? The explanation (Matsuura et al. 1978, Matsuura 1984) consists in relating this local fall directly to the hyperpolarization of

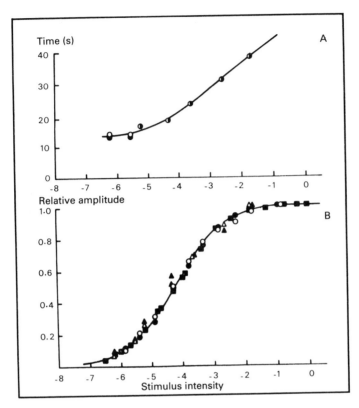

Figure 4.34
Effect of stimulus intensity on the decrease of the $[K^+]_{out}$ (KRG) and on the amplitude of wave c. Showing (A) the time in seconds taken for both functions to reach maximal value and (B) the normalized values of their amplitudes. The open symbols refer to wave c and the filled symbols to the KRG (see text). In this experiment the spectrum of the light stimulus peaked at 510 nm. (From Oakley & Green 1976)

the receptors in response to light. In the dark there exists a steady efflux of potassium from the receptors (to be discussed in more detail later) which is continually balanced by an active reabsorption of K^+ via a Na^+/K^+ pump probably localized in the inner segment of the rods (see section 3.2, below). Illumination, reducing the Na^+ permeability, reduces the passive efflux without affecting the active transport, bringing about the lowering of the external concentration of K^+.

Second, the rapid lowering of $[K^+]_{out}$ in light generates in its turn a hyperpolarization of the pigment cells, and this is the origin of the component PI (or in another classification, the component "r" of Rodiek). This hyperpolarization is explained by the fact that the pig-

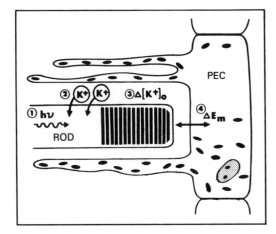

Figure 4.35
Model for the generation of the pigment epithelium hyperpolarization demonstrated by the *c* wave. Light energy is absorbed by the rod (1) and produces a loss of K^+ in the extracellular space (2, 3). This change creates the hyperpolarization (4) of the epithelial cell (PEC). (From Oakley & Green 1976)

ment cells have a high potassium permeability and thus the lowering of K^+ in their vicinity hyperpolarizes them (figure 4.35).

Third, it seems that this lowering of $[K^+]_{out}$ is not necessarily maintained throughout the duration of a prolonged light stimulus. The reasons for this recovery of $[K^+]_{out}$ are many: in particular, the bringing into play of a second K^+ diffusion, a change in the membrane potential of the rod, and finally, an inhibition of the active transport with which inward flux of K^+ is entrained.

Correspondingly, it has been shown that the pigment layer hyperpolarization decreases progressively, following very closely the recovery of $[K^+]_{out}$. In the cat, the peak of the *c* wave is attained after about 4 s of illumination.

THE VERY LATE ERG COMPONENTS

The data relating to the late ERG events have been shown to be yet more complex, particularly in recent experiments (Steinberg et al. 1983, Linsenmeier & Steinberg 1984). Effectively, the pigmented epithelium contains two layers that are relatively isolated from each other: the *basal membrane* on the choroidal side and the *apical layer* at the receptor side, separated by the subretinal space (see chapter 1, section 3). All that has been written above concerning late components in fact concerns the apical membrane which, as we have just seen, hyperpolarizes because of a lowering of $[K^+]_{out}$ and peaking near 4 s (in cat).

In some species (cat, gecko) but not in others (frog) it has been shown that the basal membrane itself also reacts to a light stimulus,

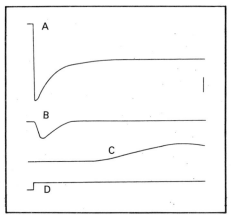

Figure 4.36
Responses at the level of the pigment epithelium. Diagram summarizing the three responses evoked by
light at the level of the pigment epithelium with their respective time
courses and relative amplitudes during the first 6 min of illumination.
A, Hyperpolarizing response at the
apical membrane with a peak at 4 s.
B, Late (peak 20 s) hyperpolarizing response at the basal membrane.
C, Very late (peak 300 s) depolarizing response at the basal membrane.
D, The light stimulus. (From Steinberg et al. 1983)

but this occurs even later and also provided that the light stimulus
is long enough. By arranging direct current recording and preferably
working on the retina in vitro, one can in fact detect two different
classes of response in the basal pigmented epithelium that appear
during a sustained illumination one after the other and later than the
apical membrane potential change (figure 4.36). *Basal late hyperpolarization* appears after 2 s of illumination and ends in the cat at around
the twentieth second of illumination. The origin of this potential is
also a local diminution of $[K^+]_{out}$. *Light peak depolarization* develops
even later, reaching its peak in the cat after around 300 s. The mechanism of this depolarization is not yet understood. These very late
waves may very well lead to understanding some observations from
direct current amplification that have been reported for the intact
human eye, but we do not have the space to discuss it here.

THE PIII SYSTEM AND IONIC MECHANISMS

Wave PIII, which we have somewhat dogmatically affirmed to be a
receptor potential (above), has also undergone a more detailed analysis (Witkovsky et al. 1975, Matsuura 1984). For optimal clarity, measurements are made on isolated retinas that have been deprived of
pigmentary epithelium to eliminate all the potentials associated with
the latter. In addition, in order to eliminate contributions from retinal
neuronal elements (bipolars, horizontal cells, and amacrines), the
preparation is treated with aspartate, which destroys them and only
allows the survival of the receptors and the Müller cells (the pigmented epithelium which itself resists aspartate having been surgically excluded).

The Operation of Retinal Receptors
249

In these somewhat special conditions, one wave recorded in response to light (PIII, so designated when it was believed to originate in the receptors; see LRP above) has in fact been found to comprise two successive components:

- *Rapid PIII*, which corresponds effectively to a summation of receptor potentials.
- *Slow PIII*, which follows it and can be dissociated from rapid PIII by treatment with Ba^{2+}, which interferes with K^+ conductance (Matsuura 1984). For this reason, slow PIII is attributed to a mechanism like that for the genesis of wave *b*, that is, the result of modifying $[K^+]_{out}$ and affecting the Müller cells.

Many uncertainties and contradictions remain unresolved. To explain the polarity of slow PIII with respect to the components *b* and *c* it may be necessary to regard the latter, particularly, as being due to a lowering of external potassium in the pigmented epithelium. It is probable that the different geometrical conditions in the more normal measuring conditions are at the root of this difference.

We have not attempted to analyze modifications of the ERG that result from changes in one or another of its components when the many variations of light stimulation are taken into account (color, duration, intensity, etc.). These would need to be considered in a complete review of the ERG, particularly one concerned with its clinical applications, but not necessarily here.

3 THE OPERATION OF RETINAL RECEPTORS

3.1 ELECTROPHYSIOLOGICAL MEMBRANE PHENOMENA

Two complementary techniques have facilitated the electrophysiological investigation of receptor (rod and cone) functional mechanisms and of the ionic changes involved: (1) traditional intracellular measurements in the receptors of the transmembrane currents and potentials and their dependence on applied voltages and currents or on intracellular injection of different substances, and so on; and (2) a method (Baylor et al. 1979) exploiting the geometry of the receptors, particularly of the rods. This consists in sucking the receptor into a transparent pipette. The suction is made at the outer or inner segment, as appropriate for the particular analysis (see figures 4.40 and 4.42). [Suction of the inner segment poses extra problems because the receptor itself must be isolated from other tissue in order to attack its basal end, which is normally solidly joined to other retinal layers.]

With this technique the investigator can directly measure the (inward or outward) transmembrane current of the segment that has been sucked into the pipette and observe its changes under the effect of some appropriate manipulation such as changing ionic environment, illumination of a precise part of the receptor, etc. [These different observations are not always made on the same source materials. These are sometimes species of fish (carp, tench), sometimes batrachians (toad, frog, necturus, amblystoma), and sometimes reptiles (turtle, gecko). This diversity explains, at least in part, some of the divergence between results, which we will not have the space to discuss in detail.

More recently, this suction electrode technique has been combined with "patch clamping," as we shall see.]

TRANSMEMBRANE POTENTIALS

A wide variety of *intracellular recordings* made in the receptors of various lower vertebrates allow us to appreciate the fundamental electrophysiological phenomena that accompany the transition from darkness to light.

In darkness, the transmembrane potential of the receptor is relatively small, having a resting value between -10 and -30 mV. This suggests the existence of a steady resting depolarization of the membrane away from the usual (more negative) intracellular values seen.

Following a light flash or a step change in illumination, the membrane hyperpolarizes by several millivolts. In general terms (ignoring detail), this hyperpolarization lasts as long as the stimulus (figure 4.37; see also Baylor & Fuortes 1970, Baylor & Hodgkin 1973). These are graded phenomena, the (linear ordinate) amplitude of which is a sigmoid function of the (log) stimulus intensity as abscissa (see figure 4.37).

The variation of this hyperpolarization (as dependent variable) as a function of incident light wavelength can be examined, taking care to maintain a constant stimulus energy. In this way the spectral light absorption by the rod pigment can be deduced.

It has also been possible to plot the sensitivity of cones in the same way (figure 4.38). This last type of experiment (exploiting appropriate preparations, in this case certain fish) once again reveals the existence of three types of cones with maximal sensitivities respectively at 462 ± 15, 529 ± 14, and 611 ± 23 nm, values that agree

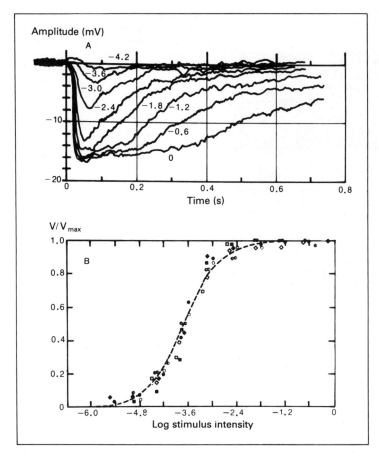

Figure 4.37
Intracellular cone responses for flashes of different intensities. *A*, Responses, superimposed on the same record, to 10 ms flashes of increasing intensity, shown in log
units for each curve. All stimuli applied at time zero. The most intense stimulus
corresponds to about $8.5 \cdot 10^6$ photons absorbable by the cone. Resting potential of
the cone about 22 mV. Deflection downward is a hyperpolarization of the cell. *B*,
Relative maximal amplitude of the hyperpolarization response as a function of the
stimulus intensity (from 10 cells). The dotted curve is the function $v/v_{max} = I/I_0 + S$,
where S is a constant. (From Baylor & Fuortes 1970)

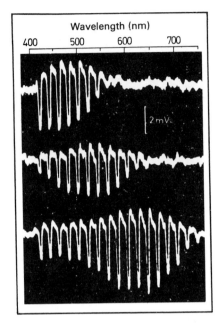

Wavelength (nm)

400   500   600   700

2 mV

Figure 4.38
Intracellular spectral responses of isolated cones of the carp retina. The spectra are explored in 20-nm steps by monochromatic stimuli of constant quantal energy $(2 \cdot 10^5$ photons/s) of identical (300-ms) duration presented every 600 ms. Downward deflection represents negativity of the intracellular electrode. (From Tomita 1972)

remarkably well with microspectrophotometric measurements in carp (Tomita et al. 1967, Tomita 1972).

TRANSMEMBRANE CURRENTS

Receptor currents have been measured using *suction micropipettes* (in the experiments to be described the suction electrode was applied to the outer segment; see Lamb et al. 1981, Matthews 1983). In darkness there is an *inward* current corresponding with the resting membrane's steady small depolarization compared with the usual intracellular hyperpolarization values. In light, this steady current is cancelled, implying a corresponding *outward* opposing current. Following impulsive stimuli, an appreciable outward transient current is seen, which is a function of the stimulus intensity and decreases progressively during the next few seconds (figure 4.39; see figure 4.41).

The maximal value of the outward current follows the stimulus intensity according to the usual sigmoid curve, saturating at about 20 pA, the luminous intensity for half saturation being about 1 photon/μm^2 (figure 4.39). [In this type of experiment it has become usual practice to specify the *intensity* in photons/μm^2 and the receptor *sensitivity* in pA/photon/μm^2.]

In diffuse illumination (thus of the whole of the outer segment)

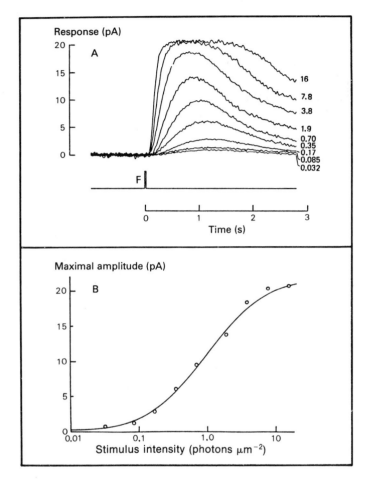

Figure 4.39
Transmembrane current responses in the outer segment to flashes of increasing intensity applied to the outer segment, measured by suction pipette (see text). *A,* Response in picoamps as a function of time for a flash (F) of 20 ms, 500 nm, at the intensities per flash shown to the right in photons · μm^{-2}. *B,* Maximal magnitude of each response as a function of stimulus intensity. Essentially the curve corresponds to a Michaelis equation, which can be written $A/A_{max} = i/(i + i_0)$ where A is the response amplitude and i is the stimulus intensity. A_{max} is 22 pA at i_0 and the intensity for half saturation is 1.0 photons · μm^{-2}. (From Lamb et al. 1981)

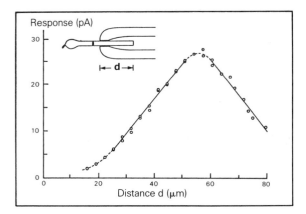

Figure 4.40
Maximal response at saturation as a function of the length d of the outer segment introduced into the measuring pipette. Flash stimulus, 20 ms, 500 nm, 64 photons · μm^{-2}, illuminating the whole segment (diffuse flash). d, distance in μm between the electrode tip and the distal extremity of the outer segment (see inset). Each point is the mean of two successive measurements. Note the linear increase of the maximal current as a function of d up to a maximum at $d = 57$ μm. Beyond this the response falls as the inner segment starts to penetrate the pipette. (From Baylor et al. 1979b)

the saturation amplitude of hyperpolarization is a practically linear function of the length of the outer segment in the pipette, which suggests that the ion channel density is about constant for the whole length of the outer segment (figure 4.40).

Using a very localized stimulation through a microslit (figure 4.41), Baylor et al. (1979b, 1984) and Lamb et al. (1981) showed that the local sensitivity ($pA/photon/\mu m^2$) is not the same from place to place along the outer segment. It is higher by about 30% in the proximal regions compared with the distal (figure 4.42).

The responses stimulated at the distal extremity are also slower (as well as smaller) than those due to the same stimulus delivered more proximally. One possible explanation (Schnapf 1983) is a longitudinal gradient of Na^+ (the ion responsible for the response) in the outer segment; another possibility is aging of the distal regions of the outer segment (this in relation to the disk renewal processes in the receptors described in chapter 1, section 3).

The use of microslits has also shown that the spread of activation (for a brief stimulus) and the spread of adaptation around a stimulus, is very restricted, probably the order of 3 to 6 μm (Lamb et al. 1981).

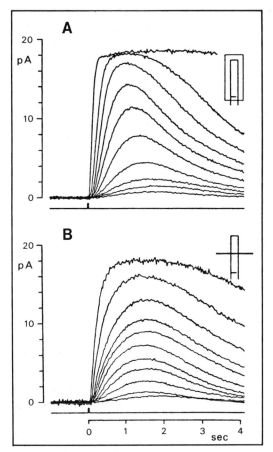

Figure 4.41
Response curves of a rod outer segment to stimuli of greater and greater luminance. The separation between successive curves corresponds to a multiplication by 2 of each flash intensity, except for the last flash in *A* and the last two flashes in *B* that correspond to increases by 4. *A*, Overall illumination of the outer segment. *B*, Illumination through a 1.7 μm wide slit. (From Lamb et al. 1981)

3.2 IONIC MECHANISMS

ROLE OF SODIUM (Na$^+$)

Research into the ionic processes accompanying these changes in membrane polarization and in membrane currents now agree on the following relevant facts: The small relative depolarization (compared with most cells) of the receptor's resting membrane potential in the dark, decreases or even disappears on reducing [Na$^+$]$_{out}$, suggesting that the depolarization is due to the existence of a *steady inward sodium current*, the ions crossing the membrane of the outer segment along their normal electrochemical sodium gradient because of a raised value of sodium transmembrane conductance (GNa$^+$). Under the same conditions of reduced [Na$^+$]$_{out}$ the response to a light stimulus

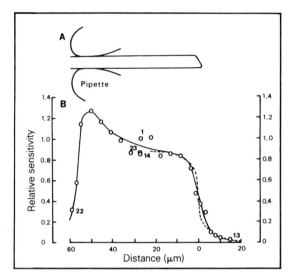

Figure 4.42
Sensitivity variation along the outer segment of a rod. A, The outer segment is enclosed in a suction pipette. B, The relative sensitivity is measured as a function of the position of a 1.7-μm illuminating slit along the outer segment. (From Lamb et al. 1981)

is reduced or abolished. Light must therefore normally generate a closure of the sodium channel (reduced GNa$^+$) in the region of the outer segment's *plasma membrane* (remember figure 4.11).

This light-dependent transmembrane current has been measured using suction electrodes but adapted to this experiment by sucking the *inner* (not outer) segment into the micropipette. This experiment allows registering the outer segment current changes (by measuring the inner segment effects) while changing the composition of the medium bathing the outer segment. In this way, Hodgkin et al. (1984) demonstrated that reducing [Na$^+$]$_{out}$ diminishes the dark current (figure 4.43A) and suppresses the responses to light. In contrast, with the first arrangement, sucking the outer segment into the pipette and treating the inner segment, a comparable lowering of [Na$^+$]$_{out}$ is without effect, showing clearly that this mechanism is located in the outer segment (figure 4.43B; see also figure 4.44).

Treating toad rods by incubating them in Ringer's solution with low calcium and chloride concentrations in the presence of ouabain, which blocks the (Na$^+$-K$^+$-ATPase) active transport, causes a suppression of the transmembrane polarization to practically zero. The electrical response of the cell to light disappears. Nevertheless, it continues to respond to light by an increase in the transmembrane *resistance*, which shows that the *light-dependent channels* have open and closed states that depend on the level of illumination and not on changes in the membrane polarization (Woodruff et al. 1982).

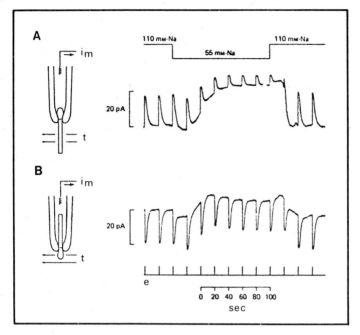

Figure 4.43
**Effect on the outer segment (*above*), and on the inner segment (*below*), of replacing
half the Na⁺ ions of a Ringer's solution bath by choline.** *Upper line,* Standard Ringer's,
110 mM of Na^+, with the dip in the line marking the time of infusion of solution poor
in Na^+ (55 nm). Flashes stimulating the responses were 20-ms duration, 78 photons ·
μm^{-2}, 500 nm. Outward current from the tip of the pipette is shown by the conventional upward deflections for trace *A* but the opposite is true for *B* since the cell's
orientation is reversed. (From Hodgkin et al. 1984)

CONTRIBUTIONS FROM OTHER ION SPECIES (Ca^{2+} AND K^+)

There is considerable experimental evidence, somewhat complex and
sometimes contradictory, showing that Na^+ is not the only ion species concerned in the transmembrane fluxes at the receptor level.
From these data it is undeniable that Ca^{2+} plays an important role.
In essence, there are two aspects of its involvement to be considered.

Fluxes at the Level of the Outer Segment
Some results from "reversed" suction electrodes (suction of the inner
segment, see above) demonstrate the influence of $[Ca^{2+}]_{out}$ bathing
the outer surface of the outer segment on the inward-going dark
current (the light-dependent sodium current). In high $[Ca^{2+}]_{out}$ the
dark current decreases and in low $[Ca^{2+}]_{out}$, on the contrary, it in-

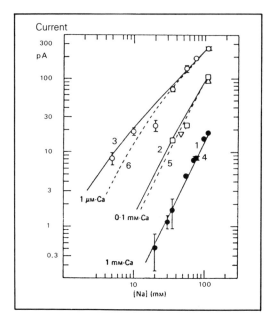

Figure 4.44
Relation between the light-stimulated current and the external concentration of Na$^+$ for three different external concentrations of Ca^{2+}. External Ca^{2+} concentrations were 1 mM, 0.1 mM, and 1 μM. Error bars represent 2 SE of the mean. (From Hodgkin et al. 1984)

creases considerably, all at constant [Na$^+$]$_{out}$ (figure 4.44). It is 3 pA at 10 mM, 300 pA at 1 μm, for example (Hodgkin et al. 1984).

The conclusion from this sort of experiment is that a complex exchange mechanism operates, in darkness, concerned with Na$^+$ and Ca^{2+} ions: Na$^+$, apart from supplying the dark current, maintains [Ca^{2+}]$_{in}$ (intracellular [Ca^{2+}]) at a low level. Any increase in [Ca^{2+}]$_{in}$, however arranged, causes a decreased light-sensitive dark current. This explains why increased [Ca^{2+}]$_{out}$ diminishes the dark current (by increasing [Ca^{2+}]$_{in}$) and why lowering [Na$^+$]$_{out}$ is involved in two ways (both by reducing the dark current by the lower external sodium concentration itself and also by allowing an increase in [Ca^{2+}]$_{in}$. In addition, this latter increase will, in turn, effectively reduce the number of available channels.

This hypothesis has been reinforced by another recent study (MacLeish et al. 1984) based on intracellular measurements on receptors combined with blocking (by appropriate treatments) any inner segment ion fluxes. Any modification of [Ca^{2+}]$_{in}$ is shown to change the current across the outer segment: Increasing the calcium concentration by intracellular Ca^{2+} injection lowers the receptor current and, conversely, reducing Ca^{2+} by intracellular injection of the chelating agent EGTA, ethylene glycol bis(β-aminoethylether)-N,N-tetracetic acid, increases it.

In summary, Ca^{2+} appears to control the Na^+ permeability of the rod plasma membrane. This control is effected by an "internal" action in the outer segment. From this it might be concluded that Ca^{2+} is a candidate for being some sort of messenger between the photoisomerization and the cell's electrical response. We will see below that this is at least partly, if not entirely, true.

Fluxes at the Level of the Inner Segment
There is a lot of evidence for the existence of an *inward* calcium dark current in the inner segment. These calcium channels are, in this case, voltage dependent, activated by depolarization (at the end of a response to light and in darkness). This Ca^{2+} entry in the dark is normally counterbalanced by an efflux of K^+, the two conductances gCa^{2+} and gK^+ being increased.

The inward flux of calcium into the inner segment has the effect of maintaining the continuous secretion of transmitter at the receptor-horizontal cell synapse or at the receptor-bipolar cell during darkness. In the light, secretion is diminished because, since Na^+ ceases to enter, the outer segment membrane hyperpolarizes and so reduces the secretion of transmitter, perhaps also because of the suppression of the calcium current and the lowering of $[Ca^{2+}]_{in}$ (Bader et al. 1982).

3.3 TOWARD A TRANSDUCTION THEORY

The absorption of a photon by Rh (with isomerization to Rh* and metarhodopsin II) sets off a cycle of events in the outer segment cytoplasm that results in a blockage of inward current flow at the plasma membrane. Assuming that we now have a reasonable picture of the ionic mechanisms in the receptors, we also need to understand how the initial stages of transduction proceed and link the absorption of a light quantum with the ensuing changes in the receptor's membrane potential.

Two ideas must dominate the search: (1) that the ionic exchanges occur at the plasma membrane of the outer segment, whereas the photochemical processes occur at the level of the disks; it will therefore be necessary to discover a mechanism by which the isomerization of Rh can be followed by a lowering of gNa^+ at a distance. (2) This action at a distance by a "second messenger" must also take into account an autoamplification process, since it is known that the isomerization of a single molecule of Rh can block the influx of approximately 10^5 Na^+ ions.

Clearly, experiments must identify—particularly at the level of the outer segment—one or more (preferably reversible) photochemical reactions, the kinetics of which must also take into account the changes in sodium conductance. There were two successive rival candidates for the role of "second messenger": Ca^{2+} ions and cyclic guanosine monophosphate (cGMP). There is no longer any real argument, as we shall see below (for a recent bibliographical source, see Lamb 1986). It is agreed that photoreceptor transduction releases a whole class of mechanisms that share in common the influence of protein G (see p. 264).

ROLE OF CALCIUM

The "calcium hypothesis" of Yoshikami and Hagins (1973) suggested that, in addition to light isomerizing rhodopsin, Ca^{2+} ions are liberated by the disk membrane also as a consequence of light absorption. These ions diffuse as an ionophore toward the plasma membrane, where they finally produce a block of the light-sensitive sodium channels by reducing GNa^+ (figure 4.45). This theory relied on several arguments but seems to be refuted at present. Of the several favorable arguments, the essential was that the sodium channels are blocked by Ca^{2+} (see above):

• Increasing external Ca^{2+} at the level of the outer segment lowers the dark current.
• Lowering external Ca^{2+} has the opposite effect.
• Injecting Ca^{2+} into the rod mimics its light response (closure of Na^+ channels).
• Injection of a chelating agent like EGTA, expected to lower the quantity of intracellular free calcium ion, has the opposite effect of desensitizing the cell to light (Brown et al. 1977).
• Ca^{2+} ions are liberated from the rods by light.

In contrast, there are also difficulties:

• It has not so far been possible directly to follow the changes in intracytoplasmic Ca^{2+} after light stimulation.
• In certain cases, a considerable Ca^{2+} entry has not caused a rapid suppression of the light-sensitive current.
• The efflux of Ca^{2+} in the light is too slow a phenomenon to be in accord with the kinetics of transduction itself.

These later observations resulted from combining suction electrode with whole-cell patch clamp techniques. This allows the cell to be

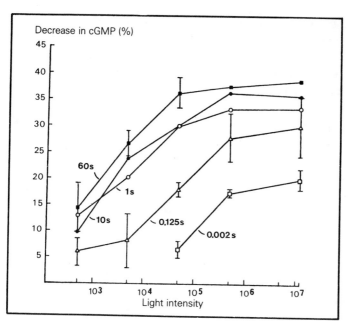

Figure 4.45
Magnitude of the decrease in cyclic GMP (cGMP) as a function of the light intensity and its duration. Outer segments were exposed for 2 ms (open squares), 125 ms (open triangles), 1 s (open circles), 10 s (filled circles), and 60 s (filled squares) at light intensities bleaching $5.0 \cdot 10^2$, $5.0 \cdot 10^3$, $5.0 \cdot 10^5$, $5.0 \cdot 10^4$, and $1.2 \cdot 10^7$ molecules of rhodopsin/external segment/s. Each point is the mean of several experiments. (From Woodruff & Bownds 1979)

voltage-clamped, while at the same time small quantities of substances (e.g., of chelator) can be injected intracellularly into the receptor (Lamb et al. 1986). Briefly, in the most strictly controlled experiments (where the chelator can be regarded as a stabilizer of the intracellular Ca^{2+}), it has been shown that the closing of the light-sensitive channels is not causally connected with an increase in free intracytoplasmic calcium ion. In contrast, light was shown to diminish Ca^{2+}.

While Ca^{2+} probably does not alone constitute the second messenger, this ion clearly plays an important role in reactions linked with cGMP, as we shall see below.

IMPORTANCE OF THE CYCLIC NUCLEOTIDE cGMP

During the last few years appreciation of the importance of guanosine-3',5'-cyclic monophosphate (cGMP) has grown, and there are strong arguments for regarding this substance as a candidate for the control of the light-sensitive membrane channels. First, the retina contains the highest concentration of cGMP in the central nervous system. Second, by measuring the concentration of cGMP in suspensions of rat outer segments, in the presence of low $[Ca^{2+}]_{out}$ (for a reason that will be described in the next section), it is possible to show that illumination of the preparation brings with it a notable *fall in the cGMP amount*, with a half-time of 125 ms (Kilbride & Ebrey 1979). The slowness of this process is nevertheless a problem, as we shall see (figure 4.45).

In the above preparation, the level of cGMP destroyed is a function of the intensity of the light stimulus. This dependence (percent lowering with respect to the level in darkness versus the log of intensity) is valid for intensities from 500 to 500,000 Rh/outer segment/second [in this sort of experiment the intensity is specified as the number of molecules of Rh isomerized per segment per second]: the concentration of cGMP falls to a value that depends on the light intensity (see figure 4.44 and Woodruff & Bownds 1979). [Extrapolating, it follows that 10^4 to 10^5 molecules of cGMP are hydrolyzed per molecule of Rh, for a light that isomerizes less than 100 molecules of rhodopsin per outer segment.]

When the light is turned off, the level of cGMP recovers progressively, in a way suggesting that for a given intensity an equilibrium is established between its breakdown and resynthesis.

An intracellular injection of cGMP into the receptor generates a membrane depolarization, which is the sign of an opening of membrane conductance channels. Such an injection reduces or even annuls the response of the rod to light (Nicol & Miller 1981, Miller 1982).

Recent studies on isolated patches of the outer rod segment cytoplasmic membrane show that the light-sensitive channels are of a particular type, called cGMP-dependent or cGMP-activated. This nucleotide-gated channel belongs to the general class of ligand-gated ion channels. The action of cGMP here is direct with no phosphorylation stage (Fesenko et al. 1985, Haynes & Yau 1990; see Kaupp 1991 for other references). The cGMP-gated channel protein from the bovine retina probably consists in a 63-kDa polypeptide forming six transmembrane segments, with an intracytoplasmic putative cGMP binding site near the carboxyl terminus. This channel is cation-selective for both monovalent alkali metals (Na^+) and also divalent

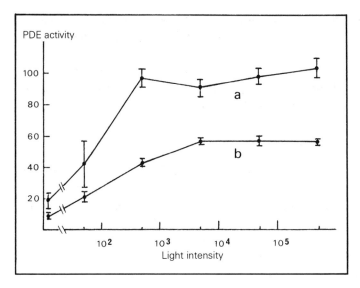

Figure 4.46
Effect of Ca^{2+} on the photosensitivity of the activation of a phosphodiesterase (PDE). In b, the outer segments were exposed to a Ringer-GTP solution with a weak concentration of Ca^{2+} (10^{-9} M). In a, the segments were prepared similarly but exposed to a solution with Ca^{2+} of 10^{-3} M. The curves are normalized and are for the means of 4 and 9 experiments, respectively. PDE activity is given as molecules of cGMP hydrolysed per molecule of rhodopsin per minute and light intensity as molecules of rhodopsin bleached per outer segment per second. (From Robinson et al. 1980)

(Ca^{2+}) ones, allowing both ions to enter the cell in the dark. In light, the cGMP channel closes, preventing the ions from penetrating the cell.

Ca^{2+} ions entering the cell have a variety of important roles (Woodruff & Fain 1982; MacLeish et al. 1984; Stryer 1986): (1) they are part of a feedback mechanism that regulates the synthesis of cGMP through guanylate cyclase; (2) they decrease the conductance of the single channel (from 20 pS down to 0.1 pS), thus reducing current noise generated by the channel itself and probably improving the probability of single photon detection; (3) they also activate the degradation enzyme of cGMP, phosphodiesterase (PDE). Previous data (Robinson et al. 1980) had already shown that in suspension of isolated rods, light increases the activity of PDE as indicated by the number of hydrolyzed cGMP molecules; this destruction of cGMP was weaker with lower doses of Ca^{2+} (10^{-9} M) than in normocalcic solutions (10^{-3} M) (figure 4.46). It has been suggested that this action of Ca^{2+}

(and of ATP) might be concerned in adaptation mechanisms and in the lowering of reactivity to successive light stimuli (Kawamura & Bownds 1981).

Finally, the action of PDE constitutes an auto-amplification process. Many hundreds of molecules of PDE are activated by a single photo-isomerization and because of this a large number of cGMP molecules are degraded $(4 \cdot 10^5)$.

THE INFLUENCE OF "G PROTEIN"

Another important advance has been identification of the importance in this context of a mechanism already well known in other systems of intracellular communication. This is the involvement of one of a family of proteins referred to as *G proteins*, that is, linked with qua-nine nucleotide. *Transducin* (T), a typical example of a G protein, comprises three subunits, α, β, and γ (see Fung et al. 1981, Stryer et al. 1981, Lamb 1986, Chabre 1985, Stryer 1986). According to the presently agreed scheme:

• The activated rhodopsin (Rh*) is linked to the α subunit of T, which is linked to GDP (definition of a G protein), the compound GDP-T* transforming to GTP-T* accompanied by a slow hydrolysis from GTP to GDP (figure 4.47).
• This will cause dissociation of protein T, and the activated fraction Tα in its turn will activate the phosphodiesterase PDE (PDE*-Tα-GTP).
• In the activated form, this PDE will lower the cytoplasmic content of cGMP in hydrolyzing it to 5'GMP.
• Finally, this cGMP depletion will in turn bring the closing of Na$^+$ channels and in consequence a hyperpolarization of the membrane.

This process is auto-amplifying; in fact, it seems that one molecule of rhodopsin can charge several hundred G protein molecules while it is activated and that each molecule of activated PDE can in its turn hydrolyze 10^3 molecules of cGMP per second. In this way, each photon absorbed can finally lead to the hydrolysis of millions of cGMP molecules per second.

Recombinant DNA methods have also allowed the sequencing in the protein T-G of its α subunit and of its tiny γ subunit. The α subunit is like that of other already well-studied G proteins (Lochrie et al. 1985).

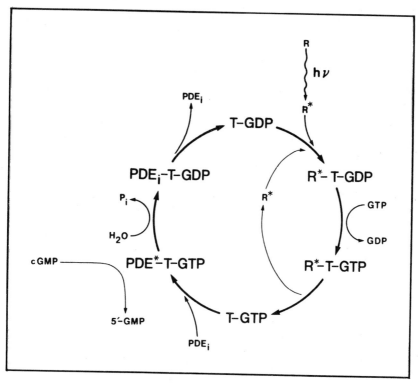

Figure 4.47
The rhodopsin cycle. hν, a light quantum; R*, photolysed rhodopsin; T-GTP, T-GDP, transducine-guanosine tri- and diphosphate complex; PDE, phosphodiesterase with its activated form PDE* and its inhibited form PDE$_i$; cGMP, cyclic GMP. (From Fung et al. 1981)

COMPLETION OF THE CYCLE

At this stage two final mechanisms become involved, one at each end of the chain. First, a deactivation of the Rh*: activated rhodopsin is probably at this stage phosphorylated by ATP (ATP → ADP) and then loses its affinity for activated transducin T*. This phosphorylation takes place on the residues of serine or of threonine close to the terminal part of the Rh, at the level of the disk membrane. This process is relatively rapid compared with another slower one, in the course of which Rh regains the 11-*cis* structure of its chromophore and will be regenerated.

The second mechanism involves an action of cGMP on the sodium channels of the plasma membrane. Here we return to a problem posed at the beginning; Is this a direct action or is there an intermediary? And what, finally, is the role of Ca^{2+}? Lamb (1986) assisted the fall from grace of the full-scale "calcium theory" while nevertheless trying to ascertain what should be considered the role of Ca^{2+}. There are various possibilities: (1) that synthesis (by cyclase) and degradation (by PDE) of cGMP are both affected by changes in calcium concentration, and (2) that calcium plays a role in the kinetics of light adaptation.

[There are yet more problems. Some studies have shown that in the outer segment of rods there is a reversible phosphorylation in darkness of two low molecular mass proteins, referred to as I and II. In the light, these two proteins are dephosphorylated in amounts that depend on the light intensity. It is notable that the light intensity that produces a 50% dephosphorylation ($5 \cdot 10^5$ quanta/outer segment/second) is the same as that which generates a 50% reduction in the light-sensitive permeability of the rod outer segment, and likewise it reduces the quantity of cGMP in the same proportion. The synthesis of these proteins seems to be linked to the activation by cGMP of a protein-kinase, catalyzing the transfer of a nucleotide-triphosphate to a protein. There is no doubt that the role of these proteins needs to be accurately assessed (see Polans et al. 1979).]

CONE MECHANISMS

Investigations recently performed on cone plasma membrane patches excised from outer segments of catfish cones indicate that basically the same type of cGMP-activated channel exists in cones as in rods, with broadly similar kinetic properties (Haynes & Yau 1990). In physiological ionic conditions, both cone and rod conductances are at least partially blocked by the divalent cations. In the absence of such cations, the cone channel has a unit conductance about twice that of the rod channel. Channel density in the cone membrane is about ten times smaller than in the rod membrane; however, since the surface membrane area in cones is about tenfold larger, the estimated total number of cGMP activated channels is comparable in both receptors (Haynes & Yau 1990).

3.4 THE QUANTUM SENSITIVITY OF RECEPTORS

A problem needing solution in various fields, for example in psychophysics, is to understand the conditions for excitation at liminal light intensities where the quantum nature of light becomes involved. Investigations have led to somewhat complex and contradictory results, some aspects of which we will now summarize.

MEAN VOLTAGE CHANGE PER PHOTON AND PER ISOMERIZATION

It is necessary to know the effect of a single photon hitting a rod and whether this effect only generates a single isomerization. There are many data available. From intracellular measurements of transmembrane potentials, the most sensitive rods in a preparation (toad rods at 520 nm) show a potential change between 3 and 6 mV for a single photoisomerization for an effective receptor surface area of 13.6 μm^2. Other experiments have shown this to be 10 to 1000 times less in cones.

Baylor et al. (1979), using the suction pipette technique, analyzed the transmembrane current response to a single photon and plotted histograms of response amplitude at a given liminal intensity. These showed two peaks, one at 0 pA (no response) and the second at 1 pA. This behavior strongly suggests that this is a matter of a quantal process with the response at 1 pA (±0.2 pA) representing the current linked to a single photoisomerization. There were, much more rarely, some responses of greater amplitude due to the arrival of several simultaneous photoisomerizations. The researchers calculated the quantum efficiency of this in vivo absorption (probability that a photon effectively causes the isomerization of one molecule of rhodopsin) as 50%. This is slightly less than Dartnall obtained for Rh in solution (figure 4.48). Increasing the stimulus intensity increases the response in a way that is also compatible with the hypothesis that one elementary quantum absorption causes a single photoisomerization.

Again using current measurement by suction electrodes on the receptor outer segment, it is possible to exploit microslits oriented perpendicularly to the long axis of the outer segment to effect a hyperfine localization of outer segment stimulation. This has shown that there is a certain scatter of isomerization, over several micrometers, representing about 50 disks, a scatter that exists in spite of all precautions (Lamb et al. 1981; see also figure 4.11).

Finally, it seems that the response to the isomerization by one photon, which we have seen is about 1 pA, will affect 1/30 the length of the OS, approximately 2 μm, or about 50 disks. This very small dispersion might be linked to a barrier resulting from the confined stacking of the disks.

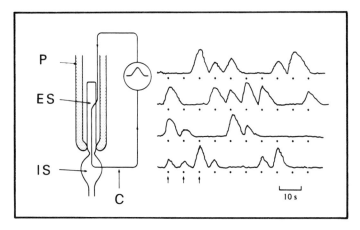

Figure 4.48
Response of a rod to the absorption of single photons. The external segment (ES) of a toad rod was sucked into a micropipette (P) and the inward current (C) measured for low intensity flashes causing a mean isomerization of 0.53. The effect is examined for 40 consecutive stimuli. As would be expected for a Poisson distribution with a mean of 0.53, a certain number of stimuli are not followed by an isomerization nor, therefore, by a response. The small amplitude responses represent a single isomerization, the larger ones represent more than one simultaneous isomerization. (From Barlow & Mollon 1982)

"PHYSIOLOGICAL NOISE" AT THE RECEPTOR LEVEL

There is experimental evidence that there are "spontaneous responses" in the dark in both rods (Schwartz 1977, Matthews 1983, 1984) and cones (Lamb & Simon 1976, Simon et al. 1975).

Baylor et al. (1979a), investigating receptor currents measured by suction electrodes on isolated receptors, have described two components in this "noise," a discrete noise and a continuous noise. The discrete events of the order of 1 pA occur randomly at a mean rate of about 1 in 50 s and are taken to represent separate spontaneous isomerizations of Rh. The continuous noise has an effective amplitude of about 0.2 pA and represents the intermediate effects of transduction. A later elaboration of the method was additionally to apply a whole-cell patch clamp to the preparation (Bodia & Detwiler 1985).

Using this improved technique and plotting the spectral density curves (in pA^2/Hz) for the continuous noise in darkness demonstrates a profile that is globally decreasing with frequency but in two quite clear sections, one at low noise frequencies (0.1 to 1 Hz), the other for higher noise frequencies (about 1 to 100 Hz). The first segment can be represented as the product of two Lorentzian functions with two distinct time constants. In contrast, the higher frequency portion (> 10 Hz) can be described by a single Lorentzian function. [In the spectral analysis of random noise, a Lorentzian function is defined by the expression

$$S(f) = S(0)/\{1 + (2\pi f\tau)^2\}$$

where $S(f)$ is the spectral density at frequency f, $S(0)$ the spectral density extrapolated to zero frequency, τ a time constant characteristic of the cell ($\tau = 1/2\pi f_c$ where f_c is the "cutoff" frequency for which $S(f_c)$ is $0.5S(0)$) and here τ is the mean duration of opening in the channel].

In summary, Bodia and Detwiler proposed the following conclusions: (1) that the low-frequency continuous noise, which is increased in low illumination, is due to a simultaneous change of state in a certain number of channels in response to a "blip" of internal messenger (whatever that might be), and (2) that the higher frequency noise is linked with changes of state in individual sodium channels. According to these authors the data are most consistent with the idea of the channel being a "pore" rather than due to an exchange mechanism in the sodium channel.

From the current measured as above in a single channel it is estimated that 200 to 300 channels contribute to a single elementary quantal event (1 pA) and that 5000 openings correspond to a current of 20 pA.

COUPLING BETWEEN RECEPTORS

The sensitivities specified above $(mV/Rh^*/OS)^{-1}$ were regarded by some as merely global figures because of the possibility of coupling between receptors. Some observations showed that although a given rod might show potential variations of the order of 400 μV/Rh*, corresponding to a single isomerization, some smaller changes are also detectable during very small stimuli that (statistically) should isomerize less than one molecule.

It appeared as if any rod could receive contributions from several others, and from this point of view it was estimated that 85% to 90% of the response recorded in a given rod might come from isomerizations taking place in other receptors in the same summation pool (Fain 1975). Other studies (in the turtle) showed that coupling between rods exists over a distance of about 100 μm (Copenhagen &

Owen 1980). In cones the maximum distance for coupling is smaller (60 μm). Only cone receptors with the same spectral sensitivity are coupled (red-red, green-green), with no crossovers. In contrast, cones can react on rods: When using wide stimuli (500 μm) the spectral sensitivity curve for the rod ceases to be that of porphyropsin (such as is obtained with small stimuli of 25 μm) but is like the curve generated by an interfering input from neighboring red cones (Schwartz 1975). This coupling does not arise at the cell bodies but, as histology suggests, via the basilar processes of the peduncles, whose tangential spread essentially agrees with the values derived experimentally (and with the fact that electron micrography has effectively shown such cone → cone and cone → rod contacts).

The question immediately arises as to the function of this sort of coupling. It is generally agreed that the effect is to reduce the stochastic noise from the receptors. Thus the dark noise is around 0.01 mV^2 when the receptors remain coupled, whereas it can attain 0.4 mV^2 in isolated receptors. This reduction in noise and in consequence some reduction in threshold variability is gained at the expense of spatial resolution but increases the absolute sensitivity by decreasing the signal-to-noise ratio.

Some histological contributions support the presence of junctions between receptors, mostly as *gap junctions*, which are regions of electrical synaptic connection. Corresponding physiological measurements have confirmed the electrical coupling between receptors in some cases, though the evidence seems to be somewhat variable, depending on which author is reporting it.

An example of a positive report, among diverse experimentation in different species, is that in the turtle of Detwiler and Hodgkin (1979), who used two intracellular microelectrodes, each penetrating a single cone (figure 4.49).

Some significant results include the following: Applying an intracellular current I to one of the cones generates a change in transmembrane potential V in the other. It is thus possible to specify a mutual resistance R between the receptors from $R = V/I$, the ratio of the resulting potential to the applied current.

[The mutual resistance is a global effect that reflects the degree of coupling between cells but does not allow a simple calculation of the resistance of the gap junction itself (in relation to the usual cell membrane resistance). Determining the gap resistance requires more elaborate techniques, including voltage clamping (Piccolino et al.

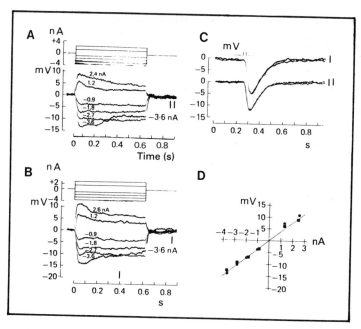

Figure 4.49

Electric coupling between cones in the turtle retina. Two neighboring cones, separated by 22 μm, are each impaled by separate microelectrodes. A rectangular current pulse is applied to one and the transmembrane voltage change is recorded in the other. *A*, Cone I is exposed to both inward going and outward going current pulses of various magnitudes. The corresponding transmembrane potential changes in cone II are shown immediately below. *B*, The opposite experiment with current applied to cone II and voltage measured in cone I. *C*, Superimposed responses to light stimulation before and after current injections in cone I (*above*) and in cone II (*below*) showing no deterioration during the experiment. Light stimulus: spot 880 μm diameter, white light, corresponding to $9.4 \cdot 10^2$ photons at 644 nm/μm². *D*, Voltage/current curves for experiment A (squares) and for experiment B (dots). The identical slope of the curves for each set of data gives a mutual coupling resistance of 4.2 MΩ. (From Detwiler & Hodgkin 1979)

1982), twin circuit voltage clamping (Giaume & Korn 1983), or even double patch clamping (Neyton & Trautmann 1985).]

This mutual resistance is a reciprocal function of the distance between the two cells (since if the cells are farther apart the leakage conductance increases). Thus the resistance is of the order 30 MΩ when the cells are very close and decreases to 0.2 MΩ when the distance between the cells is about 60 μm. These distance measurements were confirmed by extra tests using fluorescent dyes that show up the gap junctions and by using punctate stimuli to trace the spatial extent of the response for each cone.

We may therefore conclude that there are electric junctions between the receptors, probably via cone peduncles, the whole forming a network (square or hexagonal) but one that only links cones of the same color function (red-red, etc.).

3.5 QUANTUM SENSITIVITY AT THE GANGLION CELL LEVEL

The results we have just described for receptors were in fact preceded by measurements of the quantal sensitivities of the ganglion cells. A question arising from psychophysics was posed by Barlow and colleagues (1969b, 1971) concerning the minimal number of quanta needed to initiate responses in the visual system. This answer was to be derived preferably from data gained by observing a nervous system response, not a subject's perception; neither should a graduated receptor response be used but rather a retinofugal signal from the ganglion cells that, as we know, constitutes the input to the supraretinal levels of the visual central nervous system. This should yield a better defined result than some arbitrary level selected from graded potentials.

Nevertheless, determining a ganglion cell's detection threshold for a light stimulus can be more difficult than for a receptor itself because the GC has a spontaneous discharge. For that reason the estimate has to be made of the smallest intensity that generates a just-perceptible change in that spontaneous activity, namely, by using some selected change in discharge rate as a criterion.

In the following discussion of absolute threshold, the retina is assumed to be working at maximal sensitivity (i.e., in a state of complete dark adaptation). Three factors need to be considered:

• The ratio $\hat{s}$, expressing the mean number of extra quanta that must be absorbed to generate an increase in discharge rate. Experiment shows that, for low intensities, there is a linear relationship between the increase in neuronal discharge and the increase in illumination: $\hat{s}$ can thus serve to convert an increase in discharge to a corresponding increase in light energy.

• The time course of the response, which affects the time during which the single unit retinal output should be measured.

• The statistical variability of the discharge during the measuring time. Experimentally, a large number of successive tests will show that the discharge is not constant but in all situations (whether concerning the spontaneous activity in darkness or the responses to a light stimulus) follows a practically Gaussian distribution.

Thus we need to compare two Gaussian distributions established during an identical time t, one in dark adaptation, one for the light stimulus, and select some criterion to decide whether the ganglion cell has "seen" the stimulus.

For each Gaussian distribution is defined a mean value μ and a standard deviation σ (or a variance σ^2) and from these is established a criterion for "seen" (figures 4.50 and 4.51).

[Assume therefore that N_0 represents the neuronal discharge occurring during a time in darkness, with its mean μ_{N0} and its standard deviation σ_{N0}. From an examination of the Gaussian curves obtained from different experiments there arises a linear relationship between μ_{N0} and σ^2_{N0}, and this allows σ to be calculated as a function of μ, i.e., $\sigma^2 = C\mu$. This dark discharge might be considered as representing what is effectively a *dark light*.

Suppose now a weak light stimulus δI is presented, added to an intensity I to which the receptors are exposed (in principle zero in this case), there is established a new discharge with a mean μ_N and representing an increase δN over the discharge in darkness:

$$N = \delta N + \sigma_{N0}.$$

To determine a criterion for "visibility" that will lead to a definition of threshold (δN_T), the values of N_c and δN_T that N and δN must reach to attain this threshold must be defined. As before, we may write

$$N_c = \mu_{N0} + k\sigma_{N0}$$

where k is determined by the criterion proposed. Barlow selected $k = 2.88$ for which $(k \cdot \sigma)$ is that for a total of false-positive responses of 2 in 1000 (still assuming the distribution to be Gaussian).

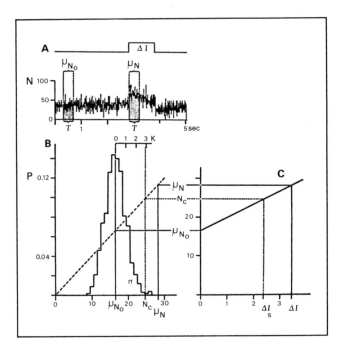

Figure 4.50
Calculation of the absolute threshold from the activity of a retinal ganglion cell in
the cat. A, Post-stimulus histograms in the temporal domain, for a weak stimulus ΔI
(*right*) and in the presence of a constant I stimulus, often in darkness ("no stimulus";
left), for identical times τ of 400 ms. N, number of impulses/s as a function of time in
seconds. The measurement leads to a mean μ_{N0} on the left and μ_N on the right.
B, Probability histogram for the number of impulses in the condition "no stimulus"
(*above, left*), for 1000 consecutive trials P, probability of a discharge vs. N. From this is
calculated μ_{N0} (16.5 discharges) and the standard deviation σ_{N0} (2.83). Similarly, for
the weak stimulus ΔI the corresponding value for N is 28.3 discharges. By constructing
the straight line C with N (as ordinate) as a function of ΔI (as abscissa) we obtain by
interpolation the liminal value ΔI_s corresponding to the value N_c given by $N_c = \mu_{N0} +$
2.88 σ_{N0} = 24.6. (Above the histogram B there is a scale of values of the coefficient k,
which allows the determination of the standard level for $N \cdot N_c$ corresponding to $k =$
2.88; see text.) This experiment refers to an ON-center unit, background illumination
22 cd/m^2, central spot 0.6° aperture. (From Barlow & Levick 1969a)

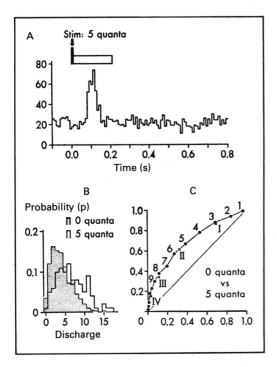

Figure 4.51
Response of a retinal ganglion cell to a mean of 5 light quanta of 507 nm reaching the cornea in 10-ms flashes. *A*, Post-stimulus histogram, class interval 10 ms, 100 repetitions. Time for counting the total number of discharges (open rectangle) is 200 ms. *B*, Results where the open histogram is for the presence of the (5-quanta) stimulation and the shaded histogram for its absence (0 quanta). *C*, "Receptor operating characteristic" (ROC) curve obtained from the data in *B*. The curve gives the probability (see text) $P = (c/S + R)$ that the criterion of c discharges or more might be attained under the influence of a stimulus added to the "random dark light" (ordinate) as a function of the probability $P = (c/R)$ of c in "dark light" alone. Arabic numbers and their corresponding points identify different experimental values of c. The roman numerals and the crosses correspond to an ideal detector in which 18% of the quanta at the cornea would be effective in the presence of a background noise equivalent to a source of 6.5 quanta at the cornea for the time of counting the discharges. The straight diagonal represents the level of equiprobability (chance) and the separation of the experimental curve from it is a way of judging the ability of the system to discriminate between the two situations, retinal noise on the one hand and retinal noise + stimulus on the other (see text). (From Barlow et al. 1971)

Finally then, we may write

$$\delta N_c = 2.88\sigma_{N0},$$

this quantity being convertible into a quantal light energy from $\hat{s}$. It is equal to

$$\hat{s} \cdot \delta N_c \text{ or } 2.88 \cdot \hat{s} \cdot \sqrt{(C \cdot \mu_{N0})}.$$

The calculation proceeds by introducing δI_T to represent the required threshold luminance (expressed in quanta) and estimating the corresponding incident energy $\delta I_T \cdot A \cdot \tau \cdot F$ where A is the area of the stimulus in degrees of solid angle, τ the duration in seconds, and F the fraction of the quanta incident on the cornea that are effectively absorbed by the rods.

Thus we may write an equation where all the values but δI_T are known. This can therefore be calculated:

$$\delta I_T \cdot A \cdot \tau \cdot F = 2.88 \cdot \hat{s} \cdot \sqrt{(C \cdot \mu_{N0})}.]$$

Barlow and collaborators' conclusions may be summarized as follows:

1. For a large number of ON ganglion cells, corresponding to the central retina and fully dark adapted, 2 or 3 quanta (at 507 nm) reaching the cornea are on average sufficient to generate a change in discharge.

2. The ratio F between the number of quanta reaching the retina and those that are effectively absorbed by the receptors is around 25% on average.

3. The mean *quantum efficiency*, which can be deduced from statistical data and is the number of quanta reaching the cornea that effectively release a discharge, is around 15%, showing that the efficiency of transduction in the receptors is very high (>50%).

4. Based on the statistics, the authors conclude that under the best conditions a *single photon* can generate several nerve impulses (about three, it is estimated).

5. An anatomical reason would account for this multiple spike output from one quantum: Such could occur because one rod might be connected to several bipolar cells, which run in parallel to connect to the same ganglion cell.

6. The spontaneous discharge in the dark has properties like those generated by light stimuli and is the result of random single-unit receptor events, each releasing several spikes.

7. A study of the variability of ganglion cell responses involves two factors: one (as in psychophysical measurements) the discontinuous nature of the stimulus itself, the number of quanta representing a sum of Poisson probabilities; the other (a contribution from physiological research) the existence of retinal noise. The ganglion cell has to detect a signal in the presence of a not inconsiderable noise and it cannot be excluded that this retinal noise limits the absolute sensitivity of the system.

8. A confirmation and stricter specification of these detection capabilities can be obtained by plotting *receiver operating characteristics* (called ROC curves; see Green and Swets 1966). A certain criterion number of discharges c is selected and, starting from two histograms of the number of discharges in the dark and during stimulation, respectively, the probability P_1 of a discharge $> c$ for a stimulus S in the presence of retinal noise R, $P_1 \Rightarrow P\{c/(S + R)\}$, is compared with the probability P_2 of generating the same number of discharges above c but in the presence of retinal noise only, $P_2 \Rightarrow P\{c/R\}$ (see figure 4.50).

The curve plotting P_1 as ordinate against P_2 as abscissa determines the discriminating power of the ganglion cell. In addition, if one considers a theoretical ideal detector and imposes criteria of ≥ 1 quantum, or ≥ 2 quanta, or ≥ 3 quanta (points I, II, and III, respectively, in figure 4.51) with a retinal noise $R = 6.5$ and assuming that 18% of the photons reaching the cornea are effectively absorbed, the theoretical receiver curve practically coincides with the preceding experimental curve. In addition, we can see that the point I corresponds with $c = 3$, II with $c = 6$, etc., in conformity with (1) above.

9. The absolute sensitivity evaluated with this physiological criterion of threshold ganglion cell response is in all cases greater than that based on psychophysical data in humans. This gives rise to the question whether this is due to species difference or whether supraretinal effects play a part. Factors such as a "central uncertainty" have been invoked for the latter possibility, depending on the channel set into activity. We will not develop further these theoretical aspects.

4 THE NEURONAL NETWORK IN THE RETINA

Here we will examine the functional characteristics of the neuronal systems of the retina, bipolar cells (Bi), horizontal cells (H), amacrines (A), and finally ganglion cells (GC). Many recent advances have been assisted by combining electrophysiological measurements with clear simultaneous cell identification using intracellular injection of markers such as horseradish peroxidase (HRP) or the fluorescent dye procyon yellow.

4.1 BIPOLAR CELL RESPONSES

Intracellular measurements have been made in bipolar cells of a variety of groups (Urodela, Pisces). These measurements show, as in the receptors, only graded potentials and no sign of propagated nerve impulses. A difference from the receptors is that the responses to light, depending on the cell, can be *either hyperpolarizations or depolarizations* (Dowling & Werblin 1969, Werblin & Dowling 1969, Wunk & Werblin 1979, Sterling et al. 1986).

Effectively, the response characteristics of Bi cells are determined by several factors:

• The type and connectivity of the receptors (REC) to which they are joined, whether rod or cone.
• The type(s) of connection(s) with the receptors (see chapter 1, section 6.1).
• The location of the stimulus with respect to the receptor.
• Where applicable, the color of the stimulus.

With the exception of the last, it is, in summary, the organization of the bipolar cell's *spatial receptive field* that matters.

In many species the retinal receptive fields have a *concentric* structure, with a central and peripheral field organization. There are two types of fields; one is *ON center*, the other *OFF center*, with each type of field having an antagonistic surround (ON center-OFF surround, OFF center-ON surround). Studying the ON- and OFF-center fields shows two fundamental types of response to a punctate stimulus applied to the center of the receptive field in Bi cells. Some respond with a graded hyperpolarization varying with stimulus intensity and lasting throughout the light stimulus. These cells, with a response very like that of the receptors are called *hyperpolarizing bipolars* (Bih).

The other bipolars, responding in the reciprocal way with a similarly graded depolarization, are referred to as *depolarizing* (Bid). Bih are OFF-center Bi; Bid are ON-center Bi. The diameter of the central field has about the same extent as the dendritic field of a Bi cell, whether Bid ON-center or Bih OFF-center. In contrast, the antagonistic surround diameter is much wider than the dendritic field: The antagonistic action of the surround on the center is determined, as we shall see,

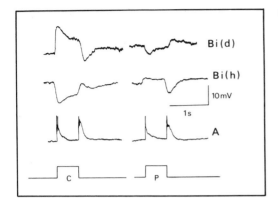

Figure 4.52
Responses of bipolar and amacrine cells. Typical responses to central (C) and (surround) peripheral (P) stimulation recorded in a depolarizing bipolar cell Bi(d), in a hyperpolarizing bipolar Bi(h) and in an amacrine cell (A). Central stimulus (C): 500 μm diameter Annular stimulus (P): 700 μm (internal) and 2000 μm (external) diameters. (From Wunk & Werblin 1979)

by more complex lateral interactions (figure 4.52). [As an example, in axolotl the central field is about 400 to 600 μm diameter and the annular surround has 700 μm (inner) and 2000 μm (outer) diameters.]

As for the present view of the synaptic actions in the direct path REC → Bi, it is known that all vertebrate photoreceptors respond with a hyperpolarization, therefore the connection REC → Bid must reverse the sign (hyperpolarization becoming depolarization), whereas the sign is conserved in the connection REC → Bih. From this there arise two problems: first, whether the functional difference is a matter of morphological differences between inverting and noninverting synapses. This sort of data (chapter 1, section 6.1) suggests that the inverting synapses might be *invaginating* and the noninverting *superficial* or *basal* types. However, as mentioned already nothing is finally settled in this respect (Miller & Schwartz 1983). The second question is whether it is a matter of what transmitter is liberated. However, the present view is as follows:

• There is only *one* transmitter, which can be either glutamate or aspartic acid (see, e.g., Miller & Slaughter 1986). [In what follows we will indicate these transmitters by Glu and Asp, respectively. Elsewhere we might use the designation EAA, excitatory amino acids, which in fact covers not only Glu and Asp but quite a series of analogous substances that are being identified in the central nervous system as subtypes of EAA; the agonists for these are N-methyl-D-aspartate (NMDA), quisqualic acid (QQ), and kainic acid (KA), respectively. Throughout the retina there seem to be receptors belonging to one of these subgroups. A wide-spectrum antagonist used is *cis*-2-3 piperidene dicarboxylic acid (PDA).]

• The transmitter is steadily excreted by the receptor in darkness and the secretion is blocked by light.
• The transmitter has opposite actions on Bih and Bid: In darkness it maintains the Bih relatively depolarized, whereas it keeps the Bid relatively hyperpolarized.
• Light causes the transmitter to be cut off, generating a hyperpolarization in the Bih and a depolarization in the Bid.

Therefore, in this mechanism the difference between the Bi cells resides in the bipolar cells themselves and not in differing transmitters (nor in their connections with the REC). As a final point, it seems that only the transmitter release at invaginated (inverting) synapses is Ca^{2+}-dependent.

Concerning the ionic mechanisms brought into play in bipolar cell function we note that the Bih suffer a reduction in their membrane conductance in response to light (like the receptors, as we have seen and as we shall see for H cells). From experiments in *Necturus* it seems that chloride ions (Cl^-), that play their part elsewhere, are not implicated here. It has been suggested that Na^+ ions may be concerned, as in the receptors and also perhaps as in H cells (see below).

The Bid, in contrast, show an increased conductance in the light. It is proposed that a Cl^- conductance increase is involved (from the behavior of Bid in Cl^--free media): In darkness GCl will be low but $[Cl^-]_{in}$ relatively high. In light, this conductance increases and because of the resulting ionic flux causes a depolarization.

The Bi responses to stimuli in the periphery of their field are essentially antagonistic to the effects of central stimuli. For an ON bipolar, an annular stimulation causes a hyperpolarization maintained during the stimulus, and for an OFF bipolar there is a similarly maintained annular depolarization (figure 4.52).

We also need to understand responses in the more complex systems, REC → Bi, where there are cones and color effects. There are now some very precise data for the carp. In this species, a considerable proportion of the Bi is affected simultaneously by rods and cones. Rods and the three types of cones are distributed more or less uniformly in the retina. The extent to which the response of a given bipolar depends on the type of receptor that is active is yet to be established. There is, in fact, evidence of three types of Bi in this species (Kaneko & Tachibana 1981, Kaneko 1983):

• Cells supplied by rods and "red" cones. Depending on their state of adaptation, these respond with different wavelengths of maximal sensitivity. In scotopic conditions they behave like the rods (sensitivity maximum at 540 nm, corresponding to porphyropsin); in photopic conditions the maximal sensitivity is at 620 nm, corresponding with the data for the red cones of this species. Some of these Bi cells are ON-center, others are OFF-center. In general, the color properties of the surround match those of the center.

• Cells that differ from the above in that, in photopic conditions (the working range of cones), the color sensitivity for the center (best response in the red) differs from that for the surround (best response in the green). They are described as *cells with single color antagonism* (e.g., center-ON-R, surround-OFF-G).

• Cells showing a *double color antagonism and a positional antagonism*, for example, with a center that in photopic conditions hyperpolarizes for red and depolarizes for green (hR-dG). Others are found with the opposite characteristic (dR-hG). The responses in the surround are once again the opposite of those in the center.

Notice that, for a white light stimulus the cells always respond as if the stimulus were red: An hR-dG cell becomes center-OFF and a dR-hG cell a center-ON (figure 4.53).

4.2 POTENTIALS IN HORIZONTAL CELLS

Other potentials measured only in the outer areas of the retina have time courses resembling those of the receptors and the Bi cells, with responses that are similarly maintained throughout a light stimulus. Intracellular marking has identified these potentials as coming from horizontal cells. [H-cell potentials have been and sometimes still are referred to as *S-potentials* after their discoverer Svaetichin; see Gouras 1972.]

It should be noted that the majority of the information on retinal cell function, including the horizontal cells, comes from lower vertebrates. For this reason, the data discussed below were acquired mainly from such animals. In section 5.3, we attempt to synthesize what is known about the cat retina.

RESPONSE CHARACTERISTICS

One of the notable response properties of the H cells is the extent of their receptive field (several millimeters around the electrode). This broad catchment area is not explained simply by the size of the cell

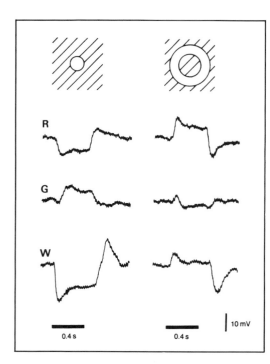

Figure 4.53
Responses of an OFF-center bipolar cell with double chromatic antagonism to a red, blue, green, and white central spot or annulus, respectively. *Left*, Responses to a central spot (diameter 100 μm), red (R) 620 nm, blue-green (G) 500 nm, and white (W). For R and G, $1.6 \cdot 10^{12}$ photons $\cdot$ cm^{-2} $\cdot$ s^{-1}, corresponding approximately to 1 log unit above the threshold for 620 nm. Intensity of W: 152 μW/cm^2. *Right*, Responses to annulus (internal diameter 0.5 mm, external 3.5 mm). Intensities of R and G $2.2 \cdot 10^{12}$ photons $\cdot$ cm^{-2} $\cdot$ s^{-1}. Intensity of W: 11.8 μW/cm^2. Stimulus duration: 400 ms. (From Kaneko 1983)

but rather by the contacts that exist between such cells, both by electrical (Lamb 1976) and chemical synapses via a cone peduncle, H → cone → H, and which are responsible for important spatial interaction effects. Figure 4.54 gives an example of one of these spatial effects: Curve *b* shows the steep change in the amplitude of the S-potential depending on whether illumination is solely in the center of the region under investigation (1) or whether the stimulus is wide enough also to affect the surround (2). This contrasts with behavior in the cones, which do not develop such lateral interactions (curve *a*; see Tomita 1972).

The S-potential amplitude increases with the intensity of the light stimulus. It is initially proportional to the log of the stimulus intensity but then reaches a saturation plateau following the classic course of a sigmoid function.

Measurements of the response as a function of wavelength (at constant spectral energy) reveal two broad classes of H cell. The first group responds by a hyperpolarization throughout the spectrum. These units were first regarded as units signaling *luminosity* because their wavelength response resembled the luminosity response of the

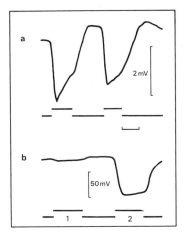

Figure 4.54
Responses to two different consecutive light stimuli. The first is sharply (diameter 0.2 mm) focused on the recording site; the second is diffuse. *a*, Responses from a carp cone. *b*, Responses from a horizontal cell showing the spatial effect. (From Tomita 1972)

(human) eye, from which arose their designation L *units* (curve *a*, figure 4.55). [In fact the situation is more complicated, since in any one species there exists L units with different wavelengths of maximal sensitivity. Using different procedures, including adaptation by colored lights of different known wavelengths, it has become clear that in *fish* there are two subassemblies of such units. Some receive signals from cones, either red or green, with different optimal wavelengths. Thus in the mullet there are H-L cells associated with red cones (H-L-R) and others with green cones (H-L-G), with maximal responses at 560 to 580 nm or at 520 nm, respectively. These H-L cells associated with cones are designated *H1* (Kaneko et al. 1982). There are also H-L scotopic cells. The envelope of their sensitivity curve is that for an optimal luminosity at 500 nm that suggests a connection with rods.

Similarly, in the *turtle*, H-L cells have been described that receive (via electronic contacts, in this particular case) simultaneous inputs from cones (R or G) and rods. In addition, there exist two sorts of contact from the receptors on the H cells, one from the red cones and rods, with these being axonal connections, and the other solely from red cones, being made on the soma of the H cell (see figure 4.31 and Norman & Pearlman 1979). Physiologically, it has been shown that these "networks" generate different sized receptive fields. There is a narrow receptive field with antagonistic surround for the network reaching the soma (called *L2*) and a wide receptive field without antagonistic surround for the network with an axonal termination (called *L1*; see Gerschenfeld et al. 1982).]

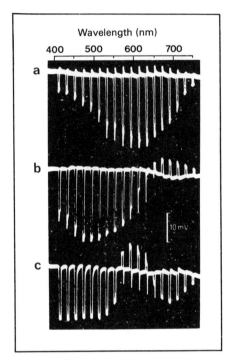

Wavelength (nm)
400   500   600   700

a

b

c

10 mV

Figure 4.55
Examples of S potentials recorded in carp retina. Potentials (hyperpolarization downward, depolarization upward) obtained in response to monochromatic flash stimuli at different wavelengths. (*a*) S potentials type L; (*b*) biphasic type C, G^+/R^-; (*c*) triphasic type c, $B^+/G^-/R^+$. (From Tomita 1963, 1972)

The second class of H cells shows hyperpolarization for some light wavelengths and depolarization for others (again without ever generating action potentials: The responses of these cells are always slow and graded). Their designation *C unit* was originally given since they were suggested to be specialized for color vision. Following recent results, it is not easy to specify the various subgroups of the *H-C units*. At present, *H2 units* that present a diphasic wavelength response envelope (curve *b* in figure 4.55) are distinguished from *H3 units* with a triphasic curve (*c* in figure 4.55). Within group *H2* there are those that hyperpolarize in red and depolarize in green (R^+/G^-), others with the opposite behavior (R^-/G^+), and yet others with antagonism between blue and green (B^-/G^+ or B^+/G^-). *H3 units* show a hyperpolarization at the two extremes of the spectrum and a depolarization between in a green-yellow (Y) intermediate band ($R^+/Y^-/B^+$). There is no evidence for any other arrangements.

These measurements have also permitted comparison of the various responses with the absorptions of the different visual pigments; in general, agreement is very good. The cell bodies of these different types of H cells are apparently not distributed randomly in the retina.

In certain species—the mullet is an example—they are layered according to the nature of their response: the red and green H-L cells (H1) are the outermost, the H2 (H-C with R/G antagonisms) and the H3 type are situated more deeply and, finally, the H-L rod cells are in the deepest parts of the outer plexiform layer (Hashimoto & Ueki 1982).

IONIC RESPONSE MECHANISMS IN HORIZONTAL CELLS

To some extent the ionic mechanisms associated with responses in H-L cells are understood, thanks to intracellular measurements. The main hypothesis is that in darkness the receptors secrete a transmitter tonically (Glu or Asp), generating thereby a steady depolarization of the postsynaptic H units, and that in the light the transmitter release is blocked and the H cell becomes hyperpolarized. This involvement of a transmitter in the interaction between the receptor and the H cell is *partly* demonstrated by the activity of bivalent cations: Increasing $[Mg^{2+}]_{out}$ hyperpolarizes the H cell in darkness and reduces its response to light. However, a reduction in $[Ca^{2+}]_{out}$, which would be expected to have the same effects (by blocking the transmitter release), is shown paradoxically to have a depolarizing action (perhaps by a direct action on the nonsynaptic membrane of the H cell).

The main discussion, however, concerns whether Na^+ or Cl^- is the main ion brought into play. In the axolotl, Waloga and Pak (1978) have shown that in the H cell, as in the receptor, the resting depolarization and the hyperpolarizing response are sensitive to a reduction in $[Na^+]_{out}$: In Na^+-free medium the H cell becomes hyperpolarized and its response to light diminishes almost to zero. This effect could certainly have been attributed to an ionic concentration effect on the receptor itself (see section 3.2) and to be none other than a secondary result on the H cell of that effect. But in fact the H cell has been demonstrated to be quantitatively more sensitive to $[Na^+]_{out}$ than the receptor, both in its membrane potential and its response, which the authors suggest indicates a direct and not just a knock-on effect and that, as in the receptor, these results arise from a local variation of GNa^+.

In *Necturus*, the conclusions of Miller and Dacheux (1976) are somewhat different, being that the depolarization in the dark is linked to a raised GCl^-, and also linked therefore with the relatively large $[Cl^-]_{in}$. The study was founded on the behavior of the isolated retina in chloride-free extracellular medium. The cell is effectively immediately depolarized in this medium and its response to light increased by outward Cl⁻ flow. Later, after "depletion" of the H cell in Cl⁻ it becomes hyperpolarized and its response is apparently abolished. More work is needed to clarify this last effect and in particular to confirm whether, as in the Bid (above), there is an essentially important role for Cl⁻ (and for the outward flux of Cl⁻).

INVOLVEMENT OF H CELL MECHANISMS IN THE RETINAL NETWORKS

Finally, we need to establish the way in which the H cells are involved in retinal mechanisms (figure 4.56; see Werblin & Dowling 1969). First of all, the H cells can exert a (backwards) influence on the receptors, particularly on the cones (in some species). Hyperpolarizing an H-L cell by intracellular current injection can cause a depolarization in a cone receptor (a sort of "inverse" effect). Essentially, the effect is neurochemical. It seems to arise from the fact that the H cells (in particular H-L) have GABA as a transmitter. Thus, isolated H cells can take up GABA; they contain GAD (glutamic decarboxylase); when they are depolarized, either by the effect of K^+ or by the receptor transmitter, they release GABA; and this release is to a large extent Ca^{2+} independent.

Behavior in these conditions suggests a *negative feedback effect*. In darkness the receptors depolarize the H cells that they make contact with and this depolarization has the effect of liberating GABA. The GABA in turn reacts on the receptors and tends to hyperpolarize them (Ayoub & Lam 1984).

Thus we might imagine there to be a sort of autoregulation circuit REC → H → REC. In the dark the cones have a depolarizing action on the H cells as we have seen: In the light, cones are hyperpolarized, as are H cells. This hyperpolarization then tends to depolarize the receptors, thus antagonizing the effect of light on them, and so on.

The H cells exert an action on the bipolars from "downstream" that is one of the two mechanisms underpinning the center-surround antagonism characteristic of receptive fields by a lateral interaction. There are many proofs of this but up to the present they have been somewhat indirect. There are powerful reasons for thinking that the action of H on Bi is the opposite of that from REC to Bi. Hyperpolarization of H produces hyperpolarization of Bid and depolarization of Bih. In other words, an ON-center bipolar, under the effect of surround illumination, will be hyperpolarized and thus not responsive to stimulus ON but responsive to stimulus OFF, and vice versa for OFF-center bipolars (Werblin 1974; see also Miller & Dacheux 1976).

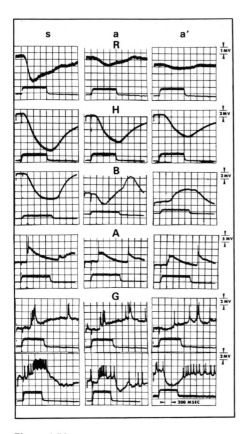

Figure 4.56
Principal response types recorded in *Necturus* **retina.** Responses to a spot stimulus
(s), to a 250-μm annulus (a), and to a 500 μm annulus (a'). The receptor cell (R) has a
small receptive field from which arises the almost total lack of response to annular
stimuli. The horizontal cell (H), in contrast, responds over a more extensive region,
with the result that illumination by an annulus with the same energy content as
the spot generates about the same response (right recording). The bipolar cell (B)
hyperpolarizes in response to the spot. If the central illumination is maintained and
then the 500-μm annulus is added (right recording), peripheral antagonism of the
central stimulation is present and generates a depolarization. For the smaller annulus
(middle recording), the excitation that it generates affects both the center and surround
fields. The amacrine cell (A) stimulated as in B shows transient ON- and OFF-
responses. The receptive fields are concentric and antagonistic, i.e., there is a greater
ON-response for the spot and a greater OFF response for the annulus. The first ganglion cell (G, *upper*) is a "transient" type, responding to ON and OFF. Its receptive
field is like that in A above. The second ganglion cell (G, *lower*) is a "sustained" type
and discharges throughout the illumination. When central illumination is maintained,
added illumination by the large annulus inhibits the discharge throughout its application (right recording). The small annulus evokes a brief depolarization and a burst of
discharge at ON and a brief hyperpolarization with discharge inhibition at OFF (middle
recording). (From Werblin & Dowling 1969)

The actual neurochemistry of the mechanisms is as yet largely un-delineated. We have just seen that in fish the H cells are most likely GABAergic, this transmitter also possibly acting jointly with Gly in the feedback H → REC and in the feedforward H → Bi (Wu & Dowling 1980). But the data are complicated by the fact (Miller et al. 1981) that in *Necturus* neither picrotoxin, bicuculline (anti-GABA), nor strychnine (anti-Gly) affect the surround antagonism at the level of the outer plexiform layer. Maybe there is a species difference.

More information is available on H cell transmitters, but the neuro-chemistry of neurotransmitters at all retinal levels presents many, often contradictory possibilities. Even the role of GABA liberated by the H cells, is currently in question.

Let us briefly address two questions that have arisen concerning H cells in particular, keeping in mind the recent structural data em-phasizing the importance of electric synapses (gap junctions) that these cells make with the receptors and with other H cells. GABA seems to control, at least in the turtle, the spread in the network REC → H cell and, more exactly, in that part affecting the axon (*L1 network*). The application of the GABA antagonist bicuculline pro-duces a retraction of the central field of L1. In other words, GABA favors spread in the L1 network. The effect appears to be paradoxical, but remember that the junctions concerned in this precise case are gap junctions and that, in fact, GABA tends thus to diminish the coupling resistance between the cells (Piccolino et al. 1982, 1985).

An influence of dopamine (DA) on the responses of H cells has also been postulated. This might increase the electrotonic coupling resistance between H cells. The DAergic receptors on H cells would be of the type D1 (blocked by substances like haloperidol and coupled with cAMP). It has been observed that DA stimulates adenyl cyclase activity in isolated carp H-L cells (cf. section 4.6 and Dowling 1986).

These effects that reduce the permeability of gap junctions, either by an anti-GABA or DA, have been confirmed histologically: The spread of Lucifer yellow, injected into an axon, toward nearby axonal terminals is significantly reduced in the presence of each of these substances.

There is much less data at our disposal concerning the mammalian HA or HB cells (defined chapter 7, section 6.2) and therefore on how they become involved in lateral spread or in the center-surround antagonistic mechanisms (cf. section 5.3).

4.3 AMACRINE CELL POTENTIALS

The amacrines (A cells) are a heterogeneous collection of cells. They
can be distinguished as A cells and properly identified as such by
their location in the innermost zone of the retina, by being bereft of
any axon, and (unlike the ganglion cells) by being *unresponsive to
antidromic stimulation of the optic nerve.*

The first category of amacrines are called *tonic.* Some are depolarized in a maintained way by light but do not develop spikes; others
are hyperpolarized (also tonically) throughout light stimulation.

A second, more interesting category comprises *phasic* or *transient
response* amacrines (Atr). They only react by a discharge at the beginning and/or end of a light stimulus. Most of them seem to be ON/
OFF types, responding therefore both at the beginning and the end
of a stepped light stimulus. Such cells can be connected to Bid and
Bih cells at the same time, which explains their dual reactivity. Other
Atr cells are of the ON type and still others are OFF types: They
make connections with the Bid and the Bih cells, respectively. Histologically, the *receptive field* of the amacrine cells is wide, unlike that
of the bipolars and the ganglion cells (see below). The dendrites of
the Atr cells are more extensive than those of the tonic amacrines;
they correspond to the "stratified amacrines," in particular to the AII
type (see chapter 1 and Murakami & Shimoda 1977).

One of the essential physiological functions of the Atr cells is to
speed up the output from the bipolar cells (figure 4.56). The potential
changes in both Bid and Bih that occur at the onset and offset of a
light stimulus occur relatively slowly. These changes are converted
in the amacrines to depolarizations with more rapid rise times, and
with *propagated impulses,* together with a return to the resting polarization (in the case of the ON effect) in spite of the continuing stimulus.
A regenerative process, occurring after the initial spike or spikes,
has been suggested to be responsible for the transient nature of the
response (Werblin 1977).

The neurochemical status of the amacrines is complex. They have
excitatory amino acid receptors at the level of their synapses with
bipolar cells. Some of them have a cholinergic excitatory action on
the ganglion cells. In the rabbit these cholinergic axons spread tangentially in the inner plexiform layer for about 500 μm (Masland et
al. 1984). There are also inhibitory actions from amacrines. Some are
mediated via GABA, some via Gly (see below).

4.4 GANGLION CELL RESPONSES

Considering the ganglion cell (GC) responses to a stepped-light stimulus (figure 4.57) reveals three fundamental response types corresponding to three types of GC: ON-GC, responding to the onset of the stimulus and in the appropriate case to its maintained value; OFF-GC, only responding at light offset; ON-/OFF-GC, responding both to light on and light off. The receptive fields are arranged concentrically in such a way that a GC responding at ON to illumination at the center of its field will respond to light OFF in the (annular) surround. We will examine these spatiotemporal integrative aspects of ganglion cell function in more detail below. For the moment let us examine some aspects of their connectivity and operation.

Intracellular GC measurements have broadly uncovered the relatively complex membrane phenomena that accompany the responses to a step stimulus:

• ON-center GC show excitatory postsynaptic potential (EPSP) and spike discharge throughout the duration of central stimulation followed by hyperpolarization at the stimulus offset. There are transient hyperpolarizations at the onset and offset of a stimulus to the surround.

• OFF-center GC show *sustained* hyperpolarization during a central stimulus with EPSP and transient spike discharge at stimulus offset. There is a sustained depolarization throughout a surround stimulation with a transient pulse of discharges at its onset and offset.

• ON-/OFF-center GC show transient depolarization and spike discharge at the beginning and end of a central stimulus. There are transient hyperpolarizations at the beginning and end of a surround stimulation.

Different experimental investigations of the radial connectivities of the GC have shown that an ON-GC is directly connected to a Bid, an OFF-GC to a Bih, and an ON/OFF-GC is connected to two bipolars, one Bid, the other Bih.

Another important characteristic is that the synapse Bi → GC always conserves sign: Injections of depolarizing current into an ON-center Bi are excitatory on the ON-center GC to which it connects, and correspondingly for the Bih cells and the OFF-center GC. The sign of the depolarizing or hyperpolarizing GC response depends therefore on the preceding REC → Bi functional connection. ON-GC

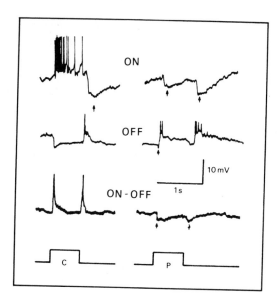

Figure 4.57
Response characteristics of the three basic types of ganglion cells in the tiger salamander retina. The responses (ON, OFF or ON/OFF) differ in the tonic (sustained) or phasic (transient) nature of their responses under the effect of central (C) or peripheral (P) illumination. Central stimulus: 500-μm diameter spot. Annular stimulus: 700-μm inner diameter and 2000-μm outer diameter. Intensities are −3 log units. The small arrows indicate hyperpolarizing responses. (From Wunk & Werblin 1979)

would therefore be expected to respond by a discharge when the receptor is hyperpolarized (by intracellular current injection) and the OFF-GC when the receptor is depolarized. This has been confirmed by Baylor and Fettiplace (1977).

Concerning synaptic actions at the ganglion cells, the EPSPs and consequently the spike discharges of the ON-GC and ON-/OFF-GC seem to be due to the release of excitatory transmitter by one or more depolarizing Bi. The Bih, on the other hand, act on OFF-GC and ON-/OFF-GC by creating hyperpolarizations in response to light. This hyperpolarization is, however, not Cl⁻ dependent; there is no inhibitory postsynaptic potential (IPSP), but rather some sort of de-facilitation. In other words, the Bid → ON-GC synapse is a mechanism that is excitatory during illumination and silent in darkness, whereas the OFF-GC synapse is excitatory in darkness but silent in the light.

The present view is that, in axolotl, the transmitter acting on the GC (as for the amacrines) is an excitatory amino acid, the receptors on the GC being "PDA sensitive" (see section 4.1). But the use of other antagonists has shown that at the GC there exist receptors belonging to all three categories of EAA receptors identified so far (by showing sensitivity to kainate, quisqualate, and N-methyl-D-aspartate, NMDA, as agonists; Miller & Slaughter 1986).

In contrast, in the cat, the differences between the classic categories

tonic GC, which respond throughout a stimulus, and the *phasic* or
transient GC (which will chiefly occupy us later) are also marked by
their neurochemical differences. But in this case the tonic GCs seem
to be effectively EAA sensitive in cat and the phasic (whether ON-
center or OFF-center) have been shown not to be sensitive but are,
in contrast, excited by Ach at nicotinic receptors. One wonders therefore whether amacrine mechanisms might also be involved in the cat.
However, there seems to be no proof of cholinergic A in the cat,
although they do exist in the rabbit, as we have mentioned (Masland
& Mills 1979).

Most axolotl GCs develop, in addition, short-duration hyperpolarizations at stimulus ON and OFF. These precede the depolarization
in an ON-GC and temporarily augment the hyperpolarization in an
OFF-GC. These particular hyperpolarizations have a clear origin:
There are Cl^--dependent IPSPs, which are due to the activity of Atr
amacrines. These Atr inhibitory effects contribute to the antagonistic
interactions that exist within each field between center and surround
(whether ON-center or OFF-center). Using GABA antagonists (bicuculline and picrotoxin) and a Gly antagonist (strychnine) demonstrates that the ON-Atr inhibit the ON-GC by GABA, whereas the
action of OFF-Atr on OFF-GC exploits a Glyergic mechanism. But
according to other authors, *all* the transient actions of Atr cells are
Glyergic and blocked by strychnine (figures 4.58 and 4.59); see
Frumkes et al. 1981, Belgum et al. 1984).

The same type of double transmitter action has been invoked to
explain inhibitions in the cat retina: GABA inhibits ON-GC and Gly
inhibits OFF-GC (whether they are tonic or phasic). Once more the
proof of this remains to be demonstrated.

4.5 ROLE OF THE INTERPLEXIFORM CELLS

Little is known about the involvement of the interplexiform cells (IP)
in retinal information transfer: Rarity has made their intracellular investigation difficult. However, among the teleosts the IP cells of the
carp family are demonstrably dopaminergic, in spite of the fact that
experimental analysis of IP cell activity tends to be mixed up with
applying dopamine to other more classic retinal elements (REC, H,
Bi, A).

Recall that the IP cells (see chapter 1) are centrifugal elements arranged so that they receive their input in the inner plexiform layer
from amacrines; their axons connect with the outer H cells (linked to

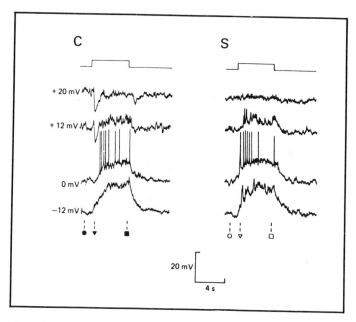

Figure 4.58
Effect of strychnine on the responses of an ON-center ganglion cell. C, Control responses. S, Responses after 13 min action of 10^{-5} M strychnine. All responses obtained by the same stimulus and with the membrane potential maintained at the values shown by current injections. The resting potential was -61 mV. Triangles indicate hyperpolarizing responses suppressed by strychnine. (From Belgum et al. 1984)

cones) and more rarely with the Bi and the H cells that control the surround inhibitory actions on the Bi and REC.

A preliminary series of studies (see Dowling 1979 for review) has shown that the application of a brief "pulse" of DA to the whole retina produces a collection of long-lasting effects (15 minutes or more). DA has practically no effect on either the membrane potential or on the response to light of the REC. In contrast, DA acts on H-L cells, in which it diminishes both the transmembrane potential and the cell's hyperpolarizing response to light. This effect is abolished by the D1 dopaminergic receptor blockers (figure 4.60, upper). DA acts in a complex way on Bi cells. For an ON-center Bid it increases both the transmembrane potential and the depolarizing response to central stimulation, whereas it diminishes the hyperpolarizing response to surround stimulation (figure 4.60, lower). DA also affects the transient (Atr) amacrines, which (as we have seen) are responsible for ganglion cell inhibition.

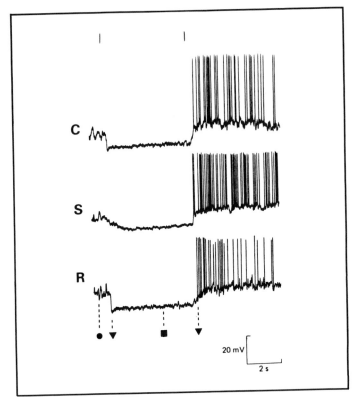

Figure 4.59
Effect of strychnine (after 12 min) on the light response of an OFF-center cell.
C, Control. S, After strychnine. R, After recovery. The first triangle indicates rapid
hyperpolarization suppressed by strychnine. The second triangle indicates depolarization accelerated by strychnine. The light was on between the vertical dashed lines
throughout. (From Belgum et al. 1984)

Other more recent studies (Mangel & Dowling quoted in Dowling
1986) investigating the action of DA on H cells in greater detail have
shown that with DA the response of the cell to a central stimulus
increases, whereas the response to a diffuse illumination over the
whole receptive field decreases. The interpretation of these observations is complex, but one of the most interesting mechanisms involves the effects of DA on the electrical coupling between cells.

This study was continued on isolated carp H cells, where it was
shown (by various manipulations) that DA reduces the receptive field
size of the H cell through cAMP as a second messenger. The effect

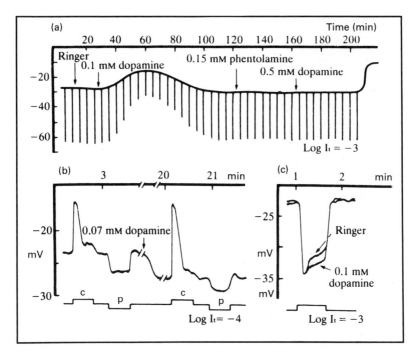

Figure 4.60
Effect of dopamine on intracellular events at the level of the outer plexiform layer of carassius (isolated retina). (*a*) Horizontal cell. Each downward vertical trace represents a response to a flash. Before the second arrow: control responses in Ringer's solution. Responses after the application of dopamine (0.1 mM) at the second arrow show depolarization of the cell and reduction of the responses to light flashes. This effect of dopamine is completely absent if it is applied (fourth arrow) after application of phentolamine (0.15 mM, third arrow). (*b*) Depolarizing bipolar cell, Bi(d). Control response to stimulation at the center of the field, depolarization for increased light (stimulus marker c below) and hyperpolarization in response to peripheral (surround) stimulation to decreasing light (stimulus marker p below). Administration of dopamine (arrow) hyperpolarizes this cell, producing an increased central depolarizing response and a reduced hyperpolarization to peripheral stimulation. (*c*) Dopamine does not significantly affect the membrane potential nor the light response of a cone. (From Dowling 1979)

of cAMP (or more stable analogues) is to reduce the diameter of the H cell receptive field. Conversely, the destruction of IP cells by the neurotoxin 60HDA increases the size of the H cell receptive field. Finally, it was also directly demonstrated that cAMP increases the resistance of the electric synapses between H cells; in other words, a decoupling of these cells occurs.

To summarize the essentials: DA acting on the dopaminergic receptors of H cells (D1 receptors that act via the adenyl cyclase system) has the net effect of reducing the capability of these cells to maintain a center/surround antagonism.

It is possible to postulate a function for this sort of mechanism if we consider what happens to a retina that has undergone prolonged dark adaptation. We know that in those conditions the actions of the surround field are much reduced or disappear completely. This long-term degradation of the surround antagonism may possibly be linked to a tonic secretion of DA by the IP cells. This could be the way the IP cells constitute regulatory elements upon the surround effects of the receptive fields. Undoubtedly, these special effects of DA via the H cells do not exhaust all the possible actions of the substance. A neuromodulation of the Bi cells (as of the amacrines) modifying the center/surround antagonism via that route is not absolutely excluded.

5 CODING OF THE SPATIOTEMPORAL CHARACTERISTICS OF LIGHT STIMULI

We examined above, to some extent in isolation, how different cellular mechanisms in the retinal network dictate the responses of the GCs. These cells provide the final common pathway output signals from the retinal network to the supraretinal visual pathways. We know that in response to a step stimulus, GC respond sometimes at stimulus ON (phasically or tonically), and sometimes at OFF. Our first analysis introduced the concept of a receptive field and briefly discussed the differences between tonic and phasic GC behavior. However, it still remains necessary to relate these response characteristics to a more truly functional view—in other words, to try to understand how the cells might provide a basis, at the retinal level, for a perception of the spatial contrast, the movement, and the temporal parameters of visual stimuli.

5.1 RECEPTIVE FIELDS: SPATIAL CONTRAST PERCEPTION

The concept of a receptive field arose when the recordings made from ganglion cells (or strictly speaking, from an axon in the optic nerve)

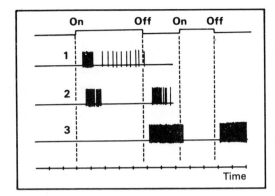

Figure 4.61
Diagram of the three typical types of neuronal signals seen in the axons of the frog optic nerve. *Upper line,* Stimulation. (*1*), ON-unit response. (*2*), ON-OFF-unit. (*3*) OFF-unit; note that in this case the OFF-response seems to be inhibited by the application of a second ON stimulus. The time axis is scaled in units of 200 ms. (From Levick 1972)

showed that the cells' activity changes when the stimulus (a pencil of light rays entering the eye and producing a point image) is turned ON or OFF. The receptive field is that area of visual space—or correspondingly of the retina—within which such effects can be observed, depending on the use of adequate stimuli (see figure 4.61; Levick 1972).

The first significant discovery was Hartline's (1938) identification in the frog of three types of optic nerve fibers (GC axons). Of these, 20% respond to the onset of a stepped light stimulus by a discharge that carries on (even if its frequency diminishes slightly) throughout the stimulus (ON-unit); 50% respond by a brief burst of spikes at the onset (ON) and end (OFF) of the stimulus (ON-/OFF-units); finally, 30% only respond at light off (OFF-units). Hartline also showed that the response of an OFF-unit could be immediately inhibited by the application of a second stimulus following the first. In addition (and this is an important point), the same sort of fiber response could be obtained wherever the light spot is positioned in the receptive field; the threshold simply increases from the center to the periphery of the field. For a spot of variable diameter, the threshold is inversely proportional to the area of the stimulus. In general terms, the receptive fields identified by Hartline were roughly circular with a diameter of about 1 mm (figure 4.61).

These observations were quickly confirmed but with an important supplementary observation that around the receptive field of activity (defined above) there is also an *inhibitory area.* When only this area is illuminated, no effect is observed (in this case, because the frog ganglion cells have no resting discharge: "silent inhibitory surround"). The inhibitory effect is revealed when measuring the re-

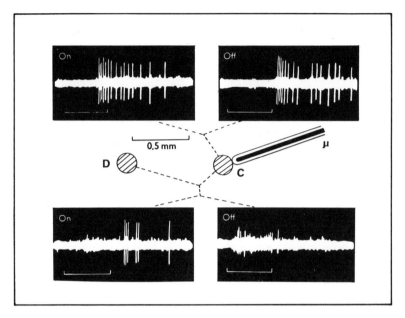

Figure 4.62
Effect of a "silent inhibitory surround" on the response of a frog ON-OFF ganglion cell. *Above,* ON- and OFF-responses to stimuli limited to the central region of the receptive field C. *Below,* Simultaneous illumination of the central region and at a point D sited lateral at 1 mm from C in the inhibitory surround. Reduction of the ON-response and suppression of the OFF-response. Time scales: 200 ms. (From Barlow 1953)

sponse while a second spot is simultaneously applied to the center of the receptive field to generate (depending on the case) either an ON- or OFF-effect. The peripheral stimulus causes an inhibition of either of these responses to field-center stimulation (figure 4.62; Barlow 1953).

The concept of a center/surround antagonism in receptive fields was considerably elaborated by observations in the cat by Kuffler (1953). In this species the receptive fields are also practically circular, but each is organized into at least two concentric functional areas (figure 4.63). The essential differences between the different types of receptive field have now become classic, with the case of the cat as the archetype.

ON-Center, OFF-Surround Field
In this type of field the onset of a step stimulus in the center generates an ON-response. The onset of a step stimulus in the surround is accompanied by an inhibition of spontaneous activity (if it exists) and

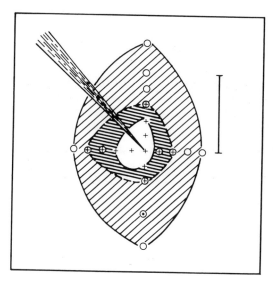

Figure 4.63
Receptive field of an ON-center ganglion cell in the cat retina. The test stimulus is 0.2-mm diameter, intensity 100 × threshold for the central region of the field. Background illumination: 25 lumen/m². Crosses, places generating ON-response; circles, OFF-responses. Note there is an intermediate ON-OFF region. (From Kuffler 1953)

above all by an OFF-response at the stimulus' end. The threshold for the surround OFF-effect is higher than for the central ON-effect. Illumination of an intermediate zone between center and surround can sometimes elicit an ON-/OFF-type of response.

Simultaneous illumination of both center and surround reveals the antagonism between the ON-center and the OFF-surround, each inhibiting the other by a "lateral inhibition" mechanism (figure 4.64). After adaptation to weak light ("in the dark"), the central response alone tends to persist (Barlow 1972, Barlow & Levick 1969a). For a wide, diffuse stimulus, the central response tends to predominate once more, in this case the ON effect.

OFF-Center, ON-Surround Field
This field has overall the opposite characteristics to the last one. Activity follows a removal of light (OFF) in the central field and the onset of a light stimulus (ON) in the surround. This time a lateral activation modifies the central response. For wide, diffuse lighting the central response once more predominates, in this case OFF.

"Luminosity Units"
This duality of retinal reception has been the object of a generalization for predicting the variety of possible variants of space perception. According to this scheme there exist in the retina two types of "luminosity units," one for brightness B and the other for darkness D (nomenclature first proposed by Jung; see Brooks & Jung 1973).

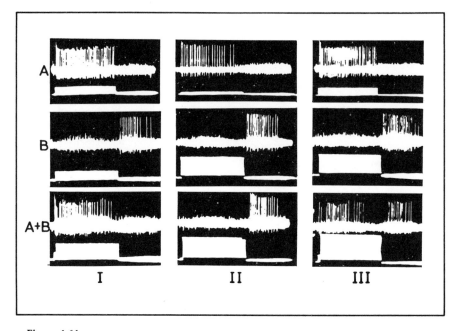

Figure 4.64
Center/surround antagonism in the receptive field of a ganglion cell of the cat retina.
A, 0.2-mm diameter flash to the center of the receptive field. B, 4-mm diameter flash
sited in the periphery. Presented separately, A shows ON-responses and B shows
OFF-responses. When presented simultaneously A + B shows: Column I, the OFF-
response is suppressed and the ON-response diminished; Column II, at reduced A
intensity and increased B intensity, the ON-response is abolished; Column III, the
stimulus intensities are adjusted so that the separate ON- and OFF-responses are
roughly equivalent and in this case both responses are reduced but neither is abolished
for simultaneous stimulation. The stimulus intensities are shown below each neural
recording. (From Kuffler 1953)

Each system has a concentric organization in which the center and
surround are antagonistic. Apart from the above considerations of
the complete onset and extinction of light, we can consider the more
general case where the reference luminosity is intermediate ("mesopic"). This allows four possibilities: onset of an illumination increment (condition $i \rightarrow i+$), suppression of the illumination increment
(condition $i+ \rightarrow i$), onset of an illumination decrement (condition
$i \rightarrow i-$), reversal of illumination deficit (condition $i- \rightarrow i$). These
four methods of stimulation also comprise (according to this scheme)
the opposite effects, which occur when they are applied to the annular surround (S) rather than the center (C). The corresponding truth
table (Table 4.2) indicates the types of response of units B and D and

Table 4.2. Response types in B and D units

	Responses			
	B units		C units	
Stimulation	Center	Surround	Center	Surround
$i \rightarrow i^+$	+	−	−	+
$i^+ \rightarrow i$	−	+	+	−
$i \rightarrow i^-$	−	+	+	−
$i^- \rightarrow i$	+	−	−	+

In the stimulation column, intensity i^+ is greater than i, intensity i^- is less than i. In the response columns, + indicates excitation, − indicates inhibition.

their excitation (+) or inhibition (−) in the center C and surround S fields.

Edge Contrast

Studies of visual perception have long tried to explain the many visual illusions in human perception; this is a good place to recall one of a set of them that depends on simultaneous contrast. One of the best known is the *edge contrast* first described by Mach in 1865, which gives rise to the *Mach bands* seen when two areas of different luminances are set side by side. The contrasts observed by Mach are the basis for understanding the essentials of contour perception (see chapter 2, section 3.1). The organization into the B and D systems has allowed an interesting interpretation of the contrast at boundaries arising from the mutual inhibitory interactions between these two units. Thus the entry of a dark edge into the surround of an ON-center GC receptive field will increase the discharge of that cell when the center is in light, compared with illumination of the same magnitude but without the contrast; conversely, this would lead to a relative inhibition when the reception field center was in the dark side of the boundary (figure 4.65; see Enroth-Cugell & Robson 1966).

General Remarks

• When a diffuse stimulus is applied, the central effect tends to predominate.
• In dark adaptation it is the surround effect that tends to disappear.
• When a retinal image is displaced (e.g., by a saccade), the systems B and D are excited simultaneously, and this can suppress all contrast information.

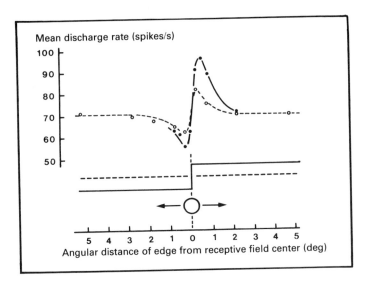

Figure 4.65
Neurophysiological interpretation of a Mach band. A step in contrast is introduced
into a uniformly illuminated field by increasing the luminance at one side of a boundary and decreasing it on the other side. This rectilinear boundary can pass through
several parts of the visual field of an ON-center X-type ganglion cell, only the center
being illustrated here. The mean discharge is measured during the period 10–20 s after
introducing the contrast "edge" at different places in the field of the cell. The filled
circles are for a contrast of 0.4 × the luminance of the uniform field. The bright side
is 1.4 × and the dim side 0.6 × the luminance of the uniform field. The open circles
are for a contrast of 0.2. Note that when the field center is just to the dim side of the
edge, the response is relatively poorer than when the center is farther away from the
edge and vice versa for the brighter side. The dotted line at 70 spikes/s is the mean
discharge of the cell in the uniform parts of the visual field. (From Enroth-Cugell &
Robson 1966)

• The field diameters for ON and OFF can vary considerably according to the retinal level. In the cat the central diameter varies from
0.5° to 8° (0.125 to 2 mm² on the retina), the smallest fields being
from the area centralis. Peripheral surround diameters vary from 6°
to 12° (1.5 to 3 mm² of retina) whatever the central diameter.
• A concentric organization of retinal fields has been found in almost
all species studied. This avoids an unnecessary elaboration of our
description. Remember, however, that the fields can be particularly
small in species with high visual acuity (birds, primates, etc.). Note
also that in primates a special complication arises from the supplementary parameter concerning antagonism between different colors
of light. We shall return to that factor later.

5.2 MOVEMENT CODING

Sensitivity to movement deserves special consideration even though it is a mechanism not universally well developed at the retinal level but rather is (more generally) a well elaborated aspect of coding at the more central stages—beyond the lateral geniculate, from the superior colliculus to the cortex. We will consider in more detail below how to establish geometrically a good definition of movement sensitivity. For the moment, we can intuitively define it as a matter of specifying the retinal excitation by a stimulus moving at a given speed and direction across a receptive field. The problem—here and more so at higher levels—is to find out to what extent such observations can be predicted by a study of the responses observed for fixed stimuli or whether some new characteristics emerge.

The classic experiments on *cat retina* (figure 4.66) show practically no preferred direction, in the sense that regardless of the displacement axis of the light spot or bar with respect to the center of the field, the response is essentially predictable. If the field is ON-center, the approach of a bar will first generate an inhibition of the resting discharge (while passing across the OFF-surround), then excitation (passing through the ON-center), followed by a second inhibition (when exiting via the further OFF-surround). If, on the other hand, the center is OFF, excitation is followed by inhibition and a further excitation. What is more, the excitation at the distal OFF-surround is found to be higher than the proximal excitation. This type of response is found whatever the axis or direction of displacement of the stimulus, since the field has circular radial symmetry (Rodieck & Stone 1965).

Having said this, we must note that if the movement is across a limited part of the receptive field (for example, within the ON area of an ON-center field), a centripetal movement would be excitatory, whereas a centrifugal movement would be inhibitory (and the opposite for an OFF-center field). That is, stimulation by moving stimuli within a zone judged to be homogeneous by exploration with fixed stimuli reveals asymmetric interactions concerned with movements relative to the geometrical center.

Finally, using drifting grating stimuli of variable orientation, Levick and Thibos (1980) discovered that there is, after all, a certain orientation selectivity in ganglion cells. In relatively peripheral visual fields (around 10°) when the place of stimulation is situated some way from the center of the retina, there is a significant preference for an

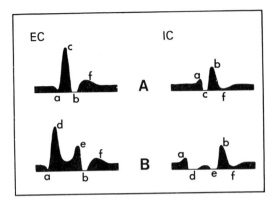

Figure 4.66
Response of retinal nerve fibers when the receptive field is crossed by a narrow (A)
or wide (B) bright bar stimulus. *Left,* Response of an excitatory center field (EC).
a, Small inhibition when the bar enters the receptive field. *b,* Larger suppression when
the bar leaves the field. *c,* Unimodal response as the narrow bar passes through the
center. *d* and *e,* Bimodal central effect, the first greater than the second, for a wide
bar. *f,* Occasional secondary excitation. *Right,* Response of an inhibitory center field
(IC). *a,* Small activation when the bar, of whatever size, enters the receptive field.
b, Greater excitation when the bar leaves the field. *c,* Unimodal inhibition when the
narrow bar passes through the central field. *d* and *e,* Bimodal inhibition frequently
seen for wide bars. *f,* Occasional secondary inhibition. (From Rodieck & Stone 1975)

orientation parallel to the straight line joining that given retinal location to the area centralis.

In the *rabbit retina,* where there are ON/OFF fields, a *directional
sensitivity* has been found ("d-selectivity") such that the movement of
a spot in one direction along a preferred axis elicits a large response,
whereas movement along the same axis but in the opposite direction
generates practically no response (figure 4.67; see Barlow et al. 1964).
This directional sensitivity is interpreted as being due to a system of
lateral inhibitory interactions—perhaps mediated by the horizontal
cells—which operates in the nonpreferred direction. By that route,
excitation of one receptor will inhibit the output channel from the
receptor stimulated immediately after it during the progress of the
moving stimulus, which gives rise to a null-response in that direction
of movement (Barlow & Levick 1965).

It is worth noting also (Oyster 1968) that if all the receptors in this
species are examined, this direction selectivity found in the rabbit
does not apply indiscriminately for all directions, but for three particular directions only. One is upward and slightly in the temporal

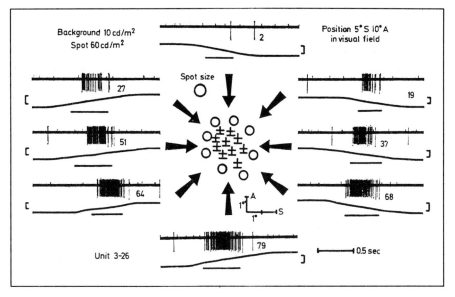

Figure 4.67
Directional sensitivity to the movement of a small spot of light in different directions
in a rabbit ganglion cell. The central receptive field is shown: ±, ON-OFF responses
evoked by a stationary spot; circles, zero responses. No response is found beyond the
0 contour. Anterior (A) and superior (S) directions within the field are shown (inset)
calibrated in 1° steps. For each recording: *Lower trace,* Movement of the spot across the
visual field in the directions indicated by the adjacent arrows (vertical calibration 5°;
horizontal line shows when the spot is within the visual field; time base marker, to
calibrate the speed, is 0.5 s). *Upper trace,* Cell's discharge, the total number of spikes
being given beside the response. Background illumination: 10 cd/m². Position of the
center of the receptive field: 5° S and 10° A. (From Barlow et al. 1964)

direction (i.e., towards the rear), another is downward and also
slightly toward the rear, and the third is horizontal and toward the
front (in the temperonasal direction therefore).

An explanation has been sought for this difference and attention
has been paid to the generality of directional sensitivities observed.
There are differences between the cat GC on the one hand and the
rabbit GC on the other that could merely be due to a species difference: Other movement sensitivities have been found in a variety of
other less evolved forms (frog, pigeon, and squirrel). But the problem
is not as simple as that since, surprisingly, the macaque also seems
to have a (limited) number of GCs specifically set into activity by
moving stimuli (Gouras 1975).

Note also in passing that circular receptive fields with center/surround antagonism do not, even in the cat, comprise the totality of retinal field types. Here and there the literature reports evidence for a small number of atypical receptive fields (nonconcentric, orientation-selective, sensitive to movement direction, etc.).

5.3 CODING BY TONIC AND PHASIC SYSTEMS

Again in the cat, in an exemplary and subtle way, it has been possible to identify another set of response characteristics for the ganglion cells. Initially, differences were discovered in the response to a stepped-light stimulus when two ways were found to code the temporal development of a signal. In general physiological terms, this is the familiar distinction between tonic and phasic receptor responses. Particularly in the visual case, these differences can take on, as we shall see, a particularly important role in information processing, and for this reason one of the first classifications made was to distinguish between *tonic GC* with a ("sustained") response, which lasts throughout the application of a long-lasting stimulus, and a *phasic GC* with a ("transient") response only occurring in the limit during temporal changes in the stimulus. These cells were respectively designated as X-cells and Y-cells. A little later a third type, W, was identified in which the responses are more complex and soon after that it became clear that there are other functional differences between X, Y, and W cells that are not solely concerned with the temporal characteristics of a response.

This new classification came to supplement the separation of GC into B and D types (above) and at that time, the two classes B and D and the X, Y, W classification were regarded as independent. All combinations of these types of response form were theoretically possible.

From a morphological point of view, it is practically certain that the three classes X, Y, and W correspond to three categories of GC distinguished morphologically in the cat and more recently in the monkey (see chapter 1, section 7.3), namely, the β, α, and γ cells. Some of these morphological differences together with some functional characteristics are specified in table 4.3 and are valid at least for the cat (Cleland et al. 1971, Ikeda & Wright 1972, Enroth-Cugell & Shapley 1973, Boycott & Wässle 1974, Fukada & Stone 1975, Dreher et al. 1976).

Table 4.3. Comparison of the properties of X, Y and W cells in the cat

	X	Y	W
I. Retinal ganglion cells			
Relative numbers	40–50%	10%	50–55%
Soma diameter	11–24 μm (β cell)	24–38 μm (α cell)	8–22 μm (γ cell)
Axon diameter	Medium	Wide	Narrow
Conduction velocity	19–24 m/s	35–45 m/s	2–18 m/s
Conduction time, retina-LGB	3.4–8.6 ms	1.8–3.0 ms	
Latency to stepped stimulus	19–24 ms	38–56 ms	
Retina site	Max. area centralis	Max. 1.5–3°	Area centralis & streak
Axon destination	A, A1, C, MIN	A, A1, C, MIN + SC	C, MIN, LGBv + SC
Response to stepped light	Tonic ("sustained") (excitatory or inhibitory)	Phasic ("transient") (excitatory or inhibitory)	Tonic or phasic
Optimal spot size	Small	Larger	
Central field diameter	0.1–1°	0.5–2.5°	0.4–2.5°
Inhibitory surround	Powerful	Weak	Nil
Center/surround interaction	Linear	Nonlinear	Not known
Movement sensitivity	Small	Considerable	Small
Field structure	Surround pure inhibition	Overlap inhibition with excitation	
Spatial resolution	Good	Poor	
Temporal resolution	Poor	Good	
Analysis of stimulus	Spatial	Temporal	Variable from cell to cell
II. Lateral geniculate body cells			
Soma diameter	Medium	Large	Small
Distribution	A, A1, and C	A, A1, C, and MIN	C parvocellular layer and MIN

Table 4.3. (continued)

	X	Y	W
Destination	Lamina IVC, VI of 17	Lamina IVA&B, VI of 17: IV, VI of 18	Lamina I, III, IV–V of 17; I, IV of 18, 19
Field structure	Relatively the same as for retina		
Movement sensitivity	Relatively the same as for retina		
Center/surround interaction	Relatively the same as for retina		
III. Cortical cells			
Field organization	Simple or complex for all classes		
Field diameter	Relative differences X, Y, W as for retina and LGB		
Movement sensitivity	Relative differences X, Y, W as for retina and LGB		
Selectivity to			
Orientation	Strong	Weak	Weak
Direction	Strong	Strong	Weak
Distribution	Chiefly 17	Most in 18	Most in 19

Based on Stone et al. (1979).

X AND Y UNITS

The situation is most clear with respect to the functional differences between the tonic X units and the Y units (see table 4.3). The X cells correspond to small GC with narrow axons of slow conduction velocity. These practically target only the lateral geniculate body. In contrast, Y units are large GCs with wide, rapidly conducting axons. Taking into account the data on the distribution of retinal GC, we conclude that X cells predominate in the area centralis where the Y cells are much more rare.

It is notable that the receptive fields of X cells (whether ON-center or OFF-center) are of small diameter with an abrupt transition between the effects in the central zone and those in the antagonistic surround, whereas the receptive fields of Y cells have a wider central region, a less powerful inhibitory zone, and a much less strongly marked sensitivity gradient between the center and periphery of the field. During a long-lasting stimulus, the X cells behave as tonic units, whereas the Y cells only respond to transient changes.

The X units, having a high spatial resolution and a poor temporal resolution, are best suited to be analyzers of spatial contrast and

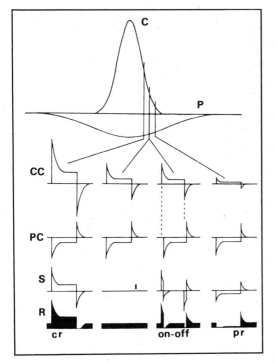

Figure 4.68
Diagram of the central and peripheral surround effects in the cat retina. C, central mechanism; P, peripheral surround mechanism; CC, central component; PC, peripheral component; S, summation; R, corresponding response. *Lowest trace, left to right:* Central response (cr), zero response, ON-OFF-response, (pr), peripheral surround response. (From Rodieck & Stone 1965)

consequently of shape and form. In contrast, the Y units, having to some extent the inverse properties, are best suited to detecting movement and temporal variations in the stimulus.

Recalling the histological data, this collection of four subassemblies of ganglion cells have the following distribution of their dendritic arborizations in the inner plexiform layer: ON-X-β and ON-Y-α cells ramify in the innermost sublayer b and the OFF-X-β and OFF-Y-α in the outermost layer a (Nelson et al. 1978; see also chapter 1, section 7.4).

The X and Y units differ even in the organization of their receptive fields, whether they are type B (ON-center) or type D (OFF-center). Suppose a particular stimulus applied to some part of the receptive field elicits *simultaneously* an excitation and an inhibition, with one of the two processes dominating in the center whether it is an ON-center or an OFF-center unit. The central response will be strong and localized, whereas the peripheral mechanism will be elicited less strongly and more spread out spatially. Figure 4.68 illustrates this hypothesis (Rodieck & Stone 1975).

The important question arises as to whether there is a *linear* summation within the receptive field of the spatially separated excitatory and inhibitory responses. The standard test of this is to present a stationary grating pattern of bright and dark bands with a sinusoidal spatial variation of luminance within the field. This grating image is switched on and off and its position in the field is progressively changed by translation movements (Enroth-Cugell & Robson 1966, Hochstein & Shapley 1976), all the other conditions remaining constant. Thus different parts of the field are successively crossed by stationary light and dark bands (figure 4.69).

Then, for X-cells it is always possible to find a certain position for the grating such that all responses at the onset or end of a stimulus are abolished. For that position, therefore, the ON-effect from one part of the field has been cancelled by the OFF-effect from another, suggesting a linear summation of spatial contrast.

However, for Y cells, such a cancelling can never be obtained whatever the position of the grating: In these cells there cannot be a linear summation of ON and OFF effects.

More recently, the distinctions between X and Y units have been further refined by considering simultaneously (figure 4.70) the variation with time, plotted along the x axis, and the spatial variation with distance from the center to periphery of the field, plotted along the y axis, using the instantaneous probability of a spike discharge as the parameter. In this way Stein et al. (1983) were able to separate four distinct *response domains:*

• A *primary excitatory* domain (PE) corresponding with the classic central response (ON for an ON-center B cell, OFF for a D or OFF-center cell)
• A *secondary excitatory* domain (SE), which represents the surround field's excitation (OFF for a B cell and ON for a D cell)
• A *secondary inhibitory* domain (SI), representing the surround inhibition that develops in the periphery at the onset of a stimulus in a B field and at its end in a D field.
• A *primary inhibitory* domain (PI), which is in fact a phenomenon arising throughout the whole field, center and surround. In a B cell this response arises at stimulus OFF and in a D cell at ON.

Notice that among these spatiotemporal domains, the first three were partially described in table 4.2, summarizing the properties of B and D units, but the fourth domain is from new data.

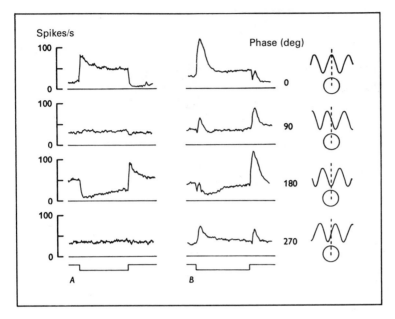

Figure 4.69
Differences between X and Y ganglion cells in the cat retina. Stimulus: Stationary grating with sinusoidal luminance variation in the field. Set up every 0.45 s and alternating with a uniform field of the same mean luminance. Contrast depth of the grating is 64% of the mean luminance (≡ contrast 0.32). *First column* (A): OFF-center X cell. *Second column* (B): OFF-center Y cell. Each column comprises: *upper trace,* discharge frequency; time calibration: a bar of 2-s duration. The lowest trace of each column is a stimulus marker, with an upward deflection designating the onset of the grating stimulus. The parameter in this experiment is the position of the grating in the field, expressed as phase angle. 0° and 360° correspond to a luminance maximum in the center of the field and each increase of 90° represents a ¼ cycle displacement of the grating toward the left in the diagram. With an X cell, two positions can be found for which the presentation or the suppression of a grating shows no response. Such positions are not found for Y cells (due to absence of linear summation within the field in the latter case). (From Enroth-Cugell & Robson 1966)

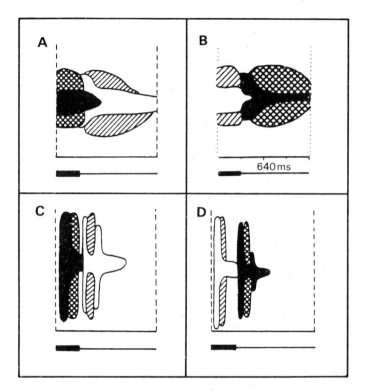

Figure 4.70
Diagram of the spatiotemporal organization of visual fields of the X and Y ganglion cells in the cat, illustrated by presenting stimuli of limited sizes. *A,* Heterogeneous ON-field. *B,* Heterogeneous OFF-field. *C,* Homogeneous ON-field. *D,* Homogeneous OFF-field. This is a schematic representation. Black areas, primary excitation; white areas, central inhibition; hatching, peripheral excitation; cross-hatching, peripheral inhibition. With x axis = time, y axis = spatial extent. Stimulus duration (marker below time scale): 320 ms. Illuminated bar: 0.5×0.25 degrees. Background illumination: $0.34 \ cd/m^2$. Stimulus luminance: $34 \ cd/m^2$.

This new multidimensional categorization allows a more exhaustive review of the properties of receptive fields and gives a striking demonstration of the differences between X and Y cells. Examining how these domains are distributed one can see that for the X cells, whether ON or OFF, different domains are encountered while passing from the center to the periphery of the field (from which arises the description *heterogeneous* that is given to them), whereas for the Y cells, these diverse domains spread throughout the length of the field, from center to its periphery (for this reason they appear *homogeneous*).

This third category is identifiable in the cat by the following character-istics: very small ganglion cells (8 to 13 μm), with axon conduction velocities less than in either X or Y cells (5 to 10 m/s). Proportionally they are 40% of the retina and are situated in the retina near the X cells (i.e., predominantly centrally); however, they have wide re-ceptive fields that resemble those of Y cells but with a more diffuse dendritic spread, as we saw above. As for their response properties, they are a heterogeneous population with some being tonic and oth-ers phasic.

Tonic W cells are either ON-center or OFF-center. Their antagonistic concentric center/surround organization allows prediction of the re-sponses to a given stimulus direction, incremental or decremental, its onset or its end, applied to the center or the periphery. The follow-ing is, however, the difference between these and the tonic X cells: While the latter obey table 4.2 with respect to B and D units, the W ganglion cells have only one mode of response (+ or −) but never both. Thus an ON-center W cell's discharge is accelerated by a light spot projected to its center field but is not inhibited when turning off the same spot stimulus. In other words, the response characteristics labeled $i+ \rightarrow i$, and $i- \rightarrow i$ (table 4.2) are not present in this case.

Phasic W cells constitute a complex subassembly that respond tran-siently either to the onset or end of a stimulus, whether central or surround, whether light or dark. Some of them have directional sen-sitivity. However, we will not elaborate on these aspects.

An attempt to define W cells by the "domains" such as were de-scribed above for the X and Y cells shows that in the case of W cells the number of excitatory and inhibitory domains is *variable,* in con-trast with the constant numbers found in the other two types of receptive field. This variability from one W cell to another illustrates very well the heterogeneity of this class of tonic and phasic cells.

PHASIC AND TONIC UNITS IN THE MONKEY

There are significant differences between the phasic and tonic GCs in a variety of species; we will not enumerate these. This general functional separation clearly has some important function in the cod-ing of stimulus characteristics.

The macaque, which has been well studied does, however, deserve special mention (Gouras 1968, 1969; Schiller & Malpeli 1977; Leven-thal et al. 1981): Both tonic (sustained) and phasic (transient) units have been found. These different units have different axonal conduction velocities, the phasic conducting faster than the tonic (3.8 m/s and 1.8 m/s, respectively, as average values). The phasic and tonic units exist throughout the retina from the fovea to 40° peripheral with a predominance of tonic cells in the center.

Other types of unit, much more scarce, have also been observed for which the axonal conduction velocity proves to be even slower. Clearly, there is a new variable to consider in this species: Some color-sensitive units must exist. We will consider these later.

There is also the question of whether it is valid to equate the monkey GC cells types M or $P\alpha$, P or $P\beta$, $P\gamma$ (described in chapter 1, section 7.3) with the feline X, Y, and W cells, respectively. There are differences, and the exact response to this question is not yet entirely clear. Some of the known differences between the M, P, and the rarer $P\gamma$ ganglion cells are morphological (cell size, axon diameter, extent of dendritic field) and were touched upon in chapter 1; in addition, we have mentioned their respective central projections. Starting from this information, we seem to be heading for the following scheme for the case of monkey GC organizations:

The P cells, projecting to the parvocellular layers of the LGB, are the color-sensitive units: When stimulated by their optimal color they give a tonic response (the characteristics of response to color will be considered in detail below). They react to a white or wide wavelength-band stimulus phasically. They have some of the characteristics of X cells but are not identical with them. Their receptive field is small but unlike in X cells, it does not increase with retinal eccentricity. Also, their sensitivity to spatial contrast, which is so high for X cells, is poor. These monkey CGs are specialized for color processing but probably not for form.

The M cells, projecting to the magnocellular LGB have chiefly X cell properties of tonic response and linear summation (Mx types) but a few of them (My types) have Y cell properties. M cells are specialized as form detectors; their power of spatial resolution decreases with increasing retinal eccentricity, while their dendritic field spread also increases, as we have seen above.

The rare $P\gamma$ cells, projecting to the superior colliculus (SC) are not yet so well defined functionally.

RETINAL CIRCUITRY IN THE CAT: NEW RESULTS AND AN ATTEMPT AT A SYNTHESIS

Given the extreme complexity of the retinal interconnections, it is obviously necessary to attain some sort of synthesized view of their operation, however provisional it might be. Here, therefore, are some aspects (Sterling et al. 1986) that take into account the histological data (already more or less covered in chapter 1) and also some functional data but which, such as they are, are only valid for the cat (figure 4.71).

Complexity of the Cone Pathways

A given ONβ-GC (i.e., X cell) receives inputs from at least two types of cone bipolars with terminals in the sublamina (b) of the inner plexiform layer. For that reason these inputs are classified as BiC-b1 and BiC-b2. Similarly, two cone bipolars terminate on a given OFFβ-GC in sublamina (a), from BiC-a1 and BiC-a2. In addition, at least one of the pair sends a collateral to a corresponding GCα (i.e., a Y cell).

These BiC cells also make gap contacts with AII amacrines, the significance of which we will summarize below.

Here we encounter one of the important aspects of this scheme: *The two types of cone bipolars connecting with a given GCβ have opponent properties, one being on the ON type (Bid) and the other OFF (Bih).* These two bipolars will be supplied by the same cone (or group of cones), and one will react with depolarization and the other with hyperpolarization for the same light stimulus to the cone. Thus an ON-GC will be excited by the first and inhibited by the second bipolar cell. This "push-pull" arrangement reinforces the effects of the stimulus and increases the dynamic range of the linear response of the GC. The same type of mechanism operates for the OFF GC.

Duality of the Rod Pathways

The "normal" pathway from the rods is to rod bipolars (RBi) via a chemical synapse; the axon from these bipolars projects to an AII amacrine. This type of amacrine cell is notable in that it has a double action: It makes numerous gap junctions with the cone bipolar BiC-b1 axons on their way to the β and α ON-GC; in addition, in sublamina (a) it makes chemical synaptic connections with the dendrites of OFF-GCβ and OFFα.

There are, therefore, two possible rod pathways:

R → RBi → AII → BiC-b1 axon → ON-GCβ and ON-GCα
R → RBi → AII ————————→ OFF-GCβ and OFF-GCα

These pathways operate in complete dark adaptation, beginning the moment when the receptive fields lose their antagonistic surround,

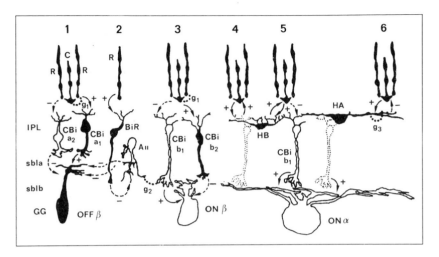

Figure 4.71
Diagram of the neural circuitry in the cat's retina. A somewhat hypothetical scheme
for the neural circuitry connecting various elements in the cat retina. 1 and 3, Connections of the cone bipolars with the OFF-(1) and ON-(3) β ganglion cells (i.e., X units).
Each cone makes contact with several types of cone bipolars (BiC), but each β ganglion
cell receives inputs from two BiC, one depolarizing Bi(d) (BiC a1 or BiC b1) and the
other hyperpolarizing BiH (BiC a2 and BiC b2). Note that BiC a1 and a2 terminate in
the sublamina s (ss1a) of the inner plexiform layer and the BiC b1 and b2 in the
sublamina b (ss1b). Thus a central light stimulus effects an excitation and disinhibition
of the ON-β ganglion cell and an inhibition and facilitation of the OFF-β ganglion cell.
The opposite effects are generated by a peripheral stimulus. In weak light the cones
cease to function but the rods can transmit a signal via the rod/cone gap junctions (g1)
in this same "push-pull" circuit. 4, 5, and 6, Influence of the horizontal cells. The BiC
b1 have an excitatory field that is wider than their dendritic spread. This enlargement
is due to lateral actions of the HB which interconnect neighboring cones (4). The
inhibitory periphery, for its part, is established by inhibitory connections of the HA
cells with the receptors (REC) (6), and then extended further by gap junctions between
HA cells (g3). 2, Circuits between rod bipolars (BiR) with ON- and OFF-β ganglion
cells. In dark adaptation, the rod/cone gap junctions cease to function (?). In contrast,
the rod signals are funnelled by the BiR (2), then by another chemical synapse to
the AII amacrines. Such an amacrine could have two effects: an inhibitory chemical
postsynaptic one via the route BiC, a1 OFF-β ganglion cell, and action via gap (g2) on
the system BiC b1 ON-β ganglion cell. The BiR do not connect with HA cells, giving
rise to the lack of peripheral inhibitory action in this case. 4, 5, and 6, Circuits of ON-α
ganglion cells (Y cells). Essentially, the ganglion cells receive inputs from BiC b1 (like
the ON-β ganglion cells above). The geometry of the connections is, however, different: ON-α cells have a large field receiving from a large number of BiC b1 (4, 5, 6).
Full arrows, excitatory actions; dashed arrows, inhibitory actions; dotted connections,
gap junctions. The cells with open contours are responsible for ON-responses (depolarizations); the filled cells are for hyperpolarizing responses to light OFF. (From Trends
in Neuroscience 1986, Vol. 9, *center page*)

when the excitatory center follows the laws of quantum summation, and when the contrast-detecting unit is transformed into a spatial summating unit. This three-neuron pathway goes via AII amacrines, which direct the bipolar signal along an excitatory path to the ON- or to the OFF-GC. The organization of center/surround antagonism is in no way the concern of the rod network proper.

Another interesting aspect is the retinal "wiring" of a different pathway for rod signals, this time relevant to twilight vision, that is, to an intermediate state of dark adaptation when the cones are just ceasing to be functional. Here the signals pass via rod gap junctions to the cones, then by the cone's own connections via cone bipolars to the corresponding cone GC. In these conditions—even though it is concerned with rod receptive field inputs—such a field retains its center surround antagonistic organization.

Horizontal Cell Action

Unlike the precise data available for the lower vertebrates, the functions of the mammalian HB and HA cells remain somewhat uncertain, or are interpretations based on merely histological data. It has been suggested that the HB cells, lacking axons, might be responsible for the size of the center of cone receptive fields (wider than the Bi dendritic field). The more widespreading HA, for their part, might control the center/surround antagonism.

5.4 CODING OF COLOR

Consider now the neurophysiological mechanisms subserving color vision at the retinal level, particularly the ganglion cell mechanisms. Clearly, this study can only be properly undertaken in those species for which color vision has been confirmed behaviorally. This limits the information to animals amenable to such experimentation such as the rabbit (non albino), the ground squirrel, and insectivores like *Tupaia* (the tree shrew) in addition to the more common primates macaque and *Saimiri*. This argument would seem tautological if in fact a collection of supposed relevant research data had not already been made in the cat, which is probably color blind. [Yet there seems to be a class of W cells that are coded for light wavelength with an antagonism of the type blue$^+$/yellow$^-$. These cells are exclusively in the pathway from cones into LGB and the superior colliculus. Perhaps these units are representatives of a frustrated color vision and are the predecessors of the organization that is found in primates

(Daw & Pearlman 1970). The other side of the argument is that the existence of units sensitive to color is not in itself a sufficient condition for the existence of color vision. We shall discuss the problem of color vision in the context of color sensitivity at cortical levels in the following chapter.]

THE ORGANIZATION OF COLOR-SENSITIVE RESPONSES: GENERAL PRINCIPLES

Our concern here is to identify ganglion cells that signal a color sensitivity with responses that are a function of light wavelength or with action spectra that are narrow and do not show a monotonic change throughout the visible spectrum. It was Granit (1947) who, investigating the GC responses in the cat, discovered some with narrow band responses that he specified as *modulators*, contrasting with others that he called *dominators* that have wide band responses and correspond with luminosity detectors. If later these considerations ran into difficulty (precisely because the cat probably has no color vision), it remains true that the question had been properly posed: It is necessary to attempt to find cells with narrow (wavelength) band responses that could be color units as distinct from wide band cells that can only be achromatic (luminosity) detectors.

However, experiment has shown that the behavior of color coding units proper is more complex, particularly beyond the retina, and seems to follow two principles. First, such a cell is excited in a certain (light-)frequency band (C) and often inhibited in another frequency band (D). This leads to defining pairs of antagonistic colors, in practice the red (R) and green (G) pair with the two possible mechanisms R^+/G^- and R^-/G^+, and the yellow (Y) and blue (B) pair with either Y^+/B^- or Y^-/B^+.

Second, a color coding can be complicated by adding a spatial coding to it, with a concentric organization (ON/OFF or OFF/ON). In this respect, a few calls can be identified as responding at the same time to a single narrow band of color but also effecting an (antagonistic) spatial coding within that same spectral band. But the majority of cells studied show a more complicated arrangement than that, with combined spatial and color contrast. Imagine the large number of a priori possibilities starting from two colors C and D with C/D antagonisms of the types shown in figure 4.72, which only shows some of them (in 2, 3, 4, and 5); note that in each case C and D can also be interchanged. Operationally then, color-sensitive mechanisms must in reality be described as *neuronal units showing color antagonisms*.

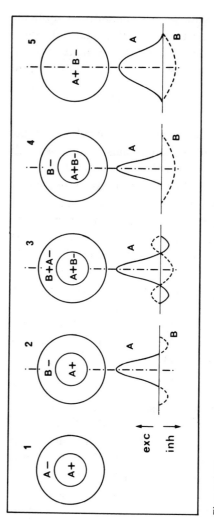

Figure 4.72
Receptive fields and color vision. Spatial arrangements of receptive field modalities in the ground squirrel for two spectral domains A and B and for response characteristics, excitatory ON (+) and inhibitory OFF (−). 1, Concentric center/surround antagonism for a single spectral region. 2, 3, 4, and 5, More complex spatial and chromatic response modalities.

In species with color vision, cells for which spatially antagonistic arrangements are not color coded can be found alongside the color-coded units, even in the foveal region. These *wide spectral band units*, as in the cat, often have a wide spectral sensitivity curve that might subserve the coding of luminance.

COLOR VISION IN THE GROUND SQUIRREL

Michael (1973), working on the ground squirrel, found that about 20% of the GC are color coded, with maximal sensitivities near 525 nm (Y or G) and around 460 nm (B) with 50% G^+/B^- and 50% G^-/G^+. Note that red and yellow act in the same way as green, which confirms the behavioral work showing that the ground squirrel is a dichromat. There are three spatial organizations in the receptive fields for the "green cones" and the "blue cones." In some (type I), the two types of cones seem to be randomly distributed throughout the field so that opponent color responses (e.g., ON-G OFF-B) are obtained throughout the field (type 5 in figure 4.72), whereas others (type II) with concentric fields have a G^+B^- organization in the center and a B^- operation in the surround (type 4), while the final third type is also concentrically organized but with G^+ in the center and B^- in the surround (type 2 in figure 4.72).

COLOR VISION IN THE MACAQUE

We now give some data on color mechanisms in the GC of rhesus retina (Gouras 1968, de Monasterio & Gouras 1975, de Monasterio et al. 1975). We will not go into great detail on the experimental methods used to classify these interactions. In essence, for each sort of response, central or surround, an action spectrum is measured as log relative threshold as a function of wavelength. Such curves are plotted in the presence of a wide field of adapting light, either white or colored, and deduced from the resulting *selective color adaptation*. The latter is effected either by using one or other of the primates R, G, B, or the colors resulting from the combinations of two primaries Y = R + G (yellow), M = R + B (magenta), or C = B + G (blue-green, "cyan"). These techniques revealed several types of GC coding, discussed below.

Color-Opponent Units
These are the most numerous (63% of the total investigated). They have a dual antagonistic field with a (+ or −) effect of one color at the center and the opposite effect (− or +) of another color in the

surround. As a general rule the responses are tonic, lasting throughout the stimulus and in this case reminiscent of X cell responses.

Selective color adaptation allowed the determination of the maximal color sensitivity in each precise range, central or peripheral, excitatory or inhibitory. Thus an inventory of many subclasses is available, enumerated here in decreasing order of importance: (G^+/R^-), (G^+/M^-), (G^-/R^+), (G^-/M^+), (R^+/G^-), (R^+/C^-), (R^-/G^+), (R^-/C^+), (Y^+/B^-), (B^+/Y^-), (B^-/Y^+).

Remembering the microspectrophotometric data that proved the existence of three types of cones R, G, and B, we can conclude after scanning this list that there must exist two types of GC: (1) some must comprise R/G units receiving only from two cones; and (2) others are quite different and receive an input (excitatory or inhibitory) from a single primary (red, green, or blue) but also have a maximal sensitivity in the antagonistic field to an intermediate color (Y, C, or M) comprised (as we have seen) of a combination of two primary colors. In other words, these GC are of three different types, green/magenta (g/M), blue/yellow (B/Y), and red/cyan (R/C), receiving an input not from two cones, one excitatory and the other inhibitory, but from *three cones,* one excitatory or inhibitory and the other an (inhibitory or excitatory) input from a combination of two other cones. It is quite clear that these ganglion cell responses show much narrower passbands than would have been expected from studying the receptors alone. This finer tuning in GC is very probably due to inhibitory interactions that occur within the retinal network. This point is important: All the data indicate that the receptors themselves constitute a trichromatic input system such as would be expected from the psychophysical data. Thus the essential message from these receptive field organizations (whether in the retina, as treated here, or in the lateral geniculate body or cortex) is that they are a first view of the visual system's antagonistic color interactions (such as Hering once proposed, followed by the recent support of Hurwich, 1985, and Jameson, 1985, among others). It is important to realize how beneath any of the apparently two/color mechanisms listed here there lies the same original trichromatic system.

Wide Spectral Band Units

These GC do not have any significant specific color sensitivity but do have a classic concentric ON/OFF spatial organization. What is more, their response is largely phasic, that is, they resemble Y cells. They comprise about 20% of the population according to Gouras (1968).

Cells with Nonconcentric Fields
These GC are rare (9%). They comprise two subgroups: (1) those with strongly phasic responses, and (2) others essentially sensitive to moving stimuli. (We have mentioned these briefly already.)

Distribution and Receptive Field Size of Color Units
In all three major categories, color units are mostly found in the central part of the retina (0° to 2°) and the wide band cells mostly in the periphery (10° to 40° eccentricity). Color opponent cells have small receptive fields (0.06° to 0.12°), which do not vary much with eccentricity. In contrast, units with a wide spectral band have wider receptive fields and a much greater variation with retinal position between the fovea (0.12°) and the periphery (>2°).

5

Mechanisms in the Central Visual Pathways

We shall not repeat the description in chapter 1 (section 7.3) of how the ganglion cell axons project more centrally but will move directly to a discussion of the results concerned with their different points of arrival.

1 THE MIDBRAIN VISUAL CENTERS

1.1 THE SUPERIOR COLLICULUS

STRUCTURE

In nonmammalian vertebrates, the superior colliculus (SC) comprises the tectum opticum (optic roof), whose organization has been the object of detailed examination that we shall not elaborate on here. Recall that the optic fibers are completely crossed (i.e., come solely from the contralateral retina), spread over the surface of the tectum, and then penetrate radially in depth to make contact with a series of neurons that are arranged in several layers, the number and size of which varies with the class of nonmammal, from the fish to the birds.

Histological Fine Structure
The *mammalian SC* follows an organizational plan, practically the same in all the diverse mammalian groups (Kanaseki & Sprague 1974, Goldberg & Robinson 1978), that shows a range of successive layers from the dorsal surface to depth, as follows:

• The *stratum zonale,* (1) in figure 5.1, has medium-sized cells whose dendrites have a tangential trajectory and remain local, and also small cells whose dendrites penetrate to depth.
• The *stratum griseum superficiale* (2) has numerous cells of different shapes and sizes, the axons of which penetrate to the deepest layers and constitute (at least some of them) an output to the thalamus.
• The *stratum opticum* (3) is essentially a layer of fibers, most of them being axons of retinal origin with some other afferent and efferent fibers also.

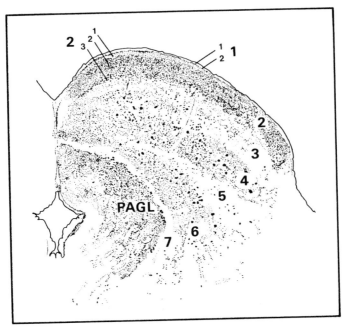

Figure 5.1
Frontal section of the superior colliculus (Nissl stain, marking cell bodies). *1, 1* and *2*: Stratum zonale and its two subdivisions. *2, 1, 2,* and *3*: Stratum griseum superficiale and its three subdivisions. *3,* Stratum opticum. *4,* Stratum griseum intermediale. *5,* Stratum lemnisci (album intermediale). *6,* Stratum griseum profundum. *7,* Stratum album profundum. PAGL, periaqueductal grey matter, pars lateralis. (From Kanaseki & Sprague 1974)

- The *stratum griseum intermediale* (4) contains the cell bodies of efferent (colliculofugal) neurons.
- The *stratum album intermediale* (5) is where some efferent axons run as well as other nonvisual axons (from the medulla or the brain stem).
- The *stratum griseum profundum* (6) also carries efferent neurons whose axons constitute the deepest layer of white matter, the *stratum album profundum* (7), that borders the SC ventrally and separates it from the mesencephalic periaquaductal grey matter.

Afferent Connections
The overall organization of the afferent connections to the SC is as follows:

Fibers from the retina, some of which are collaterals of retinogeniculate axons (see chapter 1, section 7.3), reach the SC either laterally (*lateral brachium* of the SC) or medially (*medial brachium* of the SC).

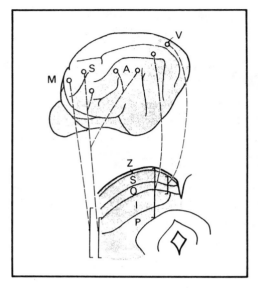

Figure 5.2
Origin and termination of the corticofugal pathways to the superior colliculus. The corticotectal pathways arise in the motor (M), somatic (S), auditory (A), and visual 17, 18, 19 areas (V). Their terminations in the layers of the tectum are different depending on their origins: Z, stratum zonale; S, stratum griseum superficiale; O, stratum opticum; I, stratum griseum intermediale; P, stratum griseum profundum. (From Sprague et al. 1973)

Most terminate in the most superficial layers (1 and 2 above; see Kaas et al. 1974, Hartling & Guillery 1976). Essentially, the distribution is retinotopic (largely confirmed electrophysiologically, as we shall see below), with the macular region projecting to the anterior, and the retinal periphery projecting to the most caudal parts of the SC. In the cat, as in the macaque, the two retinas project to each SC; however, the contralateral projection is largely predominant with the terminals in stratum 2 forming a layer that is interrupted from time to time by areas of about 200 μm diameter, these being the "spots" where ipsilateral projections arrive.

Cortical projections to the SC are numerous and constitute the majority of nonretinal afferents (Garey et al. 1968, Powell 1976). In this respect, there also seems to be a layering of these projections, those from the visual areas being the most superficial (layers 1 and 2). Those from the temporal areas, then the parietal, then finally the frontal regions project successively more deeply (layers 3 and 4). Notice (figure 5.2) that oculomotor area 8 of macaque has a considerable projection to layer 4; also, regarding area 17, there exists a topographic arrangement such that the sites of collicular and cortical projections are in register, so that each point on the retina is selectively connected retinotopically by the corresponding cortico-collicular pathway. Note that there is now known to be a deep projection from the suprasylvian area of the cat that also contains visual connections.

In addition, there are SC projections from elsewhere. Their terminations seem to obey the same general principles as those from the retina and from the cortex, in that units concerned with visual functions tend to project more superficially than those that are less directly involved with vision.

The superficial layers receive projections from the pulvinar, from the posterolateral nucleus of the thalamus, and from LGBv (pars ventralis of the lateral geniculate body). The intermediate layers likewise receive from the LGBv but also from other origins, the inferior colliculus and the pontine and bulbar reticular formation. Finally, the deep layers also receive projections from reticular afferents as well as from outputs from the fastigial nucleus of the cerebellum. There is still argument about possible pretectal projections to SC.

A projection from the pars reticulata of the substantia nigra (Chevalier et al. 1981) is also one of the afferent paths to the SC.

Efferent Connections
The SC efferents are traditionally divided into two groups which also have a certain segregation of their cells of origin in the SC depending on their destination.

The *descending efferents* arise in the deeper layers of the SC (*str. opticum* and *griseum intermediale*) and comprise:

• The tectopontine tract, projecting to the contralateral pontine nuclei. This pathway also sends off collaterals to the midbrain reticular formation and to the magnocellular division of the LGB.
• The tectoreticular tract to the ipsilateral dorsolateral midbrain reticular formation.
• The tectospinal tract (once called the "predorsal bundle") descends to the cervical spinal level C6, sending collaterals to the interstitial nucleus of Cajal, to the Darkschevich nucleus, and to certain pontine structures involved in the control of eye saccades.

Particular attention has been given recently to the detailed organization of the colliculoreticular tracts that are linked with oculomotor control (Grantyn & Grantyn 1980). In fact, monosynaptic connections are found from cells of a precise group of neurons (nucleus prepositus hypoglossi) whose activity is linked with saccadic movements. These reticular neurons (specified as "premotor for eye movements") themselves project monosynaptically on motoneurons of the oculomotor nuclei, in particular on those of the abducens nerve (VI).

The *ascending efferents*, in addition to projecting to the contralateral SC, go both to the pretectum and to the subthalamic regions (zona incerta and Forel's field) and finally to a very large number of thalamic nuclei, the dorsomedial and centrolateral (DM/CL), the pulvinar and lateral posterior nucleus, the posterior nucleus, the suprageniculate nucleus, the magnocellular region of the MGB, the dorsal and ventral regions of the LGB (LGBd and LGBv), and the ventromedial nucleus.

Some of these projections, of which most are bilateral, arise from the superficial layers, others from deeper layers of the SC. But a certain separation of function seems to exist. The nuclei that are most concerned with visual mechanisms are probably connected from the most superficial layers of the stratum griseum superficiale (LGB, pretectum and pulvinar, medial division of the posterolateral nucleus in the cat), whereas the rest connect from the deeper layers of the stratum (to the ventral division of the posterolateral nucleus in the cat and in macaque to the medial and oral pulvinar and the medial division of the posterolateral nucleus).

It is certainly interesting (Chevalier & Deniau 1984) that there are neurons that send off axon collaterals upstream and downstream ("tectospinodiencephalic" projections) that bifurcate or even trifurcate and can thus act simultaneously at both the oculocephalic and the thalamic levels of organization. Notice also that in cat some efferents enter the optic tract: The termination of these fibers (possibly retinal?) is not yet known.

FUNCTION

The structure of the SC is such that on the one hand it has clearly specified afferent inputs—visual but also, as neurophysiological exploration has shown, somatic and auditory—and on the other hand it is the source of its own typical afferents. From these data it is clearly a structure for *sensorimotor integration*. We shall now discuss some of the essential data in this respect.

Topography of the Visual Projections
Single-unit electrophysiology has broadly confirmed the anatomical data concerning the topographical representation of the visual field. The organization for the *contralateral visual hemifield* seems to be identical for species as different as the rat, cat, and monkey. The projection of the zero vertical meridian (VM) is oriented transversely and

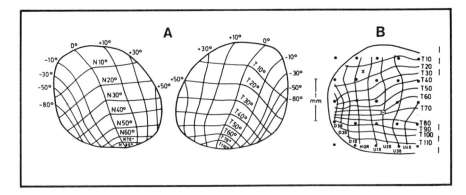

Figure 5.3
Projections of the retina to the superior colliculus of cat and rat. *A*, Projection of the visual field of the left eye to the two colliculi (cat). The colliculi are as viewed dorsally with their anterior margin above, posterior below, with the midline passing between the two structures. The horizontal meridian is indicated as the anteroposterior line marked 0°. All parts of the upper hemifield are represented medially with respect to this line (equal elevation lines +10°, +30°, +50°) and the lower hemifield is lateral (−10°, −30°, −50°, −80°). The zero vertical meridian is situated at the extreme anterior border of the colliculus. N and T indicate the nasal and temporal equal azimuth lines respectively (N10°, etc; T10°, etc.). *B*, Projection of the visual field of the right eye to the left colliculus (rat). HOR, equal elevation line 0. U10 etc., D10 etc., equal elevation lines for the upper and lower visual fields, respectively. The temporal equal azimuth lines are represented lateromedial and are marked from 10 to 110. (From Sprague et al. 1973)

mediolaterally, and situated very much anterior in the rostral region of the colliculus. The projection of the zero horizontal meridian (HM) is practically sagittal, crossing the SC more or less along the middle from anterior to posterior, with a medial representation of the upper hemifield and a lateral representation of the lower hemifield (figure 5.3; see Feldon et al. 1970, Sprague et al. 1973, McIlwain 1975).

In species with a partial chiasm separation, this projection involves at the same time the nasal hemiretina and a temporal hemiretina but with a certain predominance of contralateral representation. The SC units are thus mostly of the type "binocular with contralateral dominance."

In a number of species, including cat, squirrel, *Tupaia*, and marsupials, a considerable part of the ispilateral visual field projects equally to each SC. This projection is found in its most anterior part, in front of the zero vertical meridian; it can extend from as far as 40° in the ipsilateral visual field (figure 5.4; Lane et al. 1974). It seems to be

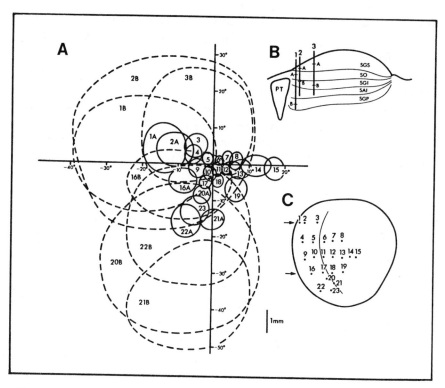

Figure 5.4
Visual field map (A) of the left superior colliculus in cat. *A*, Receptive fields of single units with respect to the horizontal and vertical zero meridians. Individual cells recorded from and marked A (small fields) are superficial while those marked B (wider fields) are deep. Notice the large representation of the ipsilateral left hemifield. *Inset C*, The sites of the penetration where the corresponding receptive fields were recorded. Arrows indicate the anterior border of the colliculus. *Inset B*, A parasagittal section of the colliculus showing the three penetrations 1, 2, and 3 in the anterior region. PT, pretectum, anterior to the colliculus; SGS, stratum griseum superficiale; SO, stratum opticum; SGI, stratum griseum intermediale; SAI, stratum album intermediale; SGP, stratum griseum profundum. (From Lane et al. 1974)

accepted that this projection arises because the fibers of the contralateral visual field cross the midline instead of staying ipsilateral (which in some way represents a persistence of the older phylogenetic organization). Another explanation for this contralateral projection of the temporal retina has postulated a crossing via the posterior (intercollicular) commissure, but this is less likely. No such projection of the ipsilateral visual field is seen in the macaque.

It is worth noticing that the projection of the contralateral retina,

even in macaque, comprises the area in which is found the discontinuity of the *blind spot*. This discontinuity is found to be preserved in
the distribution of projections in the SC by using cell markers, which
reveal a small zone where marking is entirely absent. Nevertheless,
the representation, at least in the monkey, is not registered proportionally because to some extent a "magnification factor" can be measured which shows a much more extensive projection of the central
region. In fact, a third of the (spread out) area of the colliculus is
dedicated to the central 6° of the retina.

General Characteristics of the Receptive Fields
We have already discussed above how the retinal afferent axons in
the cat are divided between the SC and the LGB. Recall that, so far
as the SC is concerned, all Y axons (from 5% of the GC) send a
collateral to the SC; some X axons (10% of the total X, the latter being
from 56% of the GC) project in a similar way, and all W axons project
to the colliculus. It seems also that the Y terminate more deeply
(stratum opticum) in SC than the W (strata zonale and griseum superficiale). Direct Y and slow W fibers drive distinct sets of collicular
neurons (stratum griseum superficiale cells for Ws, deeper layer cells
for Ys). The collicular neurons driven by some faster W fibers or by
X fibers have not been clearly identified so far (see Berson 1988 for
discussion).

In the macaque, we have so far considered two types of connections in the colliculus: one is from transient afferents (i.e., Y type)
with high axon conduction velocity; the other, rarer population has
slow conduction velocities (Pγ or W; see chapter 1, section 7.3). We
may characterize the response characteristics of the SC cells as follows: In general, the receptive fields are wider than those in the
LGB-cortex pathway. The collicular cells generally have poor response sensitivity to diffuse light, and they are more sensitive to
moving than to fixed stimuli. This sensitivity to movement can extend
to high angular velocities (800°/s). In this particular case, the same
type of response is obtained in whatever sense the contrast might
exist (bright stimulus on dark background, or the opposite; see
Straschill & Taghavy 1967).

Most cells respond uniformly to stationary local stimulation, as
ON/OFF types, throughout the whole receptive field. Concentric field
arrangements like those seen in the retina and LGB are seldom encountered. A few fields show an inhibitory surround in certain species (figure 5.5; see Dreher & Hoffmann 1973). The fields become

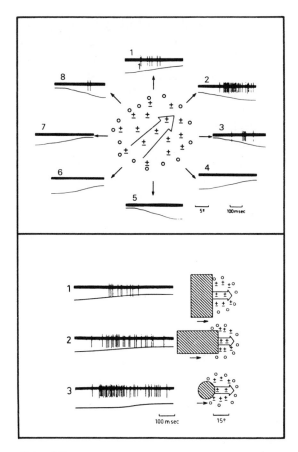

Figure 5.5
Receptive field of superior colliculus cells in the cat. *Above,* A cell with directional sensitivity. Each recording comprises the cell discharge (upper trace), the corresponding stimulus spot movement (lower trace) and an arrow indicating the direction of movement. +, − symbols: ON-OFF responses; open circles, zero responses. The large arrow crossing the whole field shows the preferred stimulus movement direction for the cell. *Below,* Peripheral inhibition in the receptive field. A dark object crosses the receptive field along the optimal direction (lower traces showing the photoelectric measure of its movement). It is evident that the widest dark object across the receptive field generates the greatest inhibition (compare 1 and 3). (From McIwain & Buser 1968)

even wider (1) the more eccentrically they are placed and (2) the deeper the cell is situated in the colliculus. The percentage of cells with phasic responses (i.e., with Y type responses) also increases the farther the cell's field is positioned in the eccentric regions of the visual field away from the area centralis (McIlwain 1976).

Cells with directional sensitivity do exist in some species. These are not often seen in the squirrel but are much more abundant in the cat, particularly so in the superficial layers of the nucleus. A good proportion of these are optimally sensitive for a horizontal movement, chiefly one that is contraversive (e.g., in the right SC for a movement from right to left). In the upper vertical quadrant they seem to be sensitive mainly to upward movement and in the lower quadrant to downward movement (figure 5.5; see McIlwain & Buser 1968).

The situation varies in primates. Macaque does not seem to have such directional responses (see figure 5.45), but in contrast the *Saimiri* and *Cebus* do seem to have a few. [Do not forget that such directional sensitivity, depending on the species, might result from a local SC mechanism or alternatively just reflect the properties carried by an input to the nucleus, with the selectivity already elaborated in the retina, perhaps.]

In the intermediate levels of the nucleus there are cells with much more extensive receptive fields than in the superficial layers, as we have underlined above. In the alert animal, these cells also show rapid adaptation properties. They may respond very well to a first stimulus but the responses become rapidly attenuated during successive presentations of the same stimulus.

We have considered the problem of color coding in SC. In principle, the information processed here is quite different from what happens in the visual cortex (see below). In fact, the results also depend on species: For example, color coding seems to be limited to the retina-LGB pathway in the squirrel, whereas it is equally well directed to the SC in *Saimiri*.

In the cat, a high proportion of collicular cells show a considerable binocular information convergence. These cells respond to stimulation from identical visual field locations, seen from one or the other eye. In these cases, the receptive fields are the same for the two eyes, but there is often a dominant excitatory influence from one eye (usually the contralateral one). In this case, a binocular stimulation is facilitatory, provided the stimuli are in exact spatial correspondence

(i.e., on "corresponding points" of the retina). Apart from the above
responses, other occlusive types of interaction may be seen. In this
respect, the SC mechanisms (like those in the cortex, as we shall see)
can code steroscopic visual characteristics, such as estimating depth
in the visual field (Berman & Cynader 1972, 1975; Cynader & Berman
1972; Berman et al. 1975).

Cortico-collicular paths have been confirmed physiologically.
(1) SC cells can be monosynaptically excited by electrical stimulation
of the cortex. (2) In the cat, such projections arrive from the striate
cortex (17) or from the Clare and Bishop (lateral suprasylvian) area,
together with a minimal input from areas 18 and 19. (3) The optimal
excitation of a given SC cell is from the region of the cortex that
represents the same part of the visual field, the spatial correspondence having already been established by anatomical topography.
(4) A few cells receive a convergent input from all three areas 17, 18,
and 19 (McIlwain 1977).

Two components of corticotectal fibers seem to exist: (1) a "slow"
corticofugal pathway, mainly originating from area 17, ending in SC
superficial layers, and (2) a "fast" pathway, from the suprasylvian
areas, ending in stratum opticum. These descending pathways seem
to be mainly driven by Y signals at the cortical level (see Berson 1988).
Correspondingly, deep collicular cells are preferentially affected by
cryogenic blockade of the suprasylvian cortex and superficial cells by
that of area 17 (Stein 1988).

The SC system is likely to play a major role in some effects of visual
cortex ablations. The main issue here is that the two SC inhibit each
other through the intercollicular commissure; see also the text references to Sprague (1966) in section 3.4 on ablations.

The Superior Colliculus and the Direction of Gaze
Perhaps the most interesting properties of the colliculus are those
that control eye movements and that determine the direction of gaze.
These mechanisms can comprise not only saccades, for example, but
also in appropriate cases some head movement. Clearly, most of
these measurements need to be carried out on the alert animal.

Surgical ablation in the superior colliculus. SC ablations pose a problem
because there is always a risk of cutting, in however minor a way,
into the pretectum (the presumed functional role of which will be
discussed below) or into the areas immediately below the grisea centralis or into the midbrain tegmentum (see figure 5.1).

Thus with some reservations we may present the following conclusions from such experiments:

In the hamster, the classic SC ablation observations of Schneider (1967) established the difficulty the animal had in orienting itself in space or toward a given target (e.g., food), while retaining some shape discrimination. We will return toward the end of this section to attempt a general presentation of the functional implications of this sort of data.

In *Tupaia* (see Appendix) the results are a little more subtle: Ablation of the superficial regions only interferes with form discrimination, but after ablation in deeper zones both shape discrimination and orientation in space are affected.

In the cat, there is a complex syndrome: lack of behavioral attention to visual stimuli ("apparent blindness"); absence of recognition of objects ("agnosia"); fixed gaze and no visual pursuit of moving objects. In contrast to this, there still remain behavioral shrinking to a threat, optokinetic nystagmus, and vestibular reactions.

In the macaque there are contradictory findings. First it was decided that there were no deficits, as determined from tasks in which only luminance differences needed to be detected, but later, changes were found particularly involving the latency of saccades, while apparently not affecting their precision (Wurtz & Goldberg 1972). These deficits can, however, soon be compensated for by the visual cortex.

Stimulation of the superior colliculus. [An older series of highly detailed experiments (Apter 1946) exploited the local application of strychnine stimulation to a given point on the colliculus and showed that the deviation of the eyes due to this stimulus was to the corresponding point in visual space.] The following effects in a variety of species (rodents, cat, macaque) have been established by surface electrical stimulation of the SC or by microstimulation of deeper layers, identifiable from its known morphology.

Stimulation can generate essentially conjugate saccadic movements of the eyes, predominantly horizontal, toward the opposite side, sometimes with an occasional upward component (figure 5.6; see Robinson 1972). In monkeys, particularly, the direction and amplitude of the saccade depend on the collicular location that is stimulated and not on the position of the eyes in the orbit: The eye fixates on a given point in space by this saccadic rotation. From these experiments, an *eye movements map* for SC can be plotted which is in register

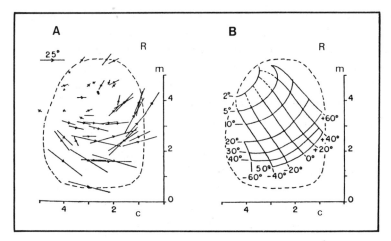

Figure 5.6
Ocular saccades initiated by collicular stimulation in the awake monkey. *A,* Diagram
of ocular saccadic movements initiated by electrical stimulation of the left collicular
surface. Each arrow shows the amplitude and direction of the movement evoked by
stimulating the points indicated by arrow heads. *B,* Map in polar coordinates of the
targets of the saccades evoked by punctate stimulation at the corresponding collicular
sites. R, c, and m indicate the rostral, causal and medial borders of the left superior
colliculus. For the identification of polar coordinates see figure 3.59. (From Robinson
1972)

with the sensory map. The deviation of the eyes is predictable from
the topography of the retino-collicular projections determined by single unit measurements. The movement deviates the visual axis toward a point in the visual field that is represented on the sensory
input map at the place stimulated.

Rotary movements of the head can also be generated in the unrestrained monkey. The latency for the start of a head movement depends on the starting position of the eyes in the orbit: When micro-
stimulating one SC, the resulting rotation of the head to the other
side begins earlier if the eyes are already turned toward that other
side (Stryker & Schiller 1975).

In the cat, the effects of electrical stimulation of SC are more complex and depend on the anterior/posterior position of stimulation on
the SC concerned (Guitton et al. 1980, Roucoux et al. 1980). [*Note:* It
has been reported that in the cat in a normal, natural environment,
movement of the head accompanies any eye movement when the
target is at an eccentricity of more than 4°. Behavior in the monkey is

quite different; much greater eye movement in the orbit is common.] Stimulation of the anterior SC invokes eye saccades (in the range 0° to 25° eccentricity) and little head movement. More caudal stimulation, however, results in a combination of head and eye movements whose net result is an orientation toward the target (in the visual angle 25° to 70°). Finally, stimulation at the extreme posterior SC evokes head movements principally and perhaps even movements of the whole body.

[Note, however, that the problem is more complex than the above suggests, since stimulation at many other brain sites elicits conjugate movements, for example, stimulation of the posterior thalamus, the hypothalamus, the midbrain tegmentum (to cite only a few subcortical levels) and certainly stimulation of the oculomotor areas of the cortex. In addition, ablation of the SC suppresses eye movements obtained by stimulating the posterior oculomotor area but not those resulting from frontal oculomotor area stimulation, (essentially Brodmann's area 8).]

Single-unit studies. The above data are broadly reinforced and confirmed by single-unit studies of the behavior of SC cells in relation to saccades. Some detailed results are now available for *macaque* (Wurtz & Goldberg 1972a,b; Goldberg & Wurtz 1972a,b; Mohler & Wurtz 1976). In the superficial layers of SC are found cells whose excitation is determined by both adequate visual stimulation and the generation of a saccade. Their particular characteristic is that their response to a stimulus appearing at a particular place in the visual field is notably increased in discharge rate and in duration if an eye saccade should be generated immediately after the presentation of the stimulus. This saccade will lead to fixation on the target. If the presentation of the stimulus is not followed by a saccade, its response to the identical stimulus remains poor or even zero. We should add, however, that these response characteristics are very sensitive to habituation and adaptation following repeated similar stimuli. An essential factor is a progressive reduction of the response discharge with respect to that at the beginning of the saccade (the latter can last 200 to 300 ms). Note also that in the superficial layers of SC the same type of saccade, generated spontaneously either in light or in darkness, generates no characteristic cell response (figure 5.7).

In the intermediate layers of SC, which is the region where move-

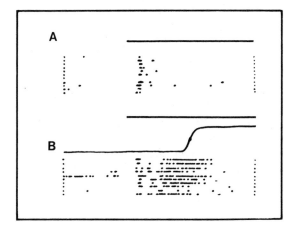

Figure 5.7
Response of a collicular cell to illumination by a light spot (1° diameter) which was either not followed (*A*) or followed (*B*) by a saccade leading to fixation of the spot stimulus. Horizontal bars, illumination of the spot stimulus. Notice in *B* the large discharge which *precedes* the saccade. The presentation is by "dotgram," or a diagram of dots each of which represents a recorded cell discharge (10 trials). Time scale: the dots are separated by 50 ms. (From Wurtz & Goldberg 1972)

ments are most easily elicited by stimulation, there are, once again, cells that are activated by saccades, which produce movement toward a certain zone in space. It is possible to define for each cell in these regions a *movement field*, a part of the visual field from which the appearance of a stimulus generates a saccade. If the cell responds to light independently of a saccade, the receptive field can be compared with the movement field: Overall, the two are similar except that the movement field is apparently wider in extent. Finally, deep cells are excited whatever the nature of the saccade, for instance, whether it is one that has arisen spontaneously in darkness or is even the rapid phase of a nystagmus.

In a detailed study, Sparks and Mays (1980) demonstrated that the cell discharges that precede a saccade do not seem to contain information relating to either the direction or the amplitude of a saccade that is about to happen. This finding is obviously partly in conflict with the idea of a movement field, but it emphasizes the fact that the behavior of the SC cells with respect to the saccade is different from that of the *premotor neurons* (which belong to the pontine and midbrain reticular formation), whose discharges precisely code the characteristics of the eye movement that is about to happen (in particular, its amplitude). In contrast, no cells have been found in this species with discharges that are clearly related to head movements. In the *cat* there are cells that discharge in response to a saccadic movement, some preceding it (as in the monkey), others discharging during its occurrence (Peck et al. 1980). In addition, the cat has cells with discharges associated with head movement.

Thus the SC appears to participate in mechanisms that direct the gaze toward a target, that is, mechanisms assuring the placing of the target's image on the retinal macula ("centralization," "foveation," "visual capture"), while the appropriate orientation is achieved by eye movements or head movements or both (Sparks & Mays 1986).

Other Noteworthy Response Characteristics
As we have just described, some of the response characteristics of SC cells are more or less directly correlated with the direction of the gaze or, if we are prepared to speculate beyond that simple behavioral description, with the focusing of attention not only in the visual domain but also in the other sensory modalities, particularly the auditory and the somaesthetic. Whereas the superficial layers are exclusively visuorecipient, the intermediate layers respond also to auditory and somesthetic stimuli, sometimes with a convergence between modalities (Stein et al. 1976).

A very interesting cell type is one that is excited by complex sounds. In some of these cells, the preferred sound stimulus is from a source moving in the direction corresponding with the optimal direction of movement for a visual target that is also an effective stimulus. We have described the observations leading to a spatial auditory map in SC in more detail elsewhere (Buser & Imbert 1992).

As for those cells that react to both visual and somesthetic stimuli, in some cases (e.g., hamster and cat) general somesthetic sensitivity and visual topography seem to be in register in some respects (Finlay et al. 1978). Thus the representation of the central visual region coincides with the somesthetic representation of the face, while more peripheral visual zones converge with more distal and caudal somesthetic representations (figure 5.8). In the monkey, the representation is such that the receptive fields for the foveal area also receive facial inputs, and the cells responding to the peripheral visual field respond to forelimb somesthetic fields.

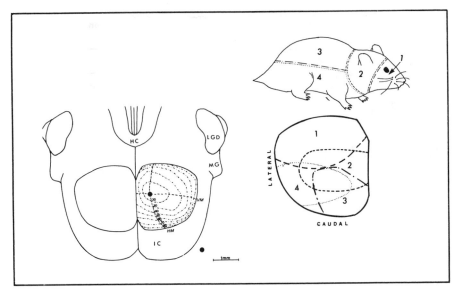

Figure 5.8
Sensory maps in the hamster superior colliculus. *Left,* Visual mapping. On the right
SC, the optic disk is shown as a dot and the horizontal meridian (HM) and vertical
meridian (VM) zeros are shown by dashed lines with the equal contours represented
as dot/dash lines (thus different from figure 5.6). IC, inferior colliculus; MG, LGD,
medial geniculate, and dorsal lateral geniculate bodies, respectively. HC, habenula.
Right, Somesthetic topography. 1, orofacial regions; 2, neck and ears; 3, dorsal and 4,
ventral parts of the body. (From Finlay et al. 1978)

1.2 THE PRETECTUM

We cannot discuss the responses of SC cells without also considering
those of the pretectum, the neighboring structure at the junction of
the midbrain and the diencephalon.

STRUCTURE

Anatomically, there are a whole series of different nuclei distinguishable at this level (the complete list borders on the tedious) that are
common to several mammalian groups (cat, Kanaseki & Sprague
1974, Avendaño & Juetschke 1980; *Saimiri,* Hutchins and Weber
1985). These neurons fall into essentially three groups (figure 5.9):

• Nuclei of the posterior commissure, with dorsal, lateral, and ventral
divisions
• A dorsolateral group of nuclei, comprising a pars lateralis and a

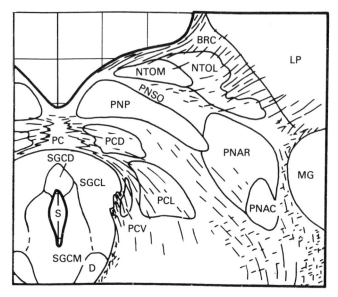

Figure 5.9
Drawing of a frontal section across the pretectum (cat). PCD, PCL, PCV, dorsal, lateral, and ventral nuclei of the posterior commissure (PC); PNP, PNAR, PNAC, posterior, anterior reticular, anterior compact pretectal nuclei; PNSO, suboptic pretectal nucleus; NTOM, NTOL, pars medialis and pars lateralis of the nucleus of the tractus opticus; BRC, brachium of the superior colliculus; LP, lateral posterior nucleus; MG, medial geniculate nucleus; D, Darkschevich nucleus; PC, posterior commissure; SGCD, SGCL, SGCM, pars dorsalis, lateralis, and medialis of the substantia grisea centralis; S, sylvian aqueduct (mid line). (From Avendaño & Juretschke 1980)

pars medialis of the nuclei of the optic tract and the pretectal olivary nucleus

• An intermediate group of nuclei comprising the posterior pretectal nuclei, the suboptic, anterior, and median

Histological (degeneration) studies have shown that the pretectal olivary nuclei, posterior and median, and the nucleus of the optic tract receive direct projections from the contralateral retina, whereas fibers from the ipsilateral retina only reach the olivary nucleus and the nucleus of the optic tract.

FUNCTION

The nucleus of the optic tract has special properties in that its cells (1) are sensitive to diffuse illumination, (2) are endowed with receptive fields often like those of the retinal GC, (3) are found to behave particularly frequently as phasic/tonic with a burst of ON discharge at the onset of the light stimulus but also by a maintained discharge throughout illumination, or (4) they are phasic/tonic OFF, only responding when the stimulus ends but with a discharge that carries on for some time. These types of activity are compatible with the long-recognized fact that this region of the pretectum is involved with control of pupil diameter: The ON type cells excite the pupillo-constrictor neurons of nerve III, whereas the OFF cells are in contrast inhibitory on these same neurons.

In the other pretectal nuclei, the response characteristics of the cells resemble those of the SC, in particular by their sensitivity to movements, especially vertical and horizontal. One population of cells responds to the movement of targets in the sagittal plane that are approaching or receding from the eye. These latter are probably concerned with another set of functions attributable to the pretectum, namely, accommodation and convergence, which are the other two components of the "fixation triad."

1.3 THE ACCESSORY OPTICAL SYSTEM

STRUCTURE

In mammals, notably in the rat, the accessory optical system arises from axons of retinal origin that separate from the normal pathway after the chiasm and comprise two bundles, one inferior, the other superior (figure 5.10; see Hayhow 1959, Marg 1973).

The *inferior tract* (AOS-IF) is formed from a group of axons that deviate from the postchiasm trajectory, that is, after crossing. These fibers run alongside the cerebral peduncle and terminate in a nucleus situated in the ventral midbrain, medial with respect to the substantia nigra, called the *medial terminal nucleus* (NTM).

The *superior tract* (AOS-S) leaves the principal optic pathway at the brachium of the superior colliculus. These fibers run along the lateral surface of the brain and comprise three components: (1) anterior fibers that rejoin the NTM, therefore having the same termination as the AOS-IF; (2) medial fibers which, having left the trajectory of the principal optical pathway in the ventroposterior region of the LGB, plunge ventrally toward the NTM, with some of them sending collaterals to another nucleus, the terminal lateral nucleus (NTL); and (3) posterior fibers coming from the edge of the brachium of the superior colliculus, with some of them ending in yet another nucleus, the terminal dorsal nucleus (NTD), and others ending in the NTM or NTL. The NTD is close to the nucleus of the optic tract (NTO).

Most of these projections come from the contralateral retina; the ipsilateral population is very sparse. Finally, note that in the primates there are only the two dorsal nuclei, NTL and NTD. The nonmammals have a simpler arrangement in this respect, since only a single collection of optical fibers has been described with a nontectal destination. It is called the *basal optic root* and terminates in a nucleus called the nucleus of the basal optic root.

The ganglion cells that innervate the AOS in the cat are the γ type (see chapter 1, section 7.3). In this case, the axons to this destination do not bifurcate. They also arrive at centers other than those belonging to the AOS. Remember, however, that (even more so in the rabbit than in the cat) the majority of cells projecting to the AOS are localized in a particular region of the retina (cf. Simpson 1984), namely, the horizontal streak in the rabbit and the area centralis in the cat. It is curious that in the pigeon they leave neither the fovea nor the "red area" (see chapter 1, section 3).

To fully understand the AOS it is worth noting that the AOS is definitely connected to the inferior olive, to the "vestibular division" of the cerebellum (uvula, paraflocculus; see Simpson et al. 1979), to the oculomotor nuclei, and to the pretectum. All these structures receive connections from the nuclei of the AOS. (Do not forget, however, that our knowledge in this respect comes chiefly from the pigeon.)

FUNCTION

Essentially these data are gained from two aspects: first, from single-unit measurements in the AOS, second from ablations of parts of the system. In a fairly general way, the responses of neurons of the NTM, NTD, and NTL nuclei can be classified as follows:

Preferred excitation is by a relatively large, textured, stimulus. Orientation selectivity is seen, with a preferred direction for optimal excitation and another direction in which an inhibition of the resting discharge is seen. The two directions (for excitation and for inhibition) are not in general collinear, that is, one is not a continuation of the other (this happens but is very uncommon). There is an optimal sensitivity for slow movements (optimal velocity between 0.5° and 10°/s for the cat). Finally, and most important, the distribution of optimal directions in both cat and rabbit is not random but certain

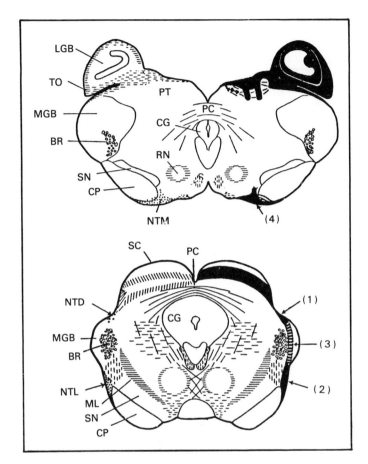

Figure 5.10
Trajectory of the accessory optic tract (TOA) in the posterior diencephalon and the
anterior mesencephalon (cat). The planes of the two frontal sections are separated by
about 2 mm. Axons that are degenerated after section of the contralateral optic tract
are shown in black. (1) indicates the origin of the TOA which has a lower trajectory
(3) that terminates (4) in the medial terminal nucleus (NTM); other terminations are in
the lateral and dorsal terminal nuclei (NTL and NTD). LGB, MGB, lateral and medial
geniculate bodies; TO, optic tract; PT, pretectal region; BR, brachium of the inferior
colliculus; SN, substantia nigra; CP, cerebral peduncle; RN, red nucleus; CG, central
grey matter; SC, superior colliculus; PC, posterior commissure; ML, medial lemniscus.
(From Hayhow 1959)

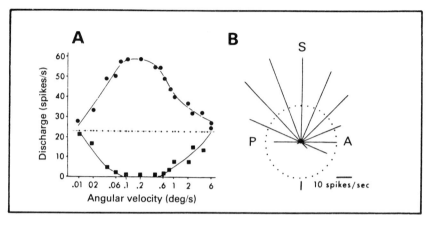

Figure 5.11
Properties of neurons in the medial terminal nucleus of the accessory optical system
in the rabbit. A, Velocity selectivity. The stimulus spot makes a vertical movement
either upward (circles) or downward (squares) at different angular velocities. Note the
optimal speed for which the discharge frequency is either maximal or minimal. B,
Directional sensitivity of the cell. For each direction of movement of the spot at the
same speed of 0.5°/s, the response is proportional to the length of the straight lines
that also show the direction. S, upward (superior); I, downward (inferior) movements;
P, movements to the rear (posterior, i.e., in a temporal direction), or A, to the front
(anterior). (From Simpson 1984)

orientations clearly predominate. Thus in the rabbit there are three
preferred directions: upward and slightly toward the rear (temporal);
downward and also slightly to the rear; horizontal and in the nasal
direction (figure 5.11).

This arrangement (particularly in the rabbit) poses two questions:
On the one hand, these preferred directions closely resemble those
already seen in the retina and there might well be in this case only an
isomorphic transfer of the retinal properties to the nucleus. However,
such orientational preferences are also seen in the cat at this level,
whereas they are scarcely discernable in its retina. Thus in the cat
there must be some local neuronal mechanism acting (possibly involving inhibitory interneurons). On the other hand, it has been proposed that these preferential directions coincide more or less with
the orientations of the three semicircular canals and that the role of
the AOS might well be some sort of proprioceptive one, detecting
movement of the animal itself with respect to the environment, a
function that would complement the role of the vestibular system by

using visual information to stabilize the head and the eyes with respect to some reference.

At present, data are lacking that can confirm or deny the above hypothetical role of the AOS in postural control. At most, there are a few hints from the fact that optikinetic nystagmus is reduced by NTM lesions in the chinchilla, as it is also in the pigeon, although in the latter by lesions of structures that are in the immediate neighborhood or are homologous (Gioanni et al. 1983).

Other functions have equally been attributed to the AOS. Earlier work suggested an involvement in neuroendocrine reflexes, in particular funnelling visual messages toward the pineal gland. More recent experiments in the monkey suggested that the AOS is the most peripheral structure in the neuroaxis that enables an animal to discriminate luminances after a concurrent ablation of both SC and the cortical visual areas (Pasik & Pasik 1982).

1.4 THE RETINOHYPOTHALAMIC PATHWAY

Finally, there are other fibers that also leave the main visual pathway to terminate in the suprachiasmic nuclei. These play an important role in the control of circadian rhythms.

2 THE LATERAL GENICULATE BODY

2.1 STRUCTURE AND PROJECTIONS

The lateral geniculate body (LGB) comprises two divisions, one dorsal (pars dorsalis, LGBd), the other ventral (pars ventralis, LGBv). Lateral and dorsal to the LGBd is a laminated structure called the perigeniculate nucleus (PG).

The LGBd constitutes the main "relay" in the visual pathway to the cortex and is the one that we will concentrate on here. The LGBv in this context has only an accessory function. The PG belongs to a collection of nuclei which, under the umbrella title of reticular nucleus (nucleus reticularis), surrounds the thalamus like an eggshell.

GENERAL MORPHOLOGY AND THE TOPOGRAPHY OF THE RETINOGENICULATE PROJECTIONS

Strictly speaking, there is no common organizational plan for the structure of the LGBd in the different groups of mammals. Therefore our discussion will be limited to some well-studied examples, those of the cat, monkey, rodents, and rabbit.

Cat

In carnivores (see, e.g., Bishop et al. 1962b, Peters & Palay 1966) the LGBd appears in frontal section as a curved structure, convex on its dorsal face, and in sagittal section as a horizontal S-shape curling downward anteriorly and upward posteriorly (figure 5.12). Adjacent and medial to the LGBd is a nuclear mass called the posterior nucleus (PO; see also figure 5.43B and Rioch 1929) to which visual projections also arrive (probably indirectly, at least in part). This nucleus may well be part of the lateral-posterior-pulvinar group of nuclei, which we shall consider again later in section 3.2 (Kingston et al. 1969).

So far, not many studies of the LGBv have been made in the cat. It is a nucleus of complex shape, squeezed between the optic tract, the perigeniculate nucleus, and another part of the nucleus reticularis. It includes a certain number of subsidiary nuclei and receives inputs from the optic tract, from the LGBd, from the SC, and from the visual cortex. In contrast, it does not seem to project to the cortex and is not therefore a relay in the main pathway to the cortex.

We now examine the projections from the retina (and the visual field) to the LGBd (Guillery 1969, Guillery et al. 1980). A first division into three principal layers may be summarized as follows (figure 5.12):

• The three principal layers, ranging dorsoventrally, called A, A1, and B (the *laminar LGB*)
• Two intermediate layers, called *interlaminar*, A-A1, A1-B
• Medially, a cellular mass, the lamination of which remains controversial, called the *medial intralaminar nucleus* (MIN)

A further elaboration divides "layer B" into several sublayers called (dorsoventrally) C, C1, C2, and C3. Layer C contains more of the larger cells (*magnocellular layer*) than layers C1 to C3, which are considered the parvocellular layers (see figure 5.16). This more detailed classification will be most often used from now on.

Each laminar LGBd receives projections corresponding to the whole contralateral hemifield, namely, the fibers from the temporal ipsilateral hemiretina (about 40%) and those from the contralateral nasal hemiretina (about 60%). One of the essential factors in this organization is that there is in general very little anatomical convergence discernable between the ipsilateral and contralateral connections. Thus: (1) layers A, C, and C2 only receive contralateral fibers, (2) layers A1 and C1 only ipsilateral fibers, (3) layer C3 has no retinal

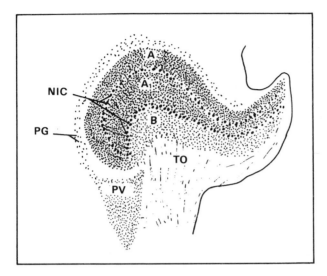

Figure 5.12
Parasagittal section of cat LGB. The front of the nucleus is to the left, the rear to the right. The lamination is shown and the layers A, A1 and B are indicated (see text for the subdivisions of B). TO, optic tract; PG, perigeniculate nucleus; PV, pars ventralis of LGB; NIC, nuclei in the central interlaminar layers (A-A1 and A1-B). (From Peters & Palay 1966)

input, and (4) only the "intralaminal" regions A-A1 and A1-C (or A1-B in the older classification) receive inputs from the two hemiretinas (and might in this respect be regarded as "binocular").

There is a topographical correspondence between the LGBd locations and places in the visual field, the latter being specified by their azimuth (a) and elevation (e) as follows (figure 5.13): Isoazimuth planes ($a = k$) are represented parasagittally and isoelevation planes ($e = k$) are transversely (i.e., parafrontally) inclined at 40° with respect to the frontal plane in the sense "superior is anterior, inferior is posterior."

The projection of the inferior hemifield ($e<0°$) in the anterior LGBd occupies a larger volume than the superior hemifield ($e>0$) does in the posterior LGBd. The lateral parts of the hemifield ($a>0$) project laterally and the central part medially. Each central zone of the visual field, namely, that near the vertical meridian zero ($a = 0$), projects to each LGB (figure 5.14; see Sanderson & Sherman 1971).

Isoazimuth contours are not equidistant for identical angular separations (90 μm/deg near the center and 50 μm/deg more laterally);

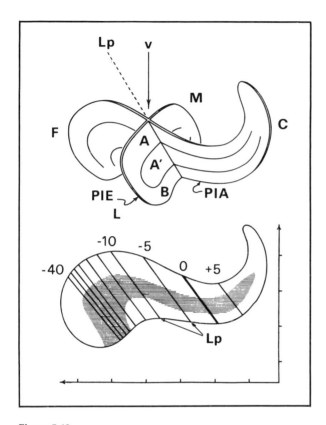

Figure 5.13
Perspective view of cat LGB. *Above:* A simplified representation of the divisions A,
A1, and B. The sections are drawn as if seen from a point situated to the rear, higher
and more lateral than the nucleus. FC (frontal, caudal) a parasagittal plane representing
a plane of isoazimuth (PIA) and a parafrontal plane LM (lateral, medial) representing
a plane of isoelevation (PIE). The intersection of the two of them essentially constitutes
the representation of the fixation point (dashed line). The lower hemifield ($e<0°$) is
represented anterior and the upper hemifield ($e>0°$) posterior. *Below:* Equal elevation
lines are shown, with their preferred directions indicated, in the lower figure, which
represents a parasagittal section of LGB, anterior to the left, posterior to the right.
Each line of projection LP in fact represents a "projection column" (PC of figure 5.15)
embracing all the cells receiving inputs from the same point in the visual field. (From
Bishop et al. 1962)

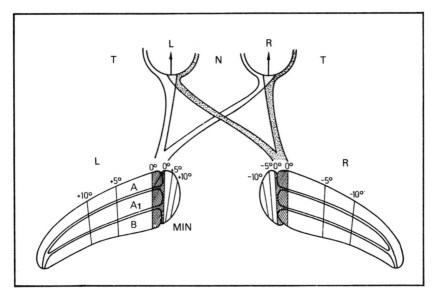

Figure 5.14
Diagram of the visual projections to LGBd proper and to the MIN nucleus (cat).
Representation of the thalamic nucleus in frontal section. The vertical lines are equal
azimuth lines (azimuth values indicated). The hatched zone represents the region of
the nasal/temporal overlap. L, R, left and right eye, then left and right LGB. T, N,
temporal and nasal retinal; A, A1, and B, see figure 5.12. (From Sanderson & Sherman
1971)

the same applies to isoelevation contours. Consequently, the central
field enjoys a more extensive representation than the space it occupies in the retina. We shall see this even more clearly in the cortex.
A *magnification factor* is defined as the amplification of the space (volume), relatively greater or less, occupied by the projection of unit
visual angle. This gives a quantitative measure of the relative importance of the projection from one part of the retinal area relative to
another.

A third dimension is specified by a *projection column,* which corresponds spatially with a given azimuth and elevation and which
crosses the various layers. Effectively, each column represents the
collection of cells receiving information from the same part of the
visual field subtending an angle of 2° to 3° (figure 5.15; see Sanderson
1977).

The layers A1 and C1 with ipsilateral projections are less extensive
than the layers A, C, and C2. This fact should be considered with

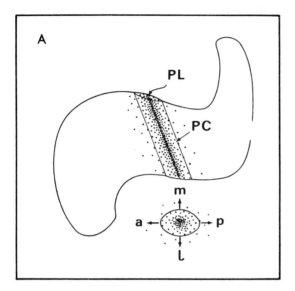

Figure 5.15
Parasagittal section in the dorsal LGB, illustrating the arrangement of all the cells
having the same receptive field for the same direction of gaze. This projection is
according to a projection line (PL) and the cells are grouped into a projection column
(PC). Below is a transverse section of such a column showing the medial (m), lateral
(l), anterior (a), and posterior (p) directions. (From Sanderson 1971)

respect to the existence in this species (as in many others) of a lateral
region of monocular vision. The results seem to confine the zone
represented in layers A1 and C1 to 45°, which suggests a binocular
field of about 90°. This is a value like that determined by other experimental approaches (see chapter 1, section 5.2).

There is also a considerable body of experiments on the special
retino-geniculate projections in feline albino mutants. In the Siamese
cat, an albino strain, a certain contingent of fibers that ought to remain ipsilateral travel apparently off-course to the contralateral
LGBd. These terminate in an area of the A1 layer (called *abA1*) that,
being part of the most lateral section of A1, should receive fibers
coming from the most lateral part of the temporal ipsilateral retina
("lateral normal segment" of Cooper et al. [1979]). This modification
does not, however, represent a simple slippage of the *line of decussation* (see figure 1.12), which separates the ipsilateral projection area
of the retina from the contralateral, but implies that in these animals
there has arisen some overlap of ipsilaterally projecting neurons with

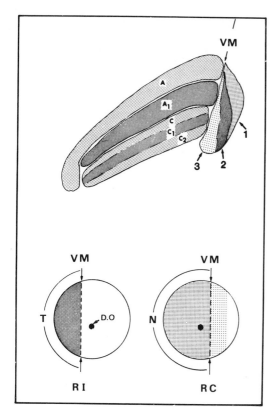

Figure 5.16
Diagram of the distribution of different retinal regions—ipsilateral retina (RI), contralateral retina (RC)—in the laminar LGB and nucleus MIN. The temporal RI (T) and the nasal RC (N) and at least 20% of the temporal RC have separate representations in the different divisions of LGB (as shown by the corresponding shading and symbols). VM, vertical meridian; DO, optic disk. For definitions of A, A1, C, C1, and C2 see text. 1, 2, and 3 mark the three distinguishably different divisions in nucleus MIN. (From Rowe & Dreher 1982)

those that project contralaterally from the lateral, temporal retinal regions.

As for the topographic distribution of projections in the medial interlaminar nucleus, or MIN (figure 5.16; see Dreher & Sefton 1978, Rowe & Dreyer 1982), it is almost universally agreed that there is no clear laminar organization in this structure. But this does not exclude in any way an "in register" arrangement of projections from the periphery (the retina). The arrangement comprises a general division into three "vertical" sections, and it is in this respect that a new

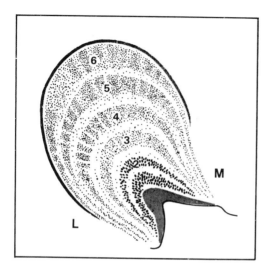

Figure 5.17
Frontal section of macaque
LGB. M, L, medial and lateral
sides. The magnocellular layers
1 and 2 are in the ventral region
with the parvocellular layers 3,
4, 5, and 6 above them (From
Szentagothai 1973)

situation arises. The most medial section receives the "usual" contralateral afferents (i.e., from the nasal part of the contralateral retina);
the intermediate section receives afferents from the temporal part of
the ipsilateral retina; and afferents from the *temporal contralateral retina*
(i.e., those concerned with the ipsilateral visual hemifield) arrive in
the third section. We will consider below with what type of retinal
afferents this crossed projection concerned with the ipsilateral visual
hemifield might correspond.

The arrangement of projections is such that contours of equal elevation are ranged from anterior (positive elevations) to posterior (negative elevations), with the equal-azimuth contours being arranged in
such a way that the central projection is sited laterally and the peripheral projection medially.

Macque

In primates, the LGBd comprises six concentric layers that are convex
dorsally and are easily seen in transverse (frontal) sections, at least
in the posterior parts of the nucleus (figure 5.17; see Szentagothai
1973). The two ventral (magnocellular) layers (1 and 2) are made up
of large cells and the other four (parvocellular) layers (3, 4, 5, and
6), more dorsal, comprise small cells. In some species (baboon, for
example), as many as eight layers may be found. The organization
of the projections in the macaque are well understood (Malpeli &
Baker 1975). They are described, based on microelectrode investiga-

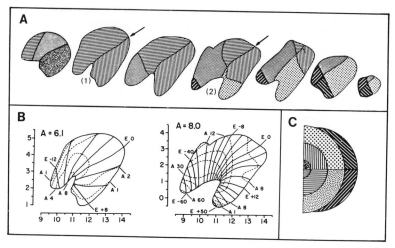

Figure 5.18
Distribution of the right visual hemifield in the left LGB in macaque. *A,* Serial frontal
sections of the LGBd from posterior (left) to anterior (extreme right). Note the projection of the fovea posterior and that of the monocular crescent anterior. *B,* Two frontal
sections, corresponding respectively to (1) and (2) in *A,* the equal azimuth lines
(dashed) and the equal elevation lines (solid curves) are shown. The arrows in *A* show
the projection of the horizontal meridian. *C,* Identification of the parts of the visual
field, which is divided into a foveal zone (up to 2.5°), a perifoveal zone (up to 17°), a
peripheral binocular zone, and finally the crescent of monocular vision. The upper
and lower quadrants are shown separately. (From Malpeli & Baker 1975)

tions, using the coordinates of elevation (*e*) and azimuth (*a*) (see chapter 2, section 8).

A discrete region of the visual field projects as a column running
between the (deep) ventral fissure and the surface (in other words,
we see that a "point" in visual space is represented by a "projection
column"). Thus the locus of points forming a line on the retina becomes a surface that crosses the LGB dorsoventrally. Therefore, a
point in the visual field defined by (*a*) and (*e*) (and situated at the
intersection of two lines corresponding to that point) will be represented by the intersection of two surfaces, one of equal azimuth, the
other of equal elevation. In summary, the representation of the visual
fields in the LGB constitutes two families of intersecting surfaces, one
for (*a*), the other for (*e*).

The lines of equal elevation constitute planes oriented anterior/
posterior, with all of them diverging from the ventral fissure like a
fan (figure 5.18). The horizontal meridian divides the LGB into two

parts, one medial and superior for negative elevations (below the horizon), the other lateral and inferior for positive elevations (above the horizon).

The equal-azimuth lines of the visual field constitute concave planes with respect to the ventral fissure of the LGB. The azimuths (a) nearest to the median plane are posterior in the nucleus and the most peripheral are anterior. In other words, the central zone of the visual field projects to the posterior third of the nucleus, the peripheral binocular field to the anterior two thirds, with the crescent-shaped monocular field being completely anterior. Here, as in the cat, the foveal region enjoys a representation that is significantly larger, relatively, than the proportion occupied by it in the retina.

With respect to the structure of LGB, there are six layers posteriorly, four layers centrally, and two layers anteriorly. Note that the layers are numbered from 1 to 6 in the ventrodorsal direction with layers 1 and 2 being magnocellular and the more dorsal layers, 3 to 6, being parvocellular. We may summarize the arrangement of a visual hemifield (ipsilateral temporal hemiretina + contralateral nasal hemiretina) as shown in table 5.1. Note that the foveal and parafoveal projections involve six layers, two magnocellular and four parvocellular, with layers 1, 4 and 6 representing the contralateral hemiretina and layers 2, 3, and 5 the ipsilateral hemiretina. The rest of the binocular visual field (for eccentricities >17°) only involves four layers (1, 6, 2, and 3) and the monocular crescent of the contralateral hemiretina only two layers (1 and 6). Notice also that, as already pointed out, the retinal discontinuity of the blind spot in the nasal hemiretina is clearly identifiable in the projection of the contralateral nasal hemiretina in layers 1, 4, and 6 by small areas of "nonprojection" that are in

Table 5.1. Laminar arrangement of a visual hemifield in primate LGB

	Laminae	
	Contralateral (Nasal Retina)	Ipsilateral (Temporal Retina)
Foveal projection (posterior third of LGB)	1, 4, 6	2, 3, 5
Eccentricity >17° (anterior two thirds of LGB)	1, 6	2, 3
Monocular crescent (anterior pole of LGB)	1, 6	

line, as would be expected from the rule of "projection column" representation of a point.

An attractive suggestion is that the the primate lamination of LGB is derived from a basic arrangement of four layers, two parvocellular and two magnocellular, the change to six layers being effected by a folding back of the parvocellular layers in the posterior parts of the nucleus to which the central part of the visual field around the fovea projects.

Finally, the macaque LGB contains, apart from the magnocellular and parvocellular layers, *interlaminar regions*, which separate the layers from each other. Note also that the *S region* has been defined in the deepest part of the nucleus near the fissure. We will see later that a zone such as this, which is very restricted in size, can nevertheless have a functional significance.

Rodents

The arrangements are different in this group since, as we know, only 5% to 10% of the fibers at the chiasm stay ipsilateral. This endows a considerable preponderance of projection from the contralateral retina compared with that from the ipsilateral retina with its limited representation. The situation may be summarized as follows, using the pigmented rat as the exemplar. There is no very clear cytoarchitectonic laminar arrangement in the nucleus. The topography of the projections is such that the representation of the lower part of the visual field (the upper retina) is chiefly posterior and lateral in the nucleus, and that of the upper field (lower retina) is anterior and on the dorsal surface.

The temporal hemifield (nasal hemiretina) projects anteriorly and ventrolateraly; the nasal hemifield (temporal hemiretina) projects posteriorly and dorsomedially.

The uncrossed fibers come from a crescent situated in the extreme lower part of the temporal retina (corresponding with a portion of the visual field sited upper nasal). The ganglion cells of this extreme temporal area of the retina do not, however, all project ipsilaterally: Only 25% of them project by the ipsilateral route, with the majority continuing to project contralaterally.

These fibers with an ipsilateral origin, which arrive in the dorsomedial part of the LGB, correspond to the upper nasal (50°, nasal, lateral) region of visual space. It is thus in the neighborhood of, or precisely within, this projection zone of the ipsilateral temporal crescent (i.e., in the dorsomedial zone of LGB) that the overlap region is found between ipsilateral and contralateral projections that can support binocular interactions (Reese & Jeffrey 1983, Lund et al. 1974). Here also, particularly in the rat and the mouse families, differences can be seen between pigmented and albino mutant strains (Dräger & Olsen 1980). In albinos there is a reduction in the projection of ipsilateral fibers and a smaller region of binocularity.

Having noted that the dorsal LGB of rat shows no lamination, cytoarchitectonically it is possible to distinguish a succession of "layers" in the dorsomedial region of the nucleus by studying terminal degenerations following pathway lesions. Hayhow et al. (1962) numbered these "layers" 2 to 6, which (unlike "layer 1," which has a purely contralateral input) are characterized by ipsilateral and contralateral overlap in their origins and could potentially subserve a bilateral innervation (see table 5.2 for a summary). The largest projection is from the median horizontal strip, that is, from the region with the greatest receptor density, in particular in the temporal retina (see chapter 1, seciton 4.2).

Rabbit
In the case of the rabbit, cytoarchitectonic studies recognize at least two zones, a peripheral one (α) and a medial one (β). But here, as in rodents, no real lamination is seen just by visually examining cell distributions.

In contrast, degeneration studies once again show series of areas sometimes characterized by a total dominance of contralateral inputs (zone 1, which practically covers zone α) and sometimes more complex regions with both ipsilateral and contralateral inputs (occupying zone β). Thus Giolli and Guthrie (1969) specify a zone 2 and a zone 4 where fibers of ipsilateral origin predominate and a zone 3 with a predominantly contralateral input (figure 5.19).

Table 5.2. Arrangements in the "layers" of rat LGB

"Layers"	Origin	Bilaterality
1	Only contralateral	Zero
2	Mainly ipsilateral	Slight
3	Mainly contralateral	Clear
4	Mainly ipsilateral	Clear
5	Mainly contralateral	Clear
6	Mainly ipsilateral	Clear

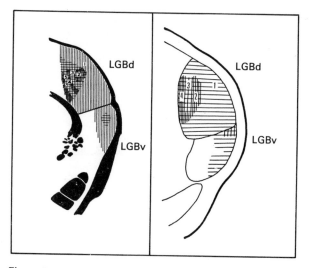

Figure 5.19
Rat (*left*) and rabbit (*right*) LGB in frontal section. Notice particularly the dorsal (LGBd) and ventral (LGBv) parts of the two nuclei as well as the terminations of the crossed and the uncrossed afferent fibers designated by the symbols (below) that alone encourage the idea of a certain "lamination" in these animals also. In the *rat*, zone 1 only comprises crossed fibers (vertical hatching) and zones 2, 4, and 6 (thin hatching) have predominantly uncrossed fibers, while regions 3 and 5 (cross-hatching) show an overlap of crossed and uncrossed fibers. In the *rabbit*, zone 1 coincides in practice with the LGBdα identified by cytoarchitectonics and only contains crossed fibers (horizontal hatching); zones 2, 3, and 4 correspond with cytoarchitectonic region β; layers 2 and 4 are predominantly uncrossed, and in zone 3 there is an overlap between crossed and uncrossed (see text). (From Hayhow et al. 1962 and Giolli & Guthrie 1969)

HISTOLOGICAL AND SYNAPTIC FUNCTIONAL ORGANIZATION

A certain amount of data is available on the fine structural organization of the LGB that help our understanding of the integrative mechanisms that are special for the nucleus. Unfortunately, the data are somewhat fragmentary for species other than the cat, for which they are relatively complete, so what follows will be largely concerned with that species and only incidentally with others.

Cat

Cell types. All researchers agree in recognizing two types of cell in the LGB: the principal cells (PC) constitute the units in the thalamocortical "relay"; the others are intrageniculate cells or interneurons, being neurons with short axons (or even some, depending on authors and species, that lack axons totally) which belong to the Golgi type II (GC) classification (see figure 5.21A).

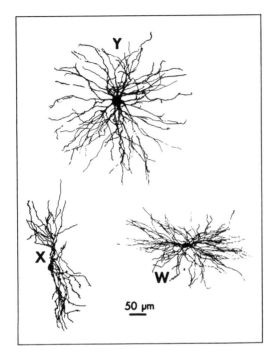

Figure 5.20
Camera lucida drawings of the cells receiving X, Y, and W inputs in LGBd. These particular cells were identified by neurophysiology and intracellular injection of HRP. The scale is parallel to the LGB lamination in which each structure is found. (From Friedländer & Sherman 1981)

Thanks to intracellular marking combined with physiological investigations, three types of PC are recognized now. The essential conclusion from these combined structural/functional experiments is that each morphological class of geniculocortical neuron receives from a given type of retinogeniculate axon, whether a functionally Y type afferent from an α GC, or an X from a β GC, or finally a W from a γ GC. From that discovery we are led to consider that the retinogeniculocortical system is organized into parallel pathways that are structurally and functionally distinct. It is thus justified to talk of geniculate X, Y, and W cells (figure 5.20; see Hoffmann & Stone 1973b, Hoffmann et al. 1972, Dreher & Sefton 1978, Friedländer & Sherman 1981, Hitchcock & Hickey 1983, Wilson 1982).

A geniculate X neuron has a small or moderate cell body and has dendrites that are predominantly arranged normal to the orientation of the geniculate lamina in which it is found. These tortuous dendrites have "grape cluster" ("en grappe") terminal swellings. A type Y geniculate neuron has a large cell body, with dendrites radiating all around it without any preferred orientation and without specialized "grape cluster" terminal swellings. The W cells have small or moderate-sized cell bodies, and their dendritic orientation is at 90° to that of the X cells, that is, tangentially with respect to the geniculate layer that contains them. The axons of these "relay" cells have been traced in their trajectory to the cortex. Their diameter, as in the projection from the retina to geniculate, is moderate for X cells, large for Y cells, and narrow for the W cells. Some axons send off collaterals, very rarely into LGB itself but usually during their traversing the PG nucleus.

It is also worth noting the distribution of the X, Y, and W cells in the different parts of LGB (A, A1, C layers and nucleus MIN). Essentially:

• Layers A and A1 have solely X and Y cells.
• Layer C has Y cells in the upper layer C (magnocellular) and W cells in the more ventral parvocellular layers C1 and C2.
• In MIN there is a clear predominance of Y cells with some X and W.

[The above classification in fact only represents the less subtle aspects of the more refined classification that some authors (initially Guillery, 1969, and then others) have provided, based on Golgi impregnation techniques. Broadly speaking, this distinguishes five cell types in LGB. We have decided not to follow this scheme rigidly here but without in any way denying its interest. The division of these classes into the X, Y, and W categories is not entirely direct. Roughly, class 1 are Y, class 2 has some X some Y, class 3 are W, class 4 has some W, and class 5 once more is Y. Discussion on the exact correspondences continues.]

Axonal terminations. There are three types of axonal termination in LGB:

1. *Retinal afferents* (Ra). These have become separate, more or less, before entering their final destination layer in LGB. Afferents corresponding to a given point in visual space terminate, as we have seen, along a column crossing all the layers A, A1, and C. The terminal arborization of each afferent occupies a practically cylindrical zone either in A, in A1, or in the C layers, depending on the ipsilateral or contralateral origin of the afferent.

[To begin with, let us summarize the distribution of the different axonal types X, Y, and W in the different divisions of LGB (recalling their possible modes of distribution to the SC). X axons terminate essentially in A, A1, and C (magnocellular region) without sending collaterals to the SC (see chapter 1, section 7.3). Y axons, in contrast, divide and send one collateral to the SC, another to the laminar LGB, and a third to nucleus MIN. The fibers from the contralateral eye (nasal retina) terminate in A, C (magnocellular region), and also C2. Fibers from the ipsilateral eye only serve A1. Note also that fibers from the contralateral temporal retina only end in MIN. W axons, for their part, reach the MIN and the C layers (essentially parvocellular regions), C and C2 for the contralateral eye, C1 for the ipsilateral. Some W fibers coming from the contralateral temporal retina end here, again exclusively in the MIN (which thus comprises about half Y afferent inputs and half W afferents; these two categories of afferents do not show any segregation here.)

Histological fine structure analysis provides an interesting index of the quantitative ratios between the numbers of retinal afferents of a given type (X, Y, or W) and the corresponding numbers of corresponding geniculate cells (X, Y, or W). Here we will discuss only the figures for X and Y cells. The retinogeniculate path comprises about 5 to 10 times more X than Y; in contrast, in the LGB that ratio is practically unity. If we now take into account that there are 4 or 5 times more neurons in the LGB than in the retina, we may conclude that each retinal X fiber innervates about 4 to 5 LGB X cells, whereas each Y input reaches 20 to 30 LGB Y cells. The nuclear system therefore enjoys a manifest amplification thanks to an abundant formation of input collaterals within LGB itself. We shall see that this process of divergence in favor of the Y cells happens once more at the cortical level.]

2. *Corticogeniculate inputs* (Cxa). In the cat, corticofugal projections have been demonstrated from area 17 to LGB (Holländer & Martinez-Millan 1975). These projections are organized topographically; however, it seems that a given cortical region sends fibers to all layers of LGB. Those coming from areas 18 and 19 are rarer and are essentially concerned with layers C.

3. *Other axonal and dendritic terminations.* There are some axon terminals from *perigeniculate nucleus cells* (PGa).

There are some axon collateral terminations from the principal cells (PCr). These do not exist in all species: they are particularly found in rat. Finally, there are possible axonal terminals from GCa interneurons; so far these have not always been formally identified by electron microscopy (EM).

Classes of synaptic connections.   EM studies have so far facilitated the identification of five types of synaptic contacts in the LGB. Founded on well agreed-upon structural criteria (degree of asymmetry of synaptic structure and shape of synaptic vesicles) these types (figure 5.21; see Szentagothei 1973) may be separately specified as follows:

• Synapses presumed to be excitatory with round, large, and pale vesicles (RLP): These constitute 10% of the total synapses in LGB and are linked with contacts from Ra retinal fibers.
• Synapses also presumed to be excitatory that have round, small, and dark vesicles (RSD). They constitute contacts from recurrent cortical inputs (Cxa) and are much more numerous than the above (50%).
• Excitatory synapses with round, large, and dark (RLD) vesicles: They belong to terminals of the collaterals of the PC (PCr).
• Synapses called F1 with flat vesicles and therefore presumed to be inhibitory: They are seen at the level of contacts with axons presumed to be from Golgi cells GCa, interneuronal axons or, according to recent studies (Montero & Scott 1981) axons from PG cells (PGa) on the dendrites of PC types.
• Paler synapses of the inhibitory type known as F2 (called "pleomorphic synapses" by some authors): These are visible on the dendrites of GCd where they contact a PCd and constitute a dendro-dendritic synapse presumed to be inhibitory. The GCd represent in this respect a *presynaptic dendrite.*

Types of intrageniculate circuitry.   Based on such data, it has been possible to suggest the types of interconnections that occur in LGB, of which figure 5.21 gives only a partial representation.

Under EM, *triad* elements are seen. In these, a retinal axon terminates by an RLP synapse simultaneously on a dendritic fold of a PC cell (PCd) and on an interneuron (GCd), the latter also elaborating an F2 dendro-dendritic contact with the PCd. The frequency of this sort of arrangement in subcortical stages of sensory systems (olfactory bulb, retina, thalamic "relay") clearly poses the question of their functional significance.

In the LGB these triads can be contained within structures of extreme complexity called glomeruli or "nests." Here, apart from Ra, are found PCd and GCd, probably axon terminals from GC (GCa) as well as corticofugal (Cxa) input terminals, others from PG (PGa), and

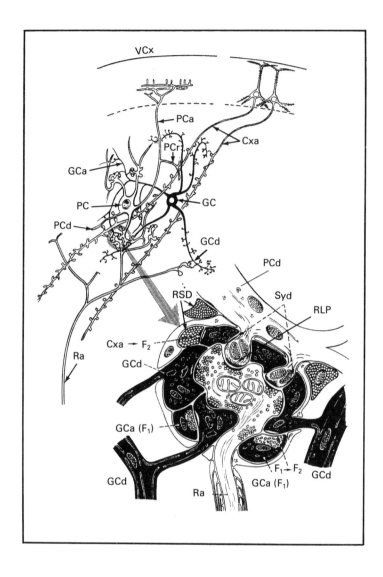

yet others that are recurrent collaterals from PC (PCx). These glomeruli have only been seen on the X type principal cells, where they are lcoated proximally on the dendrites at the level of the "grape cluster" ("en grappe") swellings. These glomeruli might well be entirely lacking among Y cells.

The X cells furnish an important system of recurrent collaterals of the PCr type, returning to the glomerulus or its vicinity and creating, via their contact on GCd, an *inhibitory* influence on the afferent system.

Y cells, more often than X cells, send collaterals to PG cells. These cells have been classified as GABAergic and make inhibitory contact with the PC.

Summary. It is clear that the LGB is far from a simple "relay," since the following functions are agreed to be present at this level: (1) negative feedback systems which for Y cells are effected via the perigeniculate system and for the X cells remain internal within the LGB itself and involving GC; (2) the possibility of feedforward inhibition via the triads; and (3) the existence of controlling influences from the cerebral cortex.

Neither is this list of controlling influences on LGB by any means complete, since it has now been shown that nonspecific inputs arising in the brainstem reticular formation also contact the LGB. These in-

---

◀ **Figure 5.21**
Histological organization of the LGB. *Above,* Diagram of a principal thalamocortical cell (PC) with its dendrites (PCd), the axon of which (PCa) terminates in the (striate) visual cortex (VCx), occasionally sending off a recurrent collateral (PCr), together with a diagram of a Golgi type II interneuron (GC) with its axon (GCa) and dendrites (GCd). Also projecting to the lateral geniculate are the axons (Cxa) of corticothalamic cells and the axons (Ra) of retinal origin. There is a certain amount of interconnection between these elements in glomeruli. *Below,* Detail of the structure of a glomerulus from EM data. A dendrite (PCd) of a principal cell can be seen with two prolongations, or spines, making contact with a retinal axon (Ra). Notice the axodendritic synapses, in general of the type round, large, pale (RLP; see text) at this level. Three interneuronal dendrites GCd also enter the glomerulus and are postsynaptic for retinal afferents (synapses Ra → GCd) but presynaptic for the dendrite PCd (dendrodendritic synapses GCd → PCd marked Syd, presumably inhibitory F2 types). Note also the triad arrangements (Ra → GCd → PCd). The axons of Golgi cells (GCa) are presynaptic on GCd dendrites (type F1 contacts, presumed inhibitory). The synaptic round, small, dark (RSD) formations are probably those of descending axons Cxa. They contact principal cells (Cxa → Pcd) but are also presynaptic on the dendrite of Golgi cells (GCd). F_1 and F_2 indicate flattened synaptic vesicles. Notice that there is no representation in this diagram of the axons of perigeniculate cells. (From Szentagothai 1973)

puts are considered to be linked to some control of selective attention processes that regulate visual information transfer from the thalamus. This reticular action could be indirect and mediated via a (cholinergic) inhibition of PG cells that are themselves inhibitory on the PC, as we have seen (Singer 1977).

Primates

Let us consider first the data on primate LGB that will finally lead to proposing a variety of parallelisms or contrasts with the feline case. We have seen above that in the macaque retina there exist essentially two types of ganglion cells, Pα and Pβ, which very likely correspond to the α and β cells in the cat and in parallel, show Y and X characteristics, respectively, in their functional properties. But it is also agreed that any third type of unit that corresponds with γ cells and W behavior is very rare or nonexistent in the primate.

That having been recognized, it is also now agreed that, as in the cat, the functional properties of the separate retinal channels with their specific (particularly temporal) characteristics for transferring visual information, are maintained throughout the pathway to the visual cortex. Thus there are, in LGB, once more found cells (Pc) with large cell bodies and wide axons as well as smaller cells with narrow axons (Dreher et al. 1976, Schiller & Malpelli 1978, Sherman et al. (1976b). As for the division of synaptic contacts between the optic fibers and the thalamocortical (Pc) cells, neurophysiological data which we shall discuss again later localizes X response units in both the parvo and magnocellular layers, whereas Y units are only found in the magnocellular layers.

2.2 FUNCTION

Functional data wil be presented chiefly with respect to the mechanisms of visual information transfer in the geniculate that are principally concerned with its spatial, temporal, and chromatic content (see, e.g., Freund 1973).

GENERAL TYPES OF SPONTANEOUS ACTIVITY

Let us take this opportunity briefly to describe the spontaneous activity that develops in darkness in the visual pathway in general (figure 5.22a; see also chapter 2, section 2.1, and chapter 3, section 3.5). The strength of this activity decreases from the optic tract (i.e., from the retinal ganglion cells), through the lateral geniculate body, and to the cortex. As some indication, the mean values of discharge rates are

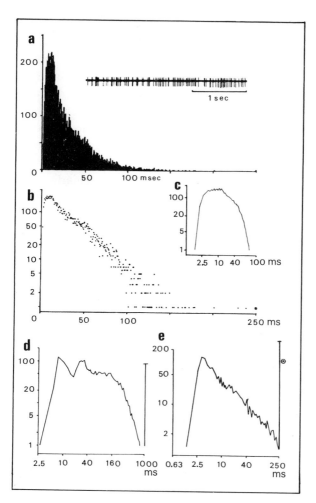

Figure 5.22
Quantitative analysis of spontaneous cell discharges in the visual pathway. *a, b, c,* Interspike interval histograms of an optic nerve fiber in the absence of stimulation (spontaneous activity), based on the measurement of 10542 intervals in 5 min. (*a*) Linear coordinates (inset, an example of a record). (*b*) Semi-log coordinates. (*c*) Log coordinates. *d*, Histogram in log coordinates for an OFF LGB cell (5887 intervals counted in 5 min); note there are three peaks. *e*, The same but for a visual cortical cell. All measurements were made under the same conditions. (From Herz et al. 1964)

around 35/s in the optic tract, 15/s in LGB, and only 5/s in the cortex, other things being equal (i.e., in the same type of preparation).

In the optic tract, activity has a random nature, since the interval distribution (as abscissa) and the probability of an event, independently of the arrival of all previous events (as ordinate) show practically a Poisson distribution, provided that account has been taken of a dead time of 5 to 15 ms that corresponds with the refractory period of the ganglion cells. In semilog coordinates this function becomes an approximately straight line. Such histograms become more complicated in the LGB and the cortex. They show, particularly in the LGB, several peaks that signify the existence of various classes of intervals, where in addition it can be seen that at this level longer intervals are rather prominent (figure 5.22d,e).

This basic spontaneous activity seen in the absence of any light originates predominantly in the ganglion cells. Retinal block or excision of the eyes reduces the spontaneous activity seen at LGB by about 60%. This does not exclude the existence of a possible modulation of activity from certain other regions such as the reticular formation (tegmentum) of the midbrain, which controls the general state of attention and, in particular, some of the responses of LGB.

SPATIAL INFORMATION: ORGANIZATION OF RECEPTIVE FIELDS

In the *cat*, the organization of LGB receptive fields has been well investigated. These recall, for the most part, those of the retinal ganglion cells. Essentially, concentric fields are found with ON-center OFF-surround or with OFF-center ON-surround (figure 5.23), but 10% of the fields have a homogeneous structure. This does not mean that their organization (figure 5.24) does not demand the consideration of a certian number of questions.

Figure 5.23
Organization of concentric receptive fields in cat LGB. Illuminated zones are in white and dark areas are shaded by dotted lines. Time scale: 400 ms. *Above*, Records 1, 2, and 3 are for an ON-center cell. Responses recorded for a stimulus that excites the ON-center but also part of the OFF-surround (each stimulation marked by a thick bar). For the cruciform stimulus (1) occupying four areas of the OFF-surround, the response is less than for a bar (2 and 3) that occupies a lesser proportion of the OFF-surround. The identity of records 2 and 3 shows the homogeneity of the OFF-region (a concentric field). *Below*, Records 4, 5, and 6 are for an OFF-center receptive field. (4) Diffuse illumination, inhibition in the light and high activity in the dark. (5) Small aperture (1°) stimulus to the OFF-center, complete inhibition of activity during illumination. (6) The same stimulus to the active ON-surround of the cell. (From Baumgartner 1978)

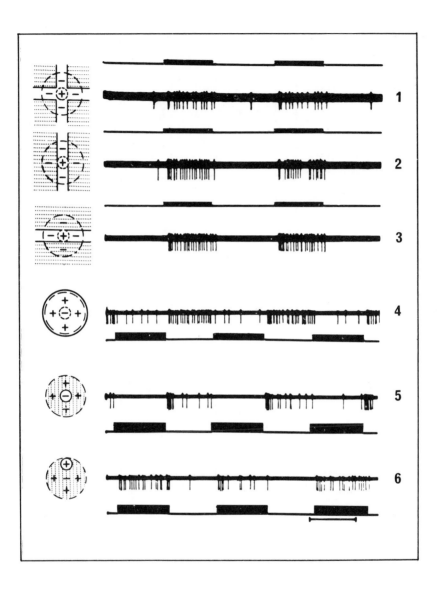

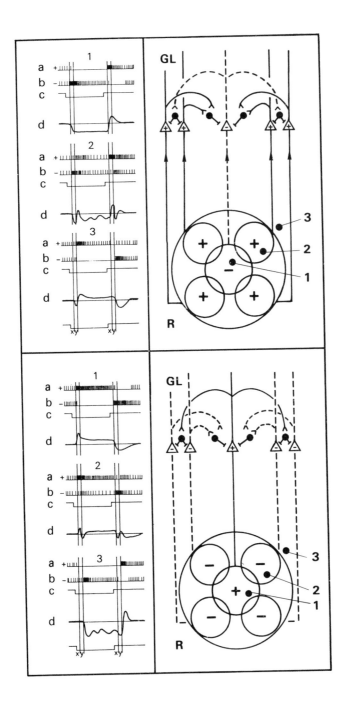

Each geniculate cell receives a small number of retinal inputs (in the lower limit one only). Retinal afferent fibers are always excitatory on geniculate cells.

The inhibitory interactions seen in the LGB between center and surround receptive fields seem to be stronger in the LGB than in the retina. This is particularly clear for the case of a simultaneous flash illumination of the center and surround; in other words, *contrast* is increased at this level.

Light and dark adaptation do not modify the LGB receptive field arrangements, unlike what is seen at the retinal level.

Close cellular measurements at the principal cells has identified exactly the hyperpolarizations and depolarizations caused by the onset and extinction of a light stimulus. These are summarized in table 5.3; note that excitation is accompanied by EPSPs and inhibition by true IPSPs. [Singer and Creutzfeld (1970) consider, in spite of all the difficulties in properly controlled intracellular measurements, that they have demonstrated the existence of real IPSPs.]

It has not been easy to imagine how to reconcile, topologically, the organization of the retina with that of the LGB network. A variety of schemes has been proposed, all of which suppose that the distribution of the retinogeniculate projections must conform with certain principles, the main one being that a given geniculate cell (for exam-

◀ Figure 5.24
Model of the organization of retinal projections to the LGB and schematic representation of the events following reception of retinal signals on an LGB cell. *Above,* An ON-center geniculate cell receives an excitatory input from an ON-center retinal cell and inhibitory inputs coming from several OFF-center retinal cells situated around the ON-center retinal cell. The inputs from these peripheral retinal cells exert their inhibitory influences via local geniculate interneurons and recurrent collaterals. The central cell exerts its influence reciprocally, inhibiting, in a similar way, the peripheral cells of the LGB. Diagrams to the left are for three positions (1, 2, and 3) of a spot (sited as shown on the right) showing (a) records from the central retinogeniculate afferent and (b) for a peripheral retinogeniculated afferent. (c) Time course of the stimulus. (d) General time course of the membrane potential changes in the central geniculate cell. The afferent (a) exerts its primary excitatory action at short latency (vertical line x). (b) The b fibers exert a secondary later inhibition (vertical line y). Notice that the membrane polarization of the geniculate cell (depolarization upward, hyperpolarization downward) is an algebraic summation of the excitatory and inhibitory retinal actions. Their time course is determined by the shorter or longer latencies of the corresponding excitatory or inhibitory retinal events. *Below,* The mirror image case of an OFF-center LGB cell: excitatory action of an OFF-center retinal cell with inhibition arising from several ON-center retinal afferents in the surround field. (From Singer & Creutzfeldt 1970)

Table 5.3. Center/surround organization of synaptic activity in ON-center and OFF-center cells

	Stimulus ON		Stimulus OFF	
	Center	Surround	Center	Surround
ON-center cell	Depolarized EPSP	Hyperpolarized IPSP	Hyperpolarized EPSP	Depolarized IPSP
OFF-center cell	Hyperpolarized IPSP	Depolarized EPSP	Depolarized EPSP	Hyperpolarized IPSP

ple, an ON-center) will receive excitatory input from an ON-center ganglion cell and inhibitory interactions from OFF-center ganglion cells that are immediate neighbors of the ON-center cell. In the LGB, these inhibitory interactions will be achieved via local interneuron collaterals. There will be, to summarize, an *isomorphic duplication* of the retinal organization at the geniculate level. In the case of an OFF-center LGB cell, the organization will be similar, mutatis mutandis.

In the *monkey*, the LGB also contains units with ON-center and OFF-center circular fields but with their organization also strongly associated with color, as will be discussed below (Derrington & Lennie 1984).

TEMPORAL AND SPATIAL INFORMATION: X AND Y UNITS

Cat

From the anatomical and histological data that have already been reported above, we have the basic knowledge of how temporal information is transmitted, recalling that in this way the geniculate (Pc) cells have been identified in the types X, Y, and W. We have also noted the excellent correlations between structure and function, in that the cells that are structurally identified as being linked to the X, Y, and W inputs, respectively, have themselves functional characteristics that correspond with what is known about their retinal counterparts (Cleland et al. 1971, Mason 1975).

Do not assume that no transformation of the receptive characteristics has taken place in the X and Y channels. Limiting discussion to the most numerous and best understood units, the following should be noted: We have seen above that the phasic Y channels in the LGB enjoy an amplification by divergence; this does not seem to exist for the X channels. However, there has been one notable change in the X channel between retina and LGB that does not appear to exist in the Y channels. This concerns a considerable diminution in their spontaneous activity. Researchers attribute this to a powerful intrageniculate inhibitory action that modulates the transfer of information in the channel (Bullier & Norton 1977, 1979; Fukuda & Stone 1976).

In considering (as in chapter 4, section 5.3) a spatiotemporal representation in four domains (PE, SE, SI, and PI), we see again at the LGB the distinctions between the X and Y type of receptive fields, with researchers concluding that the inhibitory mechanisms are not attributable to the retina but are certainly linked to processes that are *intrinsic to LGB* and achieved by local interneuronal connections (Stevens & Gerstein 1976).

Primates

The two X and Y systems have been clearly identified in macaque LGB (Shapley et al. 1981, Kaplan & Shapley 1982, Marrocco 1976, 1982). The essential criterion used by Blakemore and Vital-Durand (1986) is of spatial summation linearity, which exists in X units but which is nonlinear in Y units (as is well shown in figure 5.25). Combining this classification of spatial responses with temporal characteristics shows that the same links are seen as before between the temporal and spatial properties of X and Y cells, also essentially confirming the probably universal assumption that most "tonic" cells show linear summations and most "phasic" cells are nonlinear. But there are some exceptions.

As for the distribution of cells with X or Y characteristics in the thalamus, we have already seen that the question is probably not a simple one to answer. The proposition that all X are in the parvocellular layers and all Y are in the magnocellular layers seems to be almost certainly false.

One characteristic difference between the two geniculate zones concerns sensitivity to spatial contrast (the reciprocal of the contrast needed to generate a modulation of the response). This has been shown to be higher in the magnocellular layers (*whether for X or Y units*), whereas the X cells of the parvocellular zone show the opposite, that is, they are poor detectors of spatial contrast. In this way, there exist in monkey LGB two pairs of functional factors: one, the X and Y, that distinguishes sensitivity to temporal contrast; the other linked to parvocellular and magnocellular location, which differentiates between their capacity for spatial contrast and spatial frequency

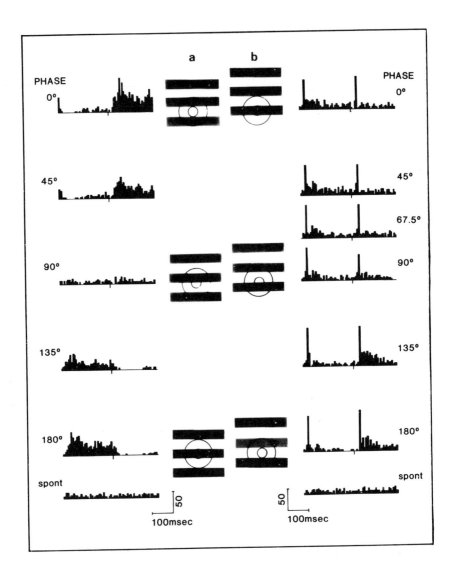

detection. These two pairs of criteria cannot be exactly superimposed in the sense that the magnocellular layers contain both X and Y types. We shall see later that this distinction is complemented by a difference in behavior with respect to stimulus color: It is in the parvocellular layers that color sensitivity is found.

MOVEMENT SENSITIVITY

In considering whether a movement sensitivity proper is found in LGB, it is necessary, as in the retina, to distinguish between movement sensitivity linked simply with the concentric topology of the receptive field and a true directional sensitivity that is not explicable by the field structure alone (such as is mapped by stationary stimuli).

In the cat, whose retina possesses no, or almost no, units with directional movement sensitivity, the discharges observed in LGB for a moving spot of whatever contrast—positive (bright spot on a dark ground) or negative (dark spot on a bright ground)—are in practice predictable and explicable from the concentric (ON-, OFF-, ON-OFF-) arrangements of the fields (Dreher & Sanderson 1973), having paid due regard to the relative sizes of the stimulus and the field (figure 5.26). But a certain directional sensitivity can also be seen, in the sense that the response is different depending whether the displacement of the spot or an edge is made in one or the opposite direction along an axis in a particular direction.

◀ Figure 5.25
Linear and nonlinear summation in the LGBd of macaque. For convenience the stimulus is drawn as a square-wave grating rather than a sinusoidal one. *Left,* The characteristics of an X cell. The stimulus phase is 0° with respect to the center of the receptive field when either the center of an illuminated (a) or dark (b) region is situated there. An ON-center cell would respond to passage of (a) but not of (b); the cell shown here is an OFF-center cell and responds to the passage of (b) with a maximal and sustained discharge. When the phase shift is 90°, half the center is stimulated by the light and half is not. Since the subdivisions of the receptive field summate linearly, the ON-responses equal the OFF-responses with a nil resultant. Thus alternating the stimulus between (a) and (b) in this position generates no response. Satisfying this so called "null test" is a characteristic of X cells. The null position is 90° away from the two phase values that give a maximal response. At intermediate positions of phase shift the response is proportionally intermediate in magnitude. The situation at 180° is the mirror image of the 0° case. *Right,* The responses of an ON-center Y cell for the same stimulus parameters. Notice that the cell responds for all phase shifts and for all alternations. In addition the response is transient, brief and intense, though a small, sustained component can also be observed. Spont. signifies the spontaneous activity in the absence of stimulation. (From Blakemore & Vital-Durand 1986).

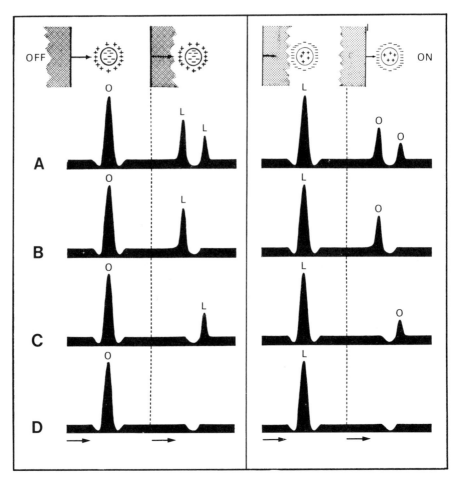

Figure 5.26
Response characteristics of cat LGB cells to the crossing of their receptive fields by a bright or dark edge. The two columns on the left are for an OFF-center cell: entry into the field of a dark (*left*) or bright (*right*) edge. The two columns on the right are for an ON-center cell: entry into the field of a bright (*left*) or dark (*right*) edge. For both the ON- and OFF-cells, A, B, C and D illustrate the different responses for each type of stimulation in the order of decreasing numbers of stimuli applied. Note in this case the same type of response is obtained whatever the direction of movement with respect to the center because of the radial symmetry of the receptive field. (From Dreher & Sanderson 1973)

Notice, therefore, that a bright or dark edge most often generates a predictable response in an ON- or OFF-center cell but can in certain circumstances demonstrate some special features (e.g., absence of an expected component; see figure 5.26). Similarly, a slit (or a bright or dark disk) in an ON- or OFF-field may produce an asymmetrical response such that the "exit" gives a larger response than the "entry" of the stimulus into the field.

In addition (still in the cat), the contribution from X and Y units can be specified. As could have been predicted in any case, type X fields seem to respond optimally to slow movements (1° to 2°/s), whereas the other type Y cells prefer rapid speeds (50° to 100°/s). In contrast, in the rabbit, the LGB clearly shows signs of directional sensitivity. However, since the rabbit retina contains exactly such units, it is not easy to decide a priori whether this is a truly geniculate mechanism or merely the projection from a retinal operation (Stewart et al. 1971).

BINOCULAR INTERACTIONS

We have seen above (for cat and no doubt also for monkey) that the projections to LGB follow a monocular arrangement with each histologically distinctive layer only receiving inputs from one half-retina (excepting the interlaminar zones). But electrophysiology now seems to have established that in the cat there are interactions between the projections of the two corresponding half-retinas, in spite of their segregation into their separate projection layers.

The experiment consists in studying the activity of a given LGB cell to determine its monocular receptive field which, predictably from the above data, is linked to either the ipsilateral or the contralateral eye, depending on the layer. Calling this the dominant input (D), the other nondominant (non-D) half-retina (contralateral or ipsilateral depending on the case) is now stimulated, say by a moving bar. The results (Susuki & Takahashi 1970, Sanderson et al. 1971) are as follows:

• In most cases there are interactions.
• They are almost always inhibitory; stimulating the non-D eye inhibits the activation of the cell by the D eye (figure 5.27).
• This inhibition is dependent on IPSP activity, presumably arising from short axon intrageniculate interneurons (figure 5.27).
• The inhibitory field of the non-D eye is wider than the excitatory field of the D eye.

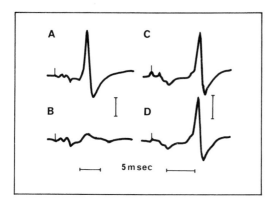

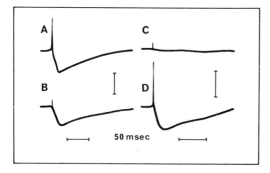

Figure 5.27
Binocular interactions in LGBd of cat. *Above,* Example of an LGB cell with binocular antagonism (A and B) and another with no binocular interaction (C and D). Extracellular recordings. *A,* Action potential of cell to stimulation of the ipsilateral optic nerve (vertical stimulus artifact is seen on the trace). *B,* The same stimulus preceded by one applied to the contralateral optic nerve 44 ms earlier. For the second cell, the response to the contralateral nerve stimulation (C), which is excitatory, is in this case unaffected by earlier stimulation of the ipsilateral nerve (D). *Below,* Intracellular responses from cells of the same types as those above. *A, B,* Cells with antagonistic interactions to combined stimulation of ipsilateral and contralateral optic nerves. *C, D,* A cell without binocular interactions. Notice, that the inhibitory stimulus in case (B) generates an IPSP in the cell, whereas in the cell with no interaction the nonexcitatory stimulus (C) does not generate any transmembrane potential change. (From Susuki & Takahashi 1970)

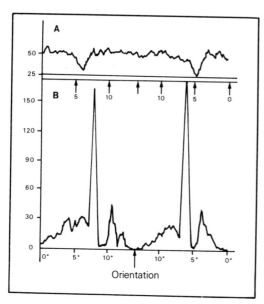

Figure 5.28
Effects of uniocular stimulation in cat LGB. Histograms of the mean discharge rate of a cell in layer A1 stimulated by slits of light displaced in one or the other direction in the orientations indicated, stimulating either the nondominant eye (A) or the dominant eye (B). A, Slit width 5.2° × 0.4°, speed of displacement 14 deg/s, traversing the receptive field (determined by the response at different abscissa values) in both directions from above to below before the central arrow, then from below to above. Note the inhibition relative to the spontaneous activity. B, Slit width 3.7° × 0.4°, displaced at the same speed but stimulating the dominant eye. The cell shows an ON-type excitation. (From Sanderson et al. 1971)

• The most significant interactions come into play between layers A and A1, and the inhibition is stronger in the direction A → A1 than in the opposite direction A1 → A. In other words, the ipsilateral projection is more inhibited by contralateral input than the contralateral projection by ispilateral input.
• The type of contrast does not seem to matter (bright stimulus on dark ground or the opposite), which suggests that inhibition involves both ON- and OFF-mechanisms together.
• The inhibition also seems to affect the spontaneous activity of the cell (figure 5.28).

These results are important since they show that LGB must constitute a first step in the domain of binocular interactions and, in other words, makes a first contribution to the operation of mechanisms for stereoscopic vision.

COLOR VISION

We have already discussed above the general principles of the doubly specific (spatial and color) organization of receptive fields in animals endowed with color vision. Here we introduce the situation in LGB to which, generally, the whole population of color-contrast ganglion cells projects (since the SC, at least in the ground squirrel and monkey, is deprived of such information. However, this question is not settled yet in the case of *Saimiri,* as already mentioned).

Considering first the work on ground squirrel, Michael (1973) found the three types of antagonism described earlier for GC in the case of B/G interactions: (1) B^+/G^- or the inverse throughout the field; (2) G^+/B^- in the center with B^- in the surround; (3) G^+ in the center and B^- in the surround. However, a new type is also described which incidentally corresponds to type III of the earlier classification scheme: G^+/B^- in the center and G^-/B^+ in the surround or the inverse combinations (these are called double color opponent cells; see section 5.4).

Considering now the case of macaque, the investigations have been both more numerous and very refined. A first study (figure 5.29) showed that there are six types of cell in the *parvocellular* layers of LGB in the regions for foveal and perifoveal projection (De Valois 1971). There are two achromatic types, called *wide spectral band fields,* with classic ON-center and OFF-center type fields, that may be regarded as subserving channels for luminance detection, B/W (black and white). There are four types of *color antagonism,* R^+/G^- and Y^+/B^- with their opposites R^-/G^+ and Y^-/B^+, respectively. These four classes are found, mixed apparently randomly, in all four *parvocellular* layers of LGB. [In many cases a distinction is made between the yellow Y and the green G; in many others, this intermediate spectral region is described globally as G.] Only achromatic cells with wide spectral bandwidth have been found in the *magnocellular layers.*

The work of Wiesel and Hubel (1966) has been further elaborated. It is now possible to specify (as in the ground squirrel) cells with doubly arranged spatial- and color-antagonisms. Three types of cells have been recognized in the foveal or parafoveal projection zones in the parvocellular layers (figure 5.30):

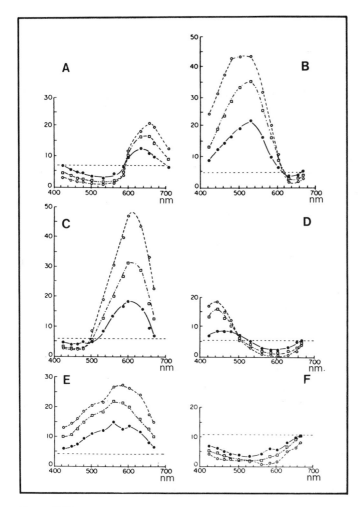

Figure 5.29
Mean spectral shape of the discharge characteristics in several types of LGB cell in
macaque as a function of color. Cells with spectral contrast: A, R + /G−; B, G + /R−;
C, Y + /B−; and D, B + /Y−. Cells lacking spectral contrast: E, W + Bl−; F, Bl + /W−.
For each cell, responses are illustrated for different wavelengths (nm) and at three
different luminance levels. (From De Valois 1973)

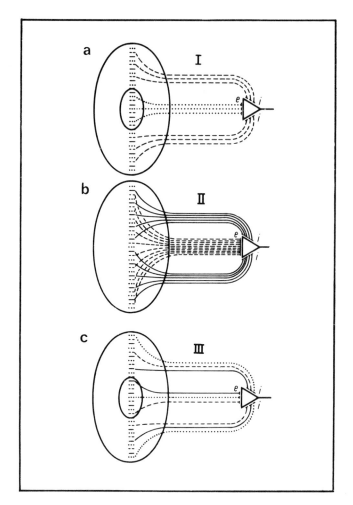

Figure 5.30
Diagram of the organization of chromatic (I and II) and achromatic (III) receptive
fields in macaque LGB. *a*, Type I: chromatic and spatial antagonism. Dots, excitatory
R+ central input; dashes, inhibitory G− antagonistic surround. *b*, Type II: ON-OFF
chromatic antagonism without spatial contrast. Dashes, excitatory G+ input; full lines,
inhibitory G− input. *c*, Type III: spatial antagonism lacking color antagonism. The
three types of color receptor (R, G, B) are similarly involved in both the central and
surround field. (From Wiesel & Hubel 1966)

• *Type I.* These, the most numerous, are shown by adaptation experiments to have a concentric spatial organization: ON- or OFF-center with the surrounds appropriately antagonistic and with *different spectral sensitivities.* Color-specific adaptation suggests that they are connected to one type of cone in their center and to another type in their surround. Five subclasses have been distinguished that have, in decreasing relative proportions, R, G, and B as their characteristic colors (see table 5.4). When stimulated by white light, these units behave like feline ON- or OFF-units.

• *Type II.* These do not have an antagonistic concentric spatial organization but respond in different ways at different wavelengths, receiving over their entire receptive field from two different types of cone. Two subclases predominate, G^+/B^-, on the one hand, and G^-/B^+, on the other. A type with G/R antagonism is seen, but only rarely.

• *Type III.* These have concentric spatial antagonism but with the identical spectral sensitivity throughout the whole receptive field. They are, in effect, wide spectral band cells. Unlike the previous examples these cells receive inputs from three types of cones in both center and periphery.

The data are summarized in figure 5.30, with the sometimes excitatory, sometimes inhibitory actions from the different types of cone to the LGB sketched in.

The data concerning the dimensions of the fields in types I, II, and III cells may be summarized as follows: *Type I* field diameters range between 2 min and 1°. The ON-fields (1/32 to 1/6 deg, mode 1/8 deg) tend to be smaller than the OFF- (mode 1/4 deg). *Type II* fields are between 1/4 and 1 deg. *Type III* cells range between 1/8 and 1 deg with a mode of 1/2 deg.

By observing dark adaptation, the existence of a Purkinje effect (wavelength slippage of the sensitivity maximum) suggests possible connections with rods in the most peripheral of these units (in addition of course to their cone inputs). The data in this respect are a little limited and uncertain: Only type II have exclusively cone connections but at least some of the type I and type II receive rod inputs in addition.

The location and temporal transfer functions of these color-sensitive cells should be investigated also. We have seen above that the P ganglion cells provide input to the parvocellular layers and they have essentially X-cell properties, whereas the magnocellular layers receive X and Y inputs. But measurements in macaque geniculate show that this dichotomy is more complex: Parvocellular cells are sometimes Y types, of which some are color-sensitive and others are not (Marrocco 1976, Blakemore & Vital-Durand 1986), whereas magnocellular layers contain mainly postsynaptic X units and a few Y.

Two types of receptive field have been identified in the ventral magnocellular layers: type III fields, and other fields known as type IV that are concentric ON-center/OFF-surround types with a very wide surround field having a spectral sensitivity in longer wavelengths that is relatively dominant over the central action. For such units, diffuse illumination with red or even with white light produces an inhibition of their spontaneous activity, which in this type of cell is very large.

Turning now to describing how color-sensitive geniculate cells are arranged with respect to their divisions into X and Y types and into parvocellular and magnocellular layer cells, it is generally found that narrow spectral band cells with color contrast are tonic and apart from that are sited in the parvocellular layers. These are thus X units. Conversely, wide spectral band cells are usually phasic and are localized in the magnocellular layers. They are generally Y units (Dreher et al. 1976). These classifications which, in addition, mainly fit into what is known of the monkey retina, of course have all sorts of exceptions such as the existence of wide spectral band X cells and luminosity detectors and, reciprocally, the existence of color-sensitive elements with transient responses, which are thus of the Y type (Marrocco 1976).

A different classification for color perception mechanisms in the parvocellular macaque LGB has recently been suggested by Creutzfeld et al. (1979). By using colored and white light stimuli, appropriately adjusted in luminance, these researchers have been able to identify a relatively larger number of types of unit than earlier workers:

• Narrow band cells excited by the short wavelengths (<475 nm) and inhibited by white light (*NS units*).
• Wide band units responding at longer wavelengths 475 to 525 nm but also excited by white light (*WS units*).
• Other wide band cells but this time with a maximal response at 600 nm (*WL units*).
• Narrow band cells with maximal response at wavelengths >675 nm and inhibited by white light (*NL units*).

Table 5.4. Response properties as a function of the spatial and color parameters of the stimulus in macaque LGB in Type I and Type II cells

Center		Surround		
ON	OFF	ON	OFF	%
		Type I		
R			G	31
	R	G		16
G			R	14
	G	R		5
B			G	1
		Type II		
G	B	G	B	
				6
B	G	B	G	

From Wiesel and Hubel (1966).

• Finally, cells inhibited by light of all wavelengths, save for a moderate excitation at the extremes of the spectrum (*LI units*).

This classification cross-checks in some measure with that of De Valois, who had also emphasized color contrast (NS ≡ B^+/Y^-; NL ≡ R^+/G^-; WS ≡ G^+/R^-; WL ≡ Y^+/B^-; LI ≡ B^+/W^-). However, it does not accommodate the strict spatial organization of the color antagonisms proposed by Wiesel and Hubel (1966) to the extent that here the excitatory and inhibitory fields are regarded as more or less superimposed. This study holds to the propositions that the original model suggested for color filtering at the LGB; but the authors propose that starting from the three types of cone, S, M, and L, the response of a geniculate cell represents the combination of excitatory action from a certain cone type plus an inhibitory action generated by *all three* cone classes and possibly by the rods also.

The results are essentially similar for other primates, except for some relative proportions. In *Saimiri* only 20% of the LGB cells recorded from have shown color sensitivity and, in another respect, the proportion of G/B cells is greater than that of R/G units (which is opposite to the situation in macaque; table 5.4).

3 THE VISUAL AREAS OF THE CORTEX

This section will cover both the structure and function of the visual cortex. First, the topographic organization of the visual cortical areas in some mammalian species will be examined, then their response properties will be introduced with respect to the stimulus characteristics (spatial, temporal, chromatic, etc.) and, finally, the effects of certain ablations will be discussed.

3.1 TOPOGRAPHIC ORGANIZATION OF VISUAL CORTICAL PROJECTIONS

In all mammals the visual pathway projects to the occipital part of the cortex. This bald observation, while globally correct, needs to be shaded in with the different details and multiplicity of projections that modern measurement has been able to reveal.

GENERAL MORPHOLOGY

In *primates*, the projection of the geniculo-cortical pathway is to Brodmann's cortical area 17, which is characterized (in the inner granular layer) by the outer band of Baillarger, which, folded, is known here as the band of Gennari. This band is visible to the naked eye as a pale stripe in sections of fresh cortex. It is from this banding and some others in this general region that the name *striate* arises for this area of the cortex. The other architectonic sectors of the occipital lobe spread, roughly speaking, around area 17. Area 18, contiguous with 17, is called *parastriate* (or *occipital, Oc*). Area 19, farther out still, is named *peristriate* (Pstr, or *preoccipital*). The morphology and the general arrangement of these territories is not identical for every group or subgroup considered.

In *humans*, (figure 5.31, lower), the projections are arranged on the median surface of the hemisphere, spreading around the lips of a sulcus (fissure) called the *calcarine sulcus* (CS), which has a quasi-horizontal trajectory until the latter curves inward and downward at its junction with the *parieto-occipital sulcus* (POS), which marks the boundary between the occipital and parietal lobes. The cortex bounded below by the CS and anteriorly by the POS constitutes the *cuneus* (CU) and the part just below CS is the *lingual gyrus* (or *lobe*, LL). Notice that area 17 spreads about equally to each side of the CS, whereas area 18 abuts 17 laterally and with 19 forms the upper part of CU and the lower part of LL. The CS does not extend very far on the lateral surface of the brain, and there is no great representation of area 17 there. At that level, areas 18 and 19 constitute concentric halos around the occipital pole making an anterior boundary on the parietal side with area 7 and the curved gyrus (area 39) and on the temporal side with the posterior temporal area 37.

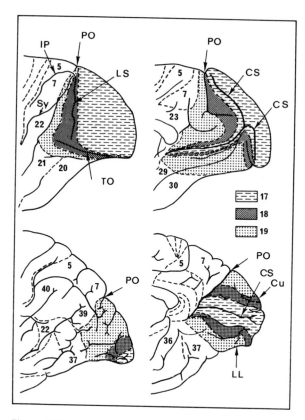

Figure 5.31
Cortical visual areas in macaque and in humans. Topography of the visual cortex (17), the paravisual cortex (18) and the perivisual cortex (19) in macaque (*above*) and in humans (*below*) mapped on the convex surface (*left*) and median plane (*right*) of the brain. PO, parieto-occipital sulcus; LS, lunate sulcus; IP, intraparietal sulcus; TO, tempero-occipital sulcus; CS, calcarine sulcus; Sy, Sylvian fissure; Cu, cuneus, LL, lingual lobe. Some of the Brodmann areas adjoining the visual areas are also indicated. The size difference between the two brains has been ignored. (From Kappers et al. 1960)

In *lower primates* (figure 5.31, upper), the situation is morphologically more complicated. On the one hand, the CS can be divided in its posterior part into an ascending and a descending branch. On the other hand, a large proportion of the striate area is sited on the convex surface of the brain bounded anteriorly by the *lunate sulcus* (LS) and the *inferior occipital* or *tempero-occipital sulcus* (TOS). Finally, the areas 18 and 19 surrounding 17 are relatively less extensive. In summary, phylogenetically, a progressive rejection of area 17 from the median surface can be observed as well as an increase in the relative importance of territories 18 and 19.

In the *cat*, the situation is quite different (see figure 5.39). Areas 17, 18, and 19 are localized on the convex surface of the *lateral gyrus* (LAT; also called *marginal*, and which is bounded by the *lateral sulcus*, SLAT), on the *posterolateral gyrus* and on the median and posterior *suprasylvian gyrus* (SSM and SSP). On the medial surface they occupy the *suprasplenial*, *splenial*, and *postsplenial gyri*. Notice here also a more or less concentric arrangement of the three areas 17, 18, and 19, at least on the lateral surface. [It can happen that, because of the shape of the gyrus, area 18 may be found more or less buried in a sulcus that can exist called the *interlateral accessory sulcus* (Otsuka & Hassler 1962].

In *rodents* (mouse, rat) and lagomorphs (rabbit), which have a smooth cortex, architectonically indicated boundaries allow the classification of an area 17 that is "typically striate" and an area of the same character as 18 more or less surrounding it; in the mouse, a lateral zone 18a and a medial zone 18b also exist (Caviness 1975). In the rabbit, the striate area (17) is bounded laterally by an occipital area, and medially by a peristriate band, each of which can be regarded as part of area 18. In both these groups, the visual cortical area does not extend to the medial plane, but is separated from it by an area with quite different characteristics (retrosplenial, area 29; figure 5.32).

TOPOGRAPHIC STUDIES

Simian Primates

In monkeys, such as the macaque, the visual projections are divided into two types. On the one hand, the striate area is the only one to receive massive inputs from the lateral geniculate body (*geniculostriate system*); on the other hand, there are areas that receive few such projections or even none at all, yet they have connections with the

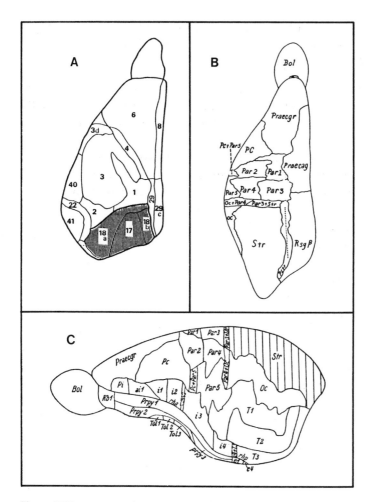

Figure 5.32
Visual cortical areas of a rodent, the mouse and the rabbit. *A,* In the mouse: the areas
are identified by Brodmann's nomenclature and the hatched regions are the 17, 18a,
and 18b divisions of the visual cortex. *B* (superior) and *C* (lateral) views in the rabbit:
the cytoarchitectonic divisions are identified by the traditional nomenclature established by the drawings of M. Rose in 1931 and utilized by O'Leary & Bishop (in 1938)
in their original definitive physiological study of the rabbit cortex. (Str, striate area 17,
bordering laterally with the so-called occipital area (Oc) and medially by the peristriate
area (Prst). Both have the characteristics of area 18. The median area (Rsg), retrosplenial, does not belong to the visual system. The areas Str and Oc are bounded in the
anterior direction by the parietal areas (Par 3,4), which are transitional zones. T1, 2,
and 3, temporal regions; i1 to i4, insular regions; PC, postcentral regions; Praecgr,
precentral granular region; Praecag, precentral agranular regions; Bol, olfactory bulb;
Prpyr 1 to 3, prepyriform areas. (*A* from Caviness 1975; *B* from Rose 1931)

other thalamic nuclei implicated in vision, more particularly those belonging to the lateral-posterior group and pulvinar. These constitute the *extrastriate system.*

The striate cortex. Retinotopicity has been studied in area 17 in macaque, baboon, and *Saimiri.* The visual fields found experimentally are sometimes presented in perimetry coordinates and sometimes in the parallels/meridians system (see chapter 3, section 8.1).

1. *Overview of topography* (figure 5.33). As we know, each visual hemifield projects to the contralateral area 17. The central parts of the field project to the anterior convex surface regions of the striate area, and the peripheral parts of the field are arranged more posteriorly and continue on the medial surface (Weller & Kass 1983). To be more detailed, the projection of the vertical meridian is curved and ranges along the anterior border of area 17 (i.e., in part of the lunate sulcus). The projection of the horizontal meridian (180° for the right hemifield and 0° for the left hemifield, see chapter 3, section 8.1) is roughly anterior-posterior on the convex brain surface. As a consequence, the fovea projects to the most anterior part of area 17.

As described above concerning the organization of the retina, there is some overlap of the ganglion cell projections to one hemisphere and the other. That type of distribution clearly finds its continuation in the arrangement of the cortical projection of the vertical meridian, which for this reason contains a projection that extends slightly into the ipsilateral field (Bunt et al. 1977).

The lower quadrant of the hemifield (corresponding to the upper quadrant of the retina) projects to the upper half of the cortex and the upper quadrant of the field to the lower half of the cortex (notice in particular the projections of the 45° and 315° meridians for the left hemifield and of the 225° and 135° meridians for the right hemifield).

For morphological reasons (sinuous course of the calcarine sulcus), the organization of the peripheral field on the medial surface is complicated.

2. *Quantitative data: the "magnification factor."* Studying the quantitative relationships between visual space and its cortical representation, Daniel and Whitteridge (1961), Cowey (1964), and Rolls and Cowey (1970) introduced a ratio (called variously the *magnification* or *amplification coefficient* or *factor [A]*). It was first defined as the distance on the cortical surface corresponding to one degree of visual angle and has more recently, by other researchers, been defined as the cortical

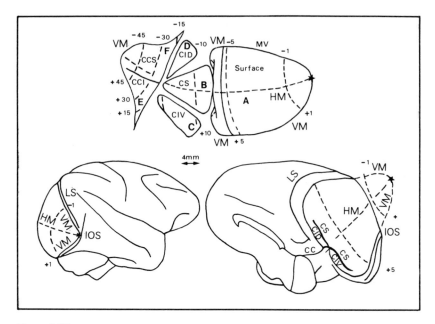

Figure 5.33
Striate area 17 of macaque. *Below,* Lateral *(left)* and median *(right)* views of the brain. On the convex surface are marked the lunate sulcus (LS), the inferior occipital sulcus (IOS), and the representations of the vertical and horizontal meridians (VM, HM). On the median surface, the same abbreviations are used where applicable. Note the calcarine sulcus with its common rim (CC) and its ascending and descending branches, with their superior (CS) and inferior rims, dorsal (CID) and ventral (CIV). Note also that the projection of the VM has been continued beyond the edge of the brain (dashed lines) including the star that marks the projection of the fovea. *Above,* An "exploded" diagram, showing the whole of area 17 as a "flattened" projection. A, lateral surface; B, superior rim of the calcarine sulcus (CS); C, inferior ventral part (CIV); D, inferior dorsal part (CID); E, inferior rim (CCI) of the common calcarine (CC); F, superior rim (CCS) of CC. Also shown are the representations of the vertical and horizontal meridians (VM, HM) and the projection of the fovea (star). (From Weller & Kaas 1983)

area representing one degree of solid angle (initially, therefore, in mm/deg and now mm^2/deg^2; see Tusa et al. 1978).

Figure 5.34 shows how A, or its reciprocal $1/A$ which is the number of degrees per unit cortical area, varies in the monkey with retinal eccentricity. This latter value (which becomes smaller the larger the cortical spread for a single degree of angle) is minimal at the fovea and increases monotonically toward the periphery. This confirms the evidence that the area occupied by the projection from the center of the retina is relatively much larger than that occupied by the projection from the periphery. The following numbers illustrate that fact: In macaque, 1° of central retina projects to 6 to 8 mm of cortex, and the central 10° around the fovea occupies 90% of area 17, the total surface area of which in this species is 1300 mm^2; in *Saimiri*, 1° of the foveal retina occupies 5 to 6 mm, and the area occupied by its visual projection is 720 mm^2.

It is worth comparing the variation with eccentricity of this cortical "magnification" with the corresponding variation with eccentricity of the density of retinal ganglion cells. Remember, as in figure 5.34, that the density of the receptors diminishes monotonically toward the periphery, whereas that of the ganglion cells shows a relative "hole" at zero eccentricity where no retinal neuron is present (the "central foveal depression"). When comparing these peripheral densities with the amplification factor A as a function of eccentricity, it appears that A is effectively proportional to the density of the cones. This is true also for the ganglion cells, but only for eccentricities greater than 10°; at lesser eccentricities, the presence of the foveal depression removes any significance in that comparison.

A systematic study of the corresponding numerical densities at the retinal level and at the cortical representation nevertheless shows that the central visual field representation at the cortex is more extensive than might be predicted from the ganglion cell counts: The proportion of cortical cell numbers devoted to central vision exceeds the corresponding proportion of ganglion cells. This difference is partly due to a divergence of foveal fibers at the LGB, as we have seen. This divergence becomes increased once more at the cortical level in such a way that the cortical representation of the fovea finally has the particularly extensive representation that is now recognized. It is this sort of enlargment of the foveal representation and not just the distance between the receptors that now tends to be accepted as

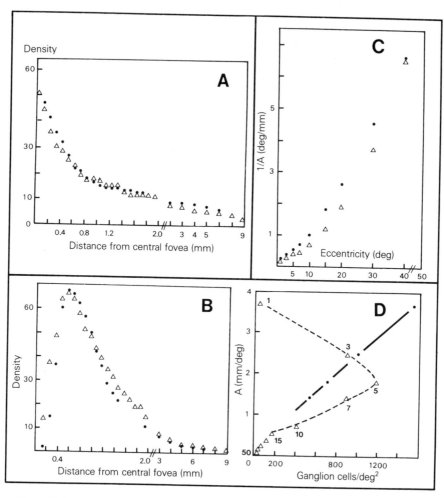

Figure 5.34

Quantitative studies of the retinocortical projections in the monkey. Variation of the cone density (A) and ganglion cell density (B) as a function of retinal eccentricity. Triangles, macaque; dots, *Saimiri*. Densities specified as number of cones and ganglion cells/600 μ^2 along the HM. C, Variation of the reciprocal of the amplification coefficient A as a function of eccentricity. D, Dashed curve and triangles, variation in *Saimiri* of the amplification coefficient A as a function of the number of *ganglion cells* per degree of solid angle. Marked on the curve are the corresponding eccentricities of the triangles (from 50° to 1°) that show the experimental observations. Note the approximate linearity to 5°, then for smaller eccentricities the foveal pit. The straight line shows the variation in A as a function of the *cone* density for small eccentricities (<7°). In this case the relationship stays linear right to the fovea where the density is maximal. (From Rolls & Cowe 1970)

explaining the high visual acuity in these species (0.65 min in macaque, 0.74 min in *Saimiri;* for humans see chapter 2, section 3.2).
Another line of approach, more typically behavioral and based on
training to a task, illustrates some characteristics of the mechanisms
for monkey visual acuity. For example, after having made lesions
that are more or less extensive in laterality in the macular region of
the *retina,* the decreasing acuity as a function of the extent of the
lesion yields a curve that essentially confirms what is known of the
cone distributions and also closely resembles the acuity curves obtained in humans. In contrast (and we will return to this point later),
cortical ablations have not brought with them the loss of acuity that
might be predicted by purely taking into account the electrophysiological data on the organization of retinocortical projections.

The prestriate cortex. A series of studies (Zeki 1974, 1978b,c; van Essen
& Zeki 1978) has been devoted to those regions situated around area
17 that essentially occupy areas 18 and 19. These are referred to as
prestriate areas, peristriate areas, or the *circumstriate belt* (figure 5.35).
Thus in *area 18* have been discovered four separate areas of projection
from part or the whole of the visual field, each containing a foveal
projection. These areas themselves have distinctive functional properties and were designated by Zeki as *V2, V3, V3A,* and *V4.* They
are practically completely buried in the lunate sulcus and the inferior
occipital sulcus on the convex surface of the brain and in the parieto-

---

Figure 5.35
Visual projections in the macaque cortex. *A,* Overall view of the lateral surface of the
left hemisphere. Dashed lines show the boundaries of V1 (area 17), V2 (area 18), V3,
and V4 as well as the midtemporal region (MT). The horizontal line in V1 marks the
projection of the horizontal meridian. STS, superior temporal sulcus; LS, lunate sulcus;
IP, intraparietal sulcus; SS, sylvian sulcus; ITG, inferior temporal gyrus; IOS, inferior
occipital sulcus. (xy indicates the approximate plane of section for C. *B,* Enlarged and
more detailed diagram of areas V1, V2, V3, V3A, and V4 viewed as if the lunate sulcus
were opened and spread out. VM and HM show the projections of the zero vertical
meridian (border of V1/V2) and zero horizontal meridian, respectively. Only the projections of the lower visual quadrant are shown (the part in *A* that is above the HM
projection line). Similarly, in the other areas all projections of VM are solid lines and
of HM are dashed. In addition, corticocortical projections from area 17 to the prestriate
areas V2, V3, V3A, and V4 are shown as well as those toward the region STS (MT).
The solid circle (arrow) from which numerous projections emerge corresponds to the
foveal projection. *C,* Diagram of a horizontal section (plane xy in *A*) showing areas V1
to V5. Str, striate area; Prstr, prestriate areas V2 to V4; LS, lunate sulcus; STS, superior
temporal sulcus with V5/V5A complex; A, P, M, L, anterior, posterior, medial, and
lateral directions. (From Zeki 1978)

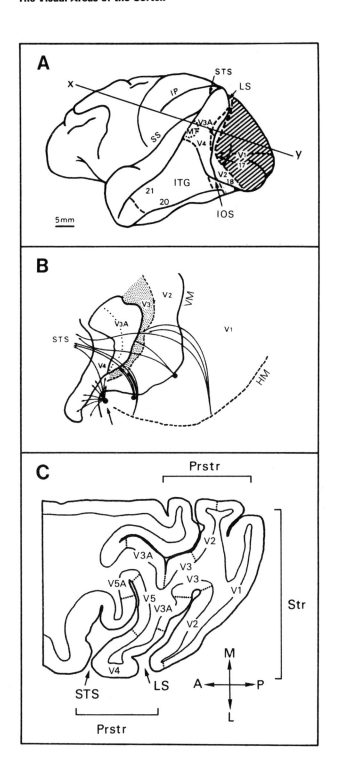

occipital sulcus on the medial face. These areas are characterized by several properties that are in some respects the opposite of those found in area 17 (which is referred to as *V1* in this classification).

As already described above, V1 has a continuous point-to-point representation of the visual hemifield. Points that are adjacent in space are represented by adjacent points on the cortex. Area V3A has a roughly similar organization.

In contrast, V2 (figure 5.36) contains a representation of the contralateral hemifield out to an eccentricity of 80°. The representation of the zero vertical meridian (VM) is contiguous with that in V1 and thus constitutes the posterior edge of this area. The representation of the horizontal meridian (HM) forms the anterior edge of V2 but is *divided* so that the representation of the lower quadrant is dorsal and that of the upper quadrant ventral. The representation of the central field is more extensive than of the peripheral. Because of this divided type of projection, two nearby ponts situated at one side or the other of the HM project to *well separated* points in V2. The authors signify this type of correspondence as a "second order representation" [also referred to as a "secondary" as opposed to "primary" projection.] This has also been found, as we shall see, in other more primitive primate species such as the *Galago* (bush baby) and the owl monkey and equally so in the cat. Apart from this, it is notable that receptive fields in area V2 are much wider than in area V1. V4 proves to be an area with much more complicated arrangements, with numerous separate representations of the same point in the visual field (Gattas et al. 1981; Gattas & Gross 1981).

Separated from these areas by the prelunate gyrus is the *superior*

Figure 5.36   ▶
Details of the topography of area V2 (*A, B*) and area MT (V5) of the superior temporal sulcus (STS) in the macaque. *A*, Lateral and *B*, medial views of the organization in V2. Insets *A'* and *B'* show, for the purposes of this description, the various fissures to have been opened up. IP, intraparietal; PO, parieto-occipital; LU, lunate; OI, inferior occipital; STS, superior temporal; LA, lateral or sylvian; CA, calcarine; TO, temporo-occipital sulci. The open squares show the projection of the vertical meridian VM and the dots the horizontal meridian HM. The stars show the fixation point (foveal projection). The lines of isoeccentricity are shown as dashes (See the inset of the visual field for reference, above right.) *C*, Site of the MT field in the depths of the STS, as if opened up, showing its superior (s), inferior (i), and deep borders (d). *D*, Detail of the visual field representation, as before. Squares, VM; dots, HM; dashed lines, isoeccentricity; U, upper and L, lower quadrant. (From Gattass et al. 1981 and Gattass & Gross 1981)

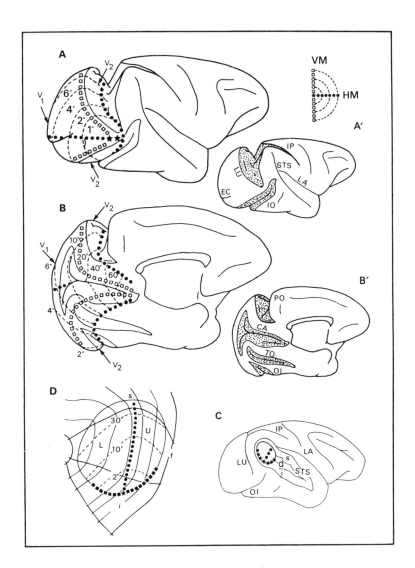

temporal sulcus (STS; Seltzer & Pandya 1978). On the lower border of this sulcus is an elliptical, limited area of projection that contains a complete representation of the contralateral visual hemisphere. The representation of VM constitutes its ventrolateral border, which ranges along the depth of the posterior bank of STS. The representation of HM is perpendicular to it, dividing area STS in two, with the representation of the superior quadrant being rostral and of the inferior quadrant caudal. This area, more recently specified as *V5-V5A* by Zeki (1990), has a representation that is thus a first order transform, as in V1. As in V1 also, the fields become larger and the amplification factor smaller as eccentricity increases. This area is within area 19 and has precise and reciprocal connections with V1 and with V2. As for its special properties, note that the fields are much wider than in V1 for a given eccentricity, and the topography is much coarser, with a great deal of it devoted to central vision. We will see that, in some other primates, researchers define a region called *medial temporal* (MT), which has been suggested to be a homologue of the zone STS-V5 (van Essen et al. 1981).

These different areas possess complex interconnections that are not hierarchical: Areas V3, V3A, V4, and V5 receive considerable projections from areas V1 and V2. The connections to V4 originate predominantly in the foveal region of V1. Areas V3, V4, and V5 are also interconnected, particularly V4 and V5. Complex convergences exist in the connections between V1 and V5 such that one place in V1 projects to several points in V5, and vice versa (Zeki 1978a, Montero 1980, Rockland & Pandya 1981, Zeki & Shipp 1988). In summary, V1 and V2 appear to be distributors of information in parallel upon areas V3, V4, and V5. The physiology of these proves to be more specialized, and they only enjoy a limited contribution that projects directly from the LGB (see below and figure 5.35).

As for callosal interconnections, these only exist in V1 for foveal projections but, in contrast, such interhemispheric tracts are equally present in the peristriate areas for peripheral fields.

We pointed out above that area 18 with its different components does not receive direct inputs from LGBd; in fact, this statement ought to be amended to include the connections from the interlaminar zones of LGB (the regions between the principal layers of the nucleus), which themselves receive inputs from SC (Kennedy & Bullier 1985).

Finally, it is noteworthy that the "specialized" areas V3, V4, and

V5 in their turn send projections to the areas often referred to as "association areas," that is, to the posterior parietal and some temporal areas, in particular the inferotemporal. We will see below how, in the macaque, these different visual regions are characterized by response properties that are specific for one or another stimulus parameter: form, orientation and size for a stationary stimulus, movement for one that is not stationary, and color.

On the whole the parameters used in such comparisons have been: binocularity, visual field size, sensitivity to orientation of a stationary stimulus, sensitivity to the direction of movement of a moving one, and color sensitivity. In this respect, note that all cells in all the areas under consideration are in practice binocular, with a possible preference for one eye. The visual fields are generally more extensive in V2 and V3 than in V1 and yet more so in V5. V1, V2, and V3 show considerable directional sensitivities, in contrast to V4 and V5. The directional sensitivity to movement is predominant in V5 ("movement area"). Differential color sensitivity is only observed in a striking way in V4. We will see below how it has been possible to make such generalizations for the global differences between the different areas.

In some ways very different functionally from these different areas is another region, the *inferotemporal area* (IT), which is an area with properties referred to as being "associative" (even though to some extent this term can seem to be devoid of any strict meaning). The characteristics of the cells are: wide receptive fields including the fovea that are often bilateral, and responses to complex stimuli that have a significance for the animal. In summary, it seems to be an area that codes strictly for operations concerned with cognition and memory.

Visual Areas in the Owl Monkey
Another series of interesting studies has been made on a small New World monkey (the owl monkey, *aotes trivirgatus*, see Appendix). This nocturnal species with highly developed eyes shares with some other primates (such as the marmoset) the advantage of having a practically smooth cortex, which facilitates topographic analysis.

Electrophysiological mapping has discovered a large number of areas of visual projection with, as in rhesus, many parallel representations of the visual field (Allman & Kaas 1971a,b, 1974a,b,c, 1975, 1976; Wagor et al. 1975). At present, the agreed inventory comprises six areas of representation of the contralateral visual hemifield. *Area V1*, which occupies Brodmann's area 17, has a classic representation of the contralateral hemifield, with adjacent points in the visual field represented as adjacent points in the visual cortex (first-order representation). The details of the represenation are as follows (figure 5.37): The fixation point is dorsolateral. Almost all the lower visual quadrant lies at the upper border of the calcarine sulcus, with the exception of the central part of the quadrant, which is on both the medial and dorsal surfaces. The upper visual quadrant spreads over the dorsolateral surface, the posterior (tentorial) surface, and the lower border of the calcarine sulcus. Its temporal periphery spreads on to the upper bank of the calcarine sulcus. The central 20° occupies almost half the striate cortex with their projections. Ninety percent of the boundary between V1 and V2 corresponds with the projection of the VM and the remaining 10% with the projection of the temporal peripheral extremity.

Area V2 is represented by a narrow band of cortex occupying area 18. The connectivity is arranged differently than in V1. In fact, beyond the central 7°, the representation of the HM is divided so that, as in the macaque, the projections from adjacent parts of the upper and lower quadrants are separated (2nd order representation).

Four other projection areas have differing organizations and seem to occupy (at least some of them) the cytoarchitectonic area 19 of Brodmann, or even more anterior regions spreading to areas 21 and 7.

[The *mid-temporal* area (MT) is in the medial temporal gyrus. It has an oval shape with its major axis rostrocaudal and its minor axis mediolateral. The HM projection crosses it along the major axis, dividing into a lateral portion, repesenting the visual upper quadrant and a medial portion, representing the lower quadrant. The fovea is represented posteriorly and the periphery anteriorly at the STS level. The topographic representation is first order, as in V1. The MT area has an equivalent area in macaque situated in the superior temporal sulcus (STS).

A *dorsolateral* crescent-shaped area (DL) embraces MT and has a topology, unlike V1 and MT, that is a second-order transform, as defined above.

A *dorsomedial* area (DM) is localized on the upper dorsal region with an extension to the adjacent medial region. This has a second-order projection, like V2 and DL.

Area M is entirely *medial;* it is not yet well understood.

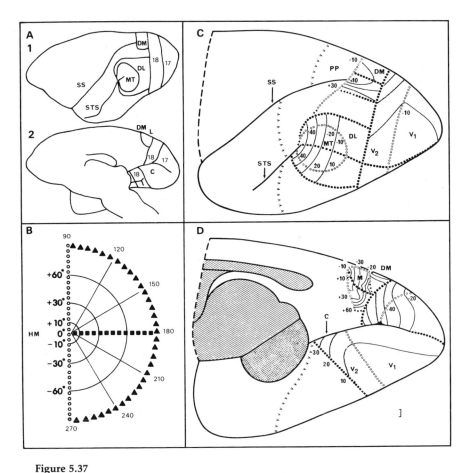

Figure 5.37
Cortical visual projections in the owl monkey. *A,* Overall view of the cerebral cortex
(1) laterally, of the convex surface of the left cortex and (2) medially, of the median
plane of the right hemisphere. Notice the boundaries of area V1 (area 17), of VII (area
18), of the dorsomedial area (DM), of the dorsolateral area (DL), and of the medial
temporal area (MT). SS, sylvian sulcus; STS, superior temporal sulcus; C, calcarine
sulcus. *B,* Boundary of the right visual field in polar coordinates. Black squares, horizontal zero meridian (HM); open circles, vertical zero meridian; black triangles, limit
L of the visual field. *C,* Details of the projection of the right hemifield on the left
hemisphere's convex surface to V1, V2, DL, MT, and DM. (Symbols for HM, VM, and
L as in *B.*) *D,* Details of the representation of the left visual field on the right median
surface. Note the projections to the median parts of V1, V2, DM, and of a supplementary zone called M, "median area." (From Allman & Kaas 1971, 1974a,b, 1976; and
Wagor et al. 1975)

Allman and Kaas (1976) propose another area (called *posterior pari-etal*, PP) which lies just anterior to DM and has its own hemifield representation.]

Clearly, very little is known at present about the reasons for these multiple representations. Data are also lacking (compared with rhesus) on the functional mechanisms that exist and must operate in parallel in these different systems. It is, however, worth noting that two areas seem to show a primary transformation in their projections (V1, V2) and two a secondary transform (MT, DL). The contrasts and the parallelisms between these two systems show up even more clearly when it is pointed out that both V1 and MT receive inputs from deeper nuclei, V1 from LGB and MT from the inferior pulvinar (the latter in this species arising in the SC). V2 and DL receive cortico-cortical inputs (from V1 and MT, respectively). Thus, in each of the two systems there is a real duality of arrangements, one of which can be sketched as LGB → V1 → V2 (geniculate system), and the other as SC → PUL → MT → DL (extrageniculate system), with the transfers V1 → V2 and MT → DL being effected in each case from a primary projection to a secondary projection.

While, as we have seen, it is traditional to propose a strict parallelism between the MT system of the owl monkey with the STS-MT system of macaque, we should remember that the multiple representations beyond V1 and V2 are relatively more prominent in this lower species than in macaque.

This leads us to consider very briefly some other species that are lower on the phylogenetic scale than the owl monkey. These studies concern the *Galago* (bush baby, a prosimian; see Appendix) and more removed still, the *Tupaia* (tree shrew); an insectivore considered to be one of the primate ancestors. Note that these two species show three of the recognized macaque areas V1, V2, and MT (Allman et al. 1973). Thus there appears to be a common plan of organization seen in the insectivores and in the Old World and New World primates, with some differences too, of course. We shall discuss later how the connections are made between thalamic nuclei and these different cortical regions.

Cortical Visual Areas in Humans

Our knowledge of the visual areas in the human species is necessarily much less detailed. Any comparison between human arrangements and the recent data on monkeys is particularly difficult since the

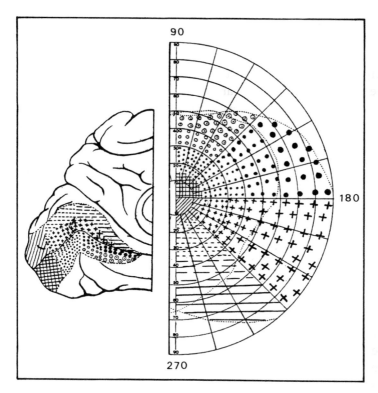

Figure 5.38
Visual cortical projections in humans. The calcarine fissure of the medial surface of the left hemisphere is drawn widely opened as if by retraction. The visual projection of the right visual hemifield is shown. Note that the macula is relatively more widely represented than the periphery. Note also the temporal crescent of monocular vision (dotted lines; cf. figure 3.60). (From Holmes 1945)

human data are generally from somewhat older experiments (figure 5.38). In our species, the foveal projection is to the tip of the occipital lobe; remember that the striate area is chiefly located medially. The periphery is also located on the median surface but more anteriorly. The calcarine fissure separates the projection of the upper quadrant of the visual field, situated below it, from the lower quadrant, located above it. Note how, as in the monkey, the foveal projection occupies a relatively large projection compared with that of the peripheral retina (figure 5.38).

In spite of the difficulties, several attempts have been made to identify (at least indirectly) functional homologues of the extrastriate visual areas of monkey. It is highly probable, if not fully proved, that areas 18 and 19 are involved in a way that is similar to the simian case. Neurophysiologically, nothing very certain is known at present because of the obvious difficulties of direct observation. Certainly, hypotheses are not lacking that attribute a visual integrative function to 18 and 19, the parastriate and peristriate areas. Some clinical data begin to prop up these hypotheses to a state of credibility.

Let us mention in passing the discussions that continue to surround the interpretation of *visual evoked potentials* in humans. As in the auditory case (see Buser & Imbert 1992), it is relatively easy to measure these from scalp electrodes (located in the occipital region) and following a repeated presentation of brief visual stimuli to observe characteristic potential changes by using summation of successive time-locked responses to extract them from the noise. Such an "evoked potential" comprises a certain number of components with essentially a triphasic complex wave formed by a negative change peaking 70 ms poststimulus (N70), followed by a positive component (P100) and another negative one (N145). These evident components can be preceded by an earlier one at 50 ms (P50) of low amplitude and also are followed by a series of other much later waves that may be very large (P200, N260, etc.). Argument continues concerning the precise origins of the principal complex N70-P100-N145: For some authors none of these components originates in area 17 but all arise in areas 18 and 19; for other authors, the first component is linked with the activity of the striate area. The very late components are now considered to be in the category of "intrinsic" responses concerned with the cognitive mechanisms associated with the stimulus' reception (see, e.g., Jeffreys & Axford 1972, Lesèvre & Joseph 1979, Haimovic & Pedley 1982).

Cortical Visual Areas in the Cat
The visual areas in this species have been the subject of many investigations. The most recent of them, which also seem to be the most comprehensive and best established, nevertheless raise the question, as in monkey, of the functional significance that can be attributed to the multiplicity of parallel pathways found to exist. The work to which we will refer (Tretter et al. 1975; Tusa et al. 1978, 1979; Tusa & Palmer 1980) has now been limited to nine different projection areas from one part or all of the contralateral hemisphere. We list these briefly below. The measurements were made by these authors

in "quasi-cartesian" visual field coordinates with azimuth specified to the right or left of the VM and with elevation (positive or negative) with respect to the HM; amplification factors A are specified in mm²/deg² (see section 3.1 and chapter 3, section 8.1).

Area 17. Area 17, defined cytoarchitectonically by the presence of the double bands of Baillarger, contains a projection of the whole contralateral hemisphere. This is illustrated by figure 5.39. Notice that (1) the projection of VM constitutes the lateral boundary of 17 on the convex surface of the brain. (2) Projections from increasingly peripheral parts of the visual field fall more and more medially on the medial surface of the brain, with the peripheral limit of the field lying on the upper lip of the splenial sulcus, near the border of the cingular gyrus. (3) The projection of the HM crosses area 17 from one side to the other, separating the (posterior) projection of the upper visual field quadrant from the anterior projection of the lower quadrant and with the projection of the area centralis sited at the intersection of VM and HM. (4) The amplification factor is maximal in the projection of the area centralis (3.6 mm²/deg² at the VM/HM intersection) and it decreases steeply toward the peripheral projections (as does the density of the retinal ganglion cells). In this species 50% of area 17 receives from the central retinal 10°, and at each eccentricity the size of the amplification factor is proportional to the density of the retinal ganglion cells. In contrast, in the monkey we saw that the proportionality is not obeyed in the fovea, where the amplification factor is very high (6.5 mm²/deg²) and that 90% of area 17 receives input from the perifoveal 10°.

Areas 18 and 19. Each of these areas, which as we know surround 17, receives a single representation of the hemifield but, compared with area 17 (1) areas 18 and 19 occupy a lesser cortical area and have a lower amplification factor (max. 0.35 mm²/deg²). (2) area 18 is limited to the representation of the central ±50° (i.e., to the zone of binocular overlap). (3) Area 19 represents a rather flattened field with a VM of only 30% but a wider extent of HM. (4) Areas 18 and 19 are essentially mirror images, with the VM constituting the extreme boundaries (at the 17-18 and 19-20 junctions). (5) In both 18 and 19 the topography of the projections is such that adjacent points in the visual field are not represented by adjacent points on the cortex. Each point on the HM projects to at least two points in these areas. These are second-order projections, as defined above.

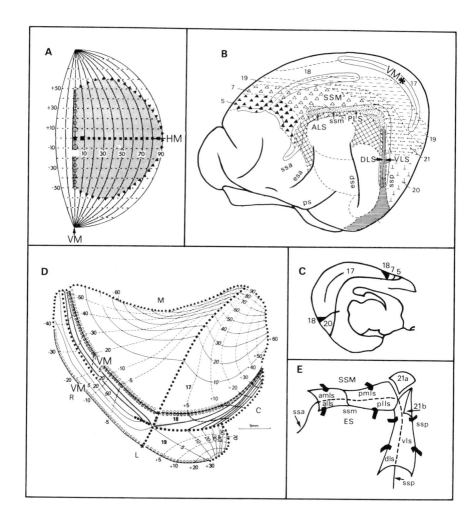

Lateral suprasylvian areas. The same group of researchers have identified the visual projections that are buried in the medial and posterior suprasylvian sulcus, sited on each bank of the sulci. It is unnecessary to enter into minute detail, but note that two areas occupy the posterior region of the lateral suprasylvian fissure, one medial (i.e., on the upper bank), the other lateral (on the lower bank). These are specified as *PMLS* and *PLLS* (posteromedial and posterolateral suprasylvian gyrus), respectively. Their topographic organization is such that one is the mirror image of the other.

There are two areas that are direct prolongations of the preceding but occupy a more anterior position on the suprasylvian sulcus. These are also organized with a mirror-image topology *AMLS* and *ALLS* (anteromedial and anterolateral suprasylvian gyrus). Two areas are in the depths of the posterior suprasylvian sulcus. Even though the latter is quasi-vertical, the distinction between them is made as more dorsal (*DLS*) and more ventral (*VLS*); dorsolateral and ventrolateral suprasylvian gyrus.

The retinotopic projections to these areas may be summarized as follows: The anterior areas AMLS and ALLS are arranged essentially

◀ Figure 5.39
Cortical visual areas in the cat. *A* illustrates the azimuth and elevation coordinates. Black squares, zero horizontal meridian (HM); open circles, zero vertical meridian (VM). Azimuth is measured from 0° to 90° with respect to VM in the right hemisphere. Elevations are positive in the upper quadrant and negative in the lower quadrant. The peripheral limits of the visual field are marked by black triangles. *B*, overall view of various cortical areas on the convex surface of the left hemisphere. Sulci: ssa, suprasylvian anterior; ssm, medial suprasylvian; ssp, posterior suprasylvian; esa, ectosylvian anterior; esp, ectosylvian posterior ps, pseudosylvian sulcus. The boundaries of areas 17 (V1), 18 (V2) and 19 (V3) are shown as well as a variety of other areas also specified by Brodmann's nomenclature (7, 5, 21, 20). The anterior boundary of 17 is marked by the projection of VM and the star shows the projection of the area centralis. The boundary 18/19 comprises the lateral sulcus (slat) (see section 3.1). All the other areas are buried in the ssm (areas ALS and PLS) or in the ssp (DLS and VLS). *C*, Schematic view of the median surface to illustrate the extent of area 17, bounded by 18 (in black). *D*, Representation of the hemifield in areas 17, 18, and 19 of the cortex, *as if unfolded.* Conventions as in *A* show HM as squares and VM as open circles. Equal azimuth lines are in solid lines and equal elevation lines are dashed (+ or −). The 20° azimuth line essentially coincides with the passage of 17 from the convex surface to the median surface, thus much of that area is on the median face. The star, as in B, shows the projection of the area centralis. *E* is as if the ssm and ssp sulci have been opened up, which allows the areas ALS medial (amls) and lateral (alls) to be seen and the two posterior areas PLS medial (pmls) and lateral (plls) as well as the two areas dls and vls. The detailed retinotopicity has not been shown here in these six areas, which are represented by lower case letters here for convenience. (From Tusa et al. 1978, 1979)

like area 17, that is, showing a first-order projection but with a smaller amplification factor. Areas DLS and VLS have a much more complicated topology. On the one hand, only HM and regions with small elevation project there, and on the other hand, a point on the retina projects as a continuous line on the cortex (*point/line correspondence*). The most extensive and most complicated areas, PMLS and PLLS, have mixed topological projections with a second-order projection for VM. This line is projected as a T, but the projection is repeated for certain ranges in an organization of the point/line variety noted above for DLS and VLS.

We are far from having provided an inventory for all the cortical visual projections. According to certain authors, some visual inputs also reach the suprasylvian areas on the convex surface of the brain (areas 5 and 7) and others project to parts of the medial surface of the brain (anterior splenial area and cingular area; see Heath & Jones 1971, Palmer et al. 1978, Mucke et al. 1982).

In addition, the thalamic areas that contribute to the channeling of different visual signals to the cortical areas remain to be specified, particularly those involving the LGB (geniculo-cortical system) and the more medial nuclei (lateral posterior-pulvinar complex). This will be examined later.

Cortical Visual Areas in the Rabbit
Recall that in lagomorphs as in rodents, the population of uncrossed afferents is limited to <10% and the eyes are very lateral (divergence of the axes being almost 160° for the rabbit and 120° for the rat and mouse).

Monocular projections. First we shall examine how each eye projects to both the ipsilateral and contralateral cortexes (figure 5.40; see Hughes & Wilson 1969, Hughes & Vaney 1982). Essentially, the main projection from a given eye is to the *contralateral cortex*, such that each point on the retina (therefore each point in the visual field) is represented in two places on the cortex, defined as *area VI* (more medial), and *area VII* (more lateral). It is agreed that areas I and II essentially coincide with the cytoarchitectonic separation into the two areas 17 and 18. Apart from this, the projections to I and II are practically mirror images, with the lines of equal elevation perpendicular to the I/II boundary and the lines of equal azimuth parallel to it. The projection of the zero HM entirely crosses the two areas, with the upper hemifield situated posterior to it and the lower hemifield ante-

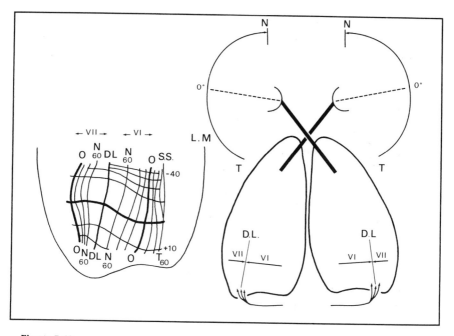

Figure 5.40
Cortical visual areas in the rabbit. *Right,* Position of areas VI and VII with their representation of the temporal (T) and nasal (N) visual hemifields with respect to the vertical meridian (shown here as passing through the entry of the optic nerve). DL, decussation lines. For simplification, the temporal retinal outputs and the noncrossed fibers that arise from them have not been shown. *Left,* Detail of areas VI and VII of the left hemisphere with the mirror image arrangement of the projections about the DL "line": nasal → 0 → temporal in the medial direction in VI, and nasal → 0 (temporal not shown) in the lateral direction in VII. SS, suprasplenial sulcus, medial limit of the visual area; LM, tracing of the medial sagittal plane. Beginning at the representation of the HM (thick mediolateral line) the lines of isoelevation correspond to the inferior quadrant anterior to −40° and the upper quadrant posterior to +10°. The binocular region is situated at each side of the DL. (From Hughes & Wilson 1969)

rior. In each area, the lines of equal azimuth are roughly parallel to the VI/VII boundary, with a representation of the VM being clearly distinguishable and with the lines of nasal azimuth (to 80° or even in principle to 90°) being very close to the I/II boundary. The lines for temporal azimuths are, in contrast, at the most peripheral borders of the visual area (most clearly seen in area I).

Each retina, however, also sends a limited projection to the *ipsilateral cortex*. Each projection is concerned with the part of the nasal field that lies between 70° and 80°, that is, from a very lateral area of the temporal retina. Single-unit recording shows the existence of units that can be excited from *both eyes* (binocular units) in the fringe area of VI/VII. This region has been described as the "line of decussation," but it is in fact an area of overlap.

Conditions for binocular vision. We have just seen that two very lateral temporal retinal zones each project to the two cortexes. However, this is not sufficient, geometrically speaking, to guarantee binocular vision. Examining the regions of binocular vision, we notice that *when the two eyes are in the resting position,* these domains do not coincide: The region of the projection of one eye to the contralateral cortex and that for the projection from the other eye to the ipsilateral cortex do not coincide in visual space. Thus binocular vision is not possible with the eyes in that position. This actual result was not predictable from examining (as we did in figure 1.11) only the simple geometry of visual fields and their forward overlap.

The horizontal separation between corresponding points seen by the eyes in those eye positions is 18°. Because of this, it is necessary to find out whether this species can make convergence movements of the eyes, which could permit binocular vision when the eyes move to directions other than the rest position. Recent studies of ocular movements have clearly shown (thanks to the present technique of measuring them with moving coils in a magnetic field) that the rabbit can in fact make such movements, with each eye turning by 9° and achieving binocularity (Zuidam & Collewijn 1979). Note that when the eyes do adopt this convergent position (described sometimes as the "primary equivalent" position) the animal that then achieves a state of binocular vision loses some lateral vision and thus part of the surveillance of the world for possible predators (Hughes & Vaney 1982).

Cortical Visual Areas in the Rodent
Using the albino mouse as an example that has been well studied recently (Wagor et al. 1980, on the C57 BL/6J strain), we once again see an area VI and a system of extrastriate areas (figure 5.41). *Area VI* is identified, as in other species, with the striate area 17 of Brodmann. It comprises a complete representation of the visual field seen by the contralateral eye. Lines of constant azimuth and elevation are practically orthogonal. The upper hemifield projects caudally and the lower rostrally, with the nasal portion represented laterally and the

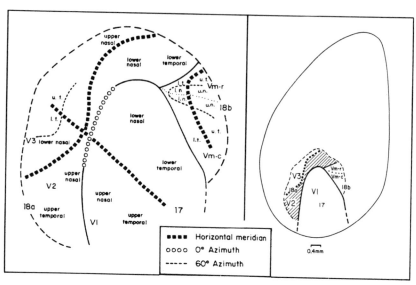

Figure 5.41
Dorsal view of the left hemisphere of mouse illustrating the relationships between the retinotopic subdivisions of the visual cortex (V1, V2, V3, Vm) and the cytoarchitectonic subdivisions (areas 17, 18a, and 18b). *Left,* Retinotopic map of the left cortex. *Right,* Relationship between retinotopic subdivisions (V1, V2, V3, Vm) and cytoarchitectonic subdivisions (17, 18a, and 18b). u.t., upper temporal; l.t., lower temporal; u.n., upper nasal; l.n., lower nasal; Vm-r, Vm-c, rostral and caudal Vm areas. Hatching, area V2. (From Wagor et al. 1980)

temporal medially. Binocular cells are encountered in the representation of the nasal 30° to 40°.

Extrastriate areas here also constitute a much more complex system that is not simply a mirror image of area VI. Multiple representations of the visual field exist in those areas. Lateral and rostral with respect to area 17 is *area 18a,* a cytoarchitectonic region that carries at least two projections. The most medial, called *V2,* surrounds V1 rostrally and laterally. The VM is on part of the boundary with area V1 and HM forms the lateral boundary. More lateral still, area 18 encompasses a second projection, apparently complete, of the whole visual field but arranged differently from V2. This field is named *V3.*

Medial with respect to area 17, a field *18b* also contains two smaller projections that are limited to the temporal field and are designated by V_{mr} (rostral) and V_{mc} (caudal).

Such multiple representations also seem to be present in other rodents, particularly rat (Montero et al. 1968), hamster (Tiao & Blakemore 1976), and guinea pig. Probably the above study on the mouse provides one of the most detailed of those available and it may be considered representative of the group.

3.2 THALAMIC CONNECTIONS WITH THE CORTICAL VISUAL AREAS

In general, the nuclei that in the cat and primates are concerned with funneling the visual signals to the cortex comprise two arrangements: either the lateral geniculate body or, alternatively, the lateral posterior-pulvinar complex (LP-PUL), together with their subdivisions (discussed below). One difficulty is that in monkeys and probably in all primates the LGB sends a considerable output only to area 17, whereas in the cat such connections are made simultaneously with areas 17, 18, and 19. There are thus differences even in the definitions of the geniculate as opposed to the extrageniculate systems. Note that a study of thalamic connectivities must also be accompanied by one concerned with the opposite connections from cortex to thalamus.

CLASSES OF LGB-CORTEX CONNECTIONS IN THE CAT

Afferent Connections
Much experimentation, using a variety of anatomical techniques, has established the cortical projections of the different parts of the LGB, including the laminar sections (layers A and A1, layers C and C1 to C3) and the medial intermediate nucleus (MIN). The essentials of the present results seem to be the following (Stone & Dreher 1973, Singer et al. 1975, Gilbert & Kelly 1975, Wilson & Stone 1975, Camarda & Rizzolatti 1976, Höllander & Vanegas 1977, Gilbert 1977, Geisert 1980, Meyer & Albus 1981, Gilbert 1983):

• The thalamo-cortical cells of layers A and A1 (i.e., all those that are not interneurons) project to 17 and 18 in the following ways: (1) 60% entirely to 17, (2) less than 10% go to both 17 and 18 by exploiting axonal bifurcation, and (3) less than 1% project only to 18. Judging by the size of the cell bodies: (1) cells projecting exclusively to 17 are X types, (2) the "branching" cells are probably Y, and (3) area 17 essentially receives X inputs, area 18 receives Y.
• The cells of the magnocellular layer C, that essentially contains only Y types, project to 17 and 18, no doubt by axonal branching.
• The parvocellular layers C1-C3, containing essentially W cells, send

60% to area 19, in part after bifurcation (or even trifurcation) to areas 17 and 18.

• The predominantly Y cells of MIN project heavily to 18 but also partly to 18 and 19. Note that at present the detail of the projections from C and MIN are less well established than those from A and A1.

• Another important matter concerns the cortical levels of termination of the different types of input X, Y, and W. Arguments continue, but essentially all these levels are found to be different. For the striate area (figure 5.42) X cells go to the deep parts of layer IV (IV C) and to VI; Y cells go to the superficial parts of layer IV (IV B) and to VI; and W cells to I, to deep III, and to VI, and perhaps to IV C.

Efferent Connections

As in other thalamocortical systems, the LGB receives a variety of connections descending from the visual cortex. Two principal assertions may be made. Corticofugal fibers from 17, 18, and 19 are, as a general rule, arranged as follows: (1) pyramidal cell efferents from layer VI project to LGB; (2) those from layer V, in contrast, go to SC; and (3) cells in layers II and III establish corticocortical connections (Szentagothai 1973, Levay & Gilbert 1976, Leventhal 1979, Bullier & Henry 1979c).

Pathways to the LGB complex itself have been carefully studied by Gilbert and Kelly (1975); their main conclusions are summarized in table 5.5.

THE LATERAL POSTERIOR COMPLEX IN THE CAT

Interest has recently been aroused in what role the collection of neurons situated medial to the LGB might play in the organization of visual signals. Essentially these neurons comprise two components, the *pulvinar nucleus* (PUL), placed dorsolaterally, and the more ventromedial *lateral posterior nucleus* (LP; figure 5.43).

Powerful opposing arguments (not yet decisive, however) have arisen among various researchers concerning the divisions of LP, while agreement is closer to unanimous concerning PUL, which constitutes a single entity. In research where the criteria first used are cytoarchitectonic in nature, there is no wide variety of data concerning such subdivisions. In contrast, investigations based on pathway analysis using (HRP) retrograde transport or (^{3}H-leucine) anterograde transport have provided much more instructive results, showing that the LP nucleus is comprised of several zones distinguished by their

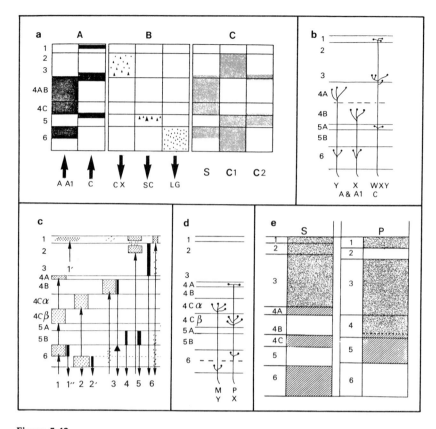

Figure 5.42
Aspects of the lamination of the visual areas, particularly of area 17. *a*, Organization
of cat area 17. The layers 1, 2, 3, 4AB, 4C, 5, and 6 are indicated to the left of the
diagram. The two A columns refer to afferents: A, A1, C, afferents having their origin
in layers A, A1, C of LGB. The three central B columns refer to corticofugal efferents:
CX to other cortical areas, SC to superior colliculus, LG to LGB. The three columns C
to the right refer to types of receptive field encountered: S sites for simple cells, C1
sites for "standard" complex fields, C2 sites for "special" complex fields defined by
the absence of summation within the field. *b*, Types of X and Y afferent terminals with
origins in layers A and A1 of LGB and also of W as well as X and Y terminals originating
in the C layers of LGB (detail for *a*, A). *c*, Laminar organization of area 17 in the
macaque. Notice that in this case layer 4 is more complicated (4A, 4B, 4Cα, 4Cβ). 1
and 1', afferents originating in the parvocellular layers of LGB; 1", efferents to LGB;
2, afferents originating in the magnocellular layers of LGB; 2', efferents to LGB; 3,
afferents originating in STS and efferents destined for that region (corticocortical connections); 4, efferents to superior colliculus; 5, afferents from the inferior pulvinar and
efferents to the same nucleus; 6, afferents from and efferents to area V2. *d*, Detail of
the routes for afferents of magnocellular (M) and parvocellular (P) origins; the first are
assumed to be Y and the second X (see text). *e*, Diagram comparing the organization
of afferents of genicular origin (hatching) and of pulvinar origin (dotted shading) in
the striate S and prestriate P areas of the macaque. ([a] from Gilbert & Wiesel 1981; [c]
from Lund 1981; [b], [d] from Lund et al. 1979; [e] from Benevento & Yoshida 1981)

Table 5.5. Corticothalamic pathways to LGB complex

From	To				
	A	A1	C, C1–C3	MIN	LGBlv
17	+	+			+
18	+	+		+	
19			+	+	

afferent and efferent connectivities and even by their acetylcholine esterase content (Graybiel & Berson 1980).

Inputs to the LP-PUL Complex

The pulvinar. This nucleus receives (1) direct retinal inputs to its lateral regions bordering MIN and LGB; (2) pretectal inputs to the rest of the nucleus; and (3) (visual) inputs from cortical areas 19 and other suprasylvian areas 20, 21, and 7. In introducing this work we can therefore no longer entirely dissociate the cortical areas that are properly visual (in the traditional sense) from neighboring suprasylvian areas that are often considered to be "association areas" (and which some of them are, effectively; see Heath & Jones 1971, Mucke et al. 1982). The above projections in (3) particularly implicate efferents from the visual suprasylvian medial areas PMLS and AMLS acting on the PUL.

The lateral posterior complex. This nuclear complex has been divided into several subassemblies, whose precise functions remain somewhat controversial. We will confine ourselves to reporting the following divisions (Updyke 1976, 1981a,b, 1983, Berson & Graybiel 1978, Rodrigo-Angulo & Reinoso-Suarez 1982, Raczkowski & Rozenquist 1983):

The lateral part, called *LPl,* to which might be added a particular supplementary nucleus PO, is called a *corticorecipient* region since it receives projections from cortical areas 17, 18, 19, 20, and 21 as well as from the visual medial suprasylvian areas PMLS and AMLS.

A medial part, called *LPm.* This is different from the above division because it is *tectorecipient,* that is, it receives powerful inputs from the superficial layers of SC. [Note that Updyke (1976, 1981a,b) distinguishes an "interjacent" LPi where there are tectal projections from a region properly medial but which contains no visual connections. We have not adopted that classification here which, moreover, differs from that of Berson & Graybiel (1978).]

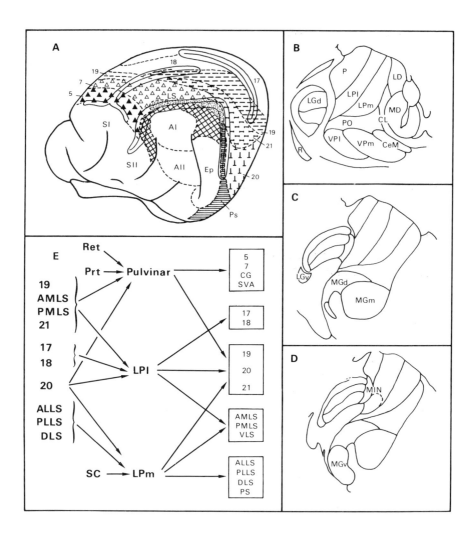

In addition, there is an accessory input from the lateral suprasyl-vian visual area ALLS and PLLS, from area 20 and from area DLS. [It has also been established recently that there are even some very sparse direct retinal inputs to different levels of the lateral posterior nucleus, particularly to the dorsomedial fringe and to the caudal region (Itoh et al. 1983).]

Outputs from the Nuclei of the PUL-LP Complex
Other studies have been directed to output projections to the cortical areas: we now summarize their layout in the lateral and suprasylvian cortical regions. Considering histological data first, we arrive at the following scheme:

• PUL projects exclusively to areas 5 and 7 as well as, on the medial surface of the brain, to the cingular gyrus and the anterior supra-splenial area.
• LPl projects exclusively to areas 17 and 18.
• LPl, PUL, and LPm project to areas 19, 20, and 21.
• LPl and LPm project to areas AMLS, PMLS, and DLS.

Figure 5.43 assembles the essentials of these data; note that the visual areas are the territories designated as AMLS and PMLS, DLS and VLS and that the other areas on the convex brain surface occu-

◀ **Figure 5.43**
Connections of the posterior lateral-pulvinar complex in the cat. *A,* To explain the connections, this diagram repeats a presentation of the cytoarchitectonic divisions of Brodmann on the convex surface of the brain. It is essentially the same as in figure 5.39, with the addition of the maps for somatic areas SI and SII, as well as for the auditory areas according to the traditional subdivisions, which have now been revised (see Buser & Imbert 1992) with AI, AII, the posterior ectosylvian area Ep, and the posterior suprasylvian area Ps. Also marked are the general contours of areas 5, 7, 17, 18, 19, 20, 21. For the suprasylvian visual areas buried in the sulci see figure 5.39. *B, C, D,* Frontal sections of the thalamus at three anterior-posterior levels establishing the location of the LGB (with its components: LGd, dorsal; LGv, ventral; and its nucleus MIN) also the pulvinar P (with its divisions: lateral LPl, medial LPm of the lateral posterior pulvinar) also other thalamic nuclei: PO, posterior nucleus; VPl, VPm, lateral and medial divisions of the ventral posterior nucleus; CeM, CL, central medial and central lateral nuclei; MD, LD, dorsomedial and lateral dorsal nuclei; MGd, MGv, MGm, dorsal, ventral, and magnocellular parts of the medial geniculate MGB; R, part of the reticular nucleus. *E,* Diagram of the afferent (left to center) and efferent (center to right) connections of the pulvinar, LPl and LPm. Ret, retina; Prt, pretectum; SC, superior colliculus. 17, 18, 19, AMLS, PMLS, ALLS, PLLS, DLS, VLS, cortical visual areas, see figure 5.39; CG, cingulate gyrus; SVA, anterior suprasplenial area. (*B, C, D* from Raczkowski & Rosenquist 1983; *E* from Updyke 1981 and Raczkowski & Rosenquist 1983)

pied by areas 5, 7, 21, and 20 are, in principle (since without demonstration of the existence at those levels of primary inputs), "association" areas. [Note that this demonstrates a correspondence to some extent between three parallel representations of the visual field in the PUL-LP region and the three projection areas of the visual pathways, one in the pulvinar, the two others in the LP (the corticoreceptive and the tectoreceptive zones, respectively)].

Two conclusions may be drawn from these histological studies: (1) The LP complex displays two main zones, one cortico(striate)-recipient (LPl), the other one tectorecipient (LPm); (2) the tectorecipient zone represents one relay for a second route for visual messages to reach the cortex, through superior colliculus with projections to various cortical areas. This second, parallel route is now commonly designated as the *extrageniculostriate system*.

Functional Properties of LP Nucleus Cells in the Cat
Some physiological investigations of feline LP nucleus cells show that the visual field is represented twice: once in the LPl, and again in the LPm, with the vertical meridian representation corresponding to the border of these two zones. Many cells in both divisions respond well to moving stimuli and many are direction sensitive. In both nuclei, cells are binocularly driven (or facilitated through binocular stimulation). The major differences between LPl and LPm were: (1) receptive field sizes significantly smaller in the corticorecipient than in the tectorecipient zone; (2) the internal receptive field organization is also different (nonhomogeneous, with distinct on and off areas in LPl, but homogeneous on-off fields in LPm); and (3) the incidence of orientation-selective neurons is higher in LPl than LPm, also with a better tuning. These functional differences may well partly reflect some of the salient properties of the striate and collicular projection neurons, respectively (Chalupa et al. 1988).

CLASSES OF LGB-CORTICAL CONNECTIONS IN THE MONKEY
In simians, as we have seen above, X and Y units are found in the retina and LGB, whereas W afferents seem to be rare if not absent. The great majority of geniculocortical afferents reach area 17. But a detailed histological study (see figure 5.42) shows that, as in the cat, X and Y project to different cortical layers. In this case, however, area IV is more complex than in the cat, since the following subdivisions can be specified in monkey: layer IV A superficially, with layer IV B

deeper and layer IV C deeper still and with two of its own subdivisions, IV Cα and IV Cβ.

The arrangement of the terminations of the geniculate afferents is essentially as follows (Lund et al. 1979, Blasdel & Lund 1983):

• Fibers with X responses, coming essentially (but not entirely) from parvocellular regions terminate in IV Cα but also tend to send collaterals to layer VI and mainly to layer IV Cβ.

• Fibers with Y responses, from the magnocellular layers, end in layer IV Cα, with possible collaterals being directed to area VI.

• The existence of direct connections from LGB to IV B is still disputed, although they seem to have been shown physiologically.

It is traditionally considered that in primates LGB only projects to area 17 (unlike the organization seen in the cat). The use of fine resolution histological marking has, however, caused a revision of that doctrine. It has been established that a variety of areas belonging to the prestriate or peristriate areas (V2 and probably V4) receive geniculate inputs. These latter are nevertheless separate from the others. They come not from the principal parvocellular or magnocellular zones but from the interlaminar regions and zone S which, as we have seen, constitutes the most ventral cellular concentration in the LGB (Benevento & Yoshida 1981, Kennedy & Bullier 1985).

These not very abundant projections only show an approximate resemblance to those of the cat. Their interest arises from the fact that the geniculate interlaminar regions and zone S themselves receive inputs from the superficial layers of the SC. In other words, this system, devoted to channeling visual signals, is distinct not only from the retinogeniculostriate system but also from the considerable extrastriate path that we discuss below, the "retinocolliculopulvino-prestriate" route. The present one is a *retinocolliculogeniculoprestriate* path, the functional significance of which is still to be discovered.

THE LATERAL POSTERIOR-PULVINAR COMPLEX IN THE MONKEY

Along with the detailed analyses of the LP-PUL complex in the cat have been others concerned with the situation in various primates at different stages of phylogenetic evolution. The new investigations confer an increasing significance on the extrageniculate pathways. This extensive comparative work between the species and the perspectives that it has opened out are very valuable; It therefore seemed worthwhile to elaborate upon this a little in this chapter, in spite of the complexity of the topic (cf. Wilson 1978).

Macaque

Histology. In this, the most evolved subject that has been studied, the LP-PUL complex is referred to as PUL alone, since the lateral-posterior nucleus, defined histologically, seems to have minimal significance. In contrast, cellular distribution studies have distinguished several divisions: *median* (PM), *lateral* (PL), *inferior* (PI), and *caudal* (PC). However, as in the cat, the basis of any functional significance comes more from studying connectivity, that is, the afferent and efferent connections of these various nuclei, than from cell cytoarchitectonic mapping. The connectivity distribution does not necessarily respect the separations suggested by cytoarchitectonic boundaries (Updyke 1983).

For a long time the pulvinar was (as was the LP nucleus of cat) regarded as an accessory nucleus in the traditional sense of not having significant connections with any main external pathway. In fact, new techniques such as retrograde HRP transport or anterograde transport of tritiated amino acids reveal this sort of connectivity in great detail.

Thanks to anatomical study of afferent inputs, a distinction can be made between two pulvinar areas: one comprises PI and the adjacent part of PL, the other the rest of the nucleus PL, PM, and PC (figure 5.44; see Benevento & Rezak 1976, Bender 1981, Benevento & Standage 1983, Ungerleider et al. 1983, Ungerleider & Mishkin 1983).

The part PI plus ventral PL (called *PIα*) is shown to project to areas 17, 18, and 19, namely, to the striate area and circumstriate band. PI-PLα receives reciprocal connections from the same three areas 17, 18, and 19 with a precise topographic correspondence, and it also receives projections from the retinorecipient superficial zones of SC, with again a well-defined organization (figure 5.44).

The other parts of the PUL (PL, PM, PC) constitute a much more extensive area that receives descending projections from areas 17, 18, and 19 but without the topographical precision of those directed to the PI-PLα. Two other subdivisions in PL, called *PLβ* and *PLγ*, receive inputs from the superficial retinoreceptive part of SC. Inputs from the pretectum (PRT) terminate in the most dorsal part of PLβ. Inputs from the nonretinoreceptive parts of SC terminate in nucleus PM. Direct afferent inputs from retinal ganglion cells, although limited in number, are found along the medial and caudal fringe of PI. These fibers belong to a bundle directed to SC and the PRT and recall the direct retinal afferents seen in cat on the dorsomedial border of LP-PUL.

Outputs from PUL to the cortex are arranged as follows: from PLβ to 17, from dorsal PLβ to (parietal) areas 5 and 7, from PC and PLγ to the inferotemporal region, from PM to 18 and 19; a crescent-shaped zone has been identified that projects to the STS region (called MT; see figure 5.35) that has been well demonstrated in macaque and in other simians and prosimians (Benevento & Rezak 1976, Benevento & Davis 1977, Rezak & Benevento 1977, Standage & Benevento 1983).

Electrophysiological research. The experimental basis for the above data was histological, either by conventional methods or by modern axonal transport marker techniques. In the parallel electrophysiological research, there are two aspects to consider. The first is studying the *correspondences between points in the visual field and electric responses in the pulvinar* or, if you wish, testing for retinotopicity of responses (whatever their origin—direct retinal, tectal, pretectal, or corticofugal). The problem is, in the thalamus as in the cortex, whether it is possible to recognize one or several visuotopic maps and whether these projections are of the *primary* or *secondary* type. We know from other parts of the visual system that the two possibilities are open, because if V2 constitutes a level of secondary projection, the other possible sources of retinotopicity in the pulvinar are known to be stages where there is a primary transformation (SC and V1 particularly). We can summarize the results as follows: The PUL contains two complete representations of the contralateral hemifield. One of them concerns a zone (also anatomically identifiable as PI and ventral PL) that enjoys corticofugal projections with a topographical organization. VM is represented dorsally and laterally, the peripheral field of view is medial, and central vision is lateral and posterior.

The other representation is entirely in PL, more or less surrounding the first. The lower visual quadrant is dorsal and the upper one is ventral and clearly separated from the former. Here a double representation of HM is found at the outer border. On the other hand, VM constitutes the boundary between the two systems of representation.

It has been concluded that the first representation is a first-order transform and the second is second order. This difference could arise from the origin of each projection to PUL, with some coming from centers with first-order representation (CS and V1 particularly) and others from those with a second-order topography.

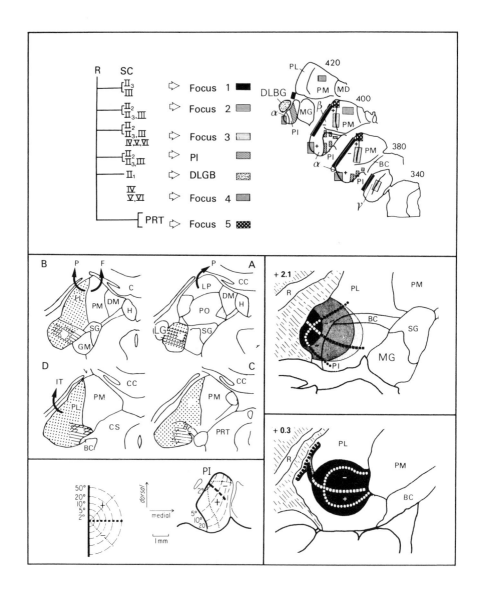

The *response properties of the cells* have also been studied but, up to the present, only in the inferior pulvinar, with the following results (Bender 1982): Most cells respond to stationary or moving spots of light over receptive fields of 1° to 5° diameter. A third of the cells have no orientation preference. In contrast, two thirds are sensitive to the orientation of both fixed and moving stimuli: Half of these respond equally well to both directions of movement of an adequately oriented strip or to its stationary counterpart, whereas the others are excited by movement in one direction and inhibited by movements in the opposite.

In summary, an exploration of the PUL reveals cell responses of the most diverse characteristics, some nonorientational, some bidirectional but also others that are specifically directional. When we recall that this thalamic region receives at the same time inputs from V1, from the various prestriate areas, V2, V3, V4, and MT, as well as from the SC, the response properties of which are themselves very

◀ **Figure 5.44**

Organization of the pulvinar in the macaque. *Above,* Foci of projection of the superior colliculus (SC) and the pretectum (PRT) on the different thalamic nuclei (shown in frontal section from anterior, above, to posterior, below). Projection of the superficial layers of SC (II and III) relayed from the retina on the PL (focus 1 in PLβ and focus 2 in PLα) to the PL/PM boundary (focus 3) upon Pl and LGB (PLα and PLβ are shown respectively as α and β). Then the retinal projection of the PRT, a retinal relay, on the dorsal PL (focus 5). *Middle left,* Serial frontal sections arranged rostrocaudally from A to D, illustrating the distribution of the different levels in the inferior pulvinar (PI) that receive collicular projections, shown hatched for the ipsilateral SC and cross-hatched for the contralateral SC. Dotted shading, areas receiving projections from 17, 18, 19. Arrows have been superimposed to indicate the projection from the dorsal PL to the parietal cortex (P), from the PM to the frontal cortex (F) and from the caudal PL to the inferotemporal cortex (IT). *Middle and lower right,* Results of a topographic study of the projections from area 17 on the pulvinar. (Middle) The first system of projections occupies part of PI and the adjacent part of PL. The central zone (0°-1°) of projection (black), the (dark gray) perifoveal region (1°-7°) and that from (7°-22°, light gray) are seen. (Lower) The second projection limited to the foveal region and entirely confined to PL is shown in a more posterior section. Dotted line, the projection of VM, line of squares, projection of HM; (−), projection of the inferior quadrant; (+), projection of the superior quadrant. *Bottom left,* Reconstruction of the visuotopic organization of PI from microelectrode exploration. Here VM is shown by a continuous line and HM by an interrupted line. BC, brachium of the superior colliculus; LP, lateral posterior nucleus; DM, dorsomedial nucleus; PI, inferior pulvinar; PL α, β, γ, lateral pulvinar; PM, medial pulvinar; DLGB, dorsal lateral geniculate body; MG, medial geniculate; sg, suprageniculate nucleus; CC, corpus callosum; PRT, pretectum; R, reticular nucleus. (From Benevento & Rezak 1976, Bender 1981, Benevento & Standage 1983, Ungerleider et al. 1983) varied, we see how difficult it is to decide on specific roles for each of these diverse sources in the modulation of pulvinar responses. Nor is it clear what role this nucleus might play in information processing on the way to the prestriate cortex: Is it purely a "relay," or does it certainly elaborate the coding of messages received from various levels?

A study by Berson (1988) provides a partial answer to this question. Subtotal striate lesions were followed by a dramatic suppression of reactivity of the cells' area of representation in PUL. After recovery, however, the cell's responsiveness suggested mediation through the superior colliculus. On the other hand, bilateral SC lesions (including both superficial and deep layers) had only a minimal effect on pulvinar receptive fields when the cortex was left intact. All receptive field types were present, in roughly the same proportions as in intact animals. Taken together, these results indicate that most inferior pulvinar neurons are dominated by inputs from the visual cortex and that the SC makes only a minor contribution to their receptive field properties. These results are hardly compatible with the view of the PUL as a thalamic relay nucleus for visual messages (at least in the anesthetized animal).

Other Primates
Here we will very briefly discuss measurements made on the thalamus of species "lower" than the macaque, starting with *Tupaia* (the tree shrew, an insectivore), the *Galago* (lemurian bush baby), then a small nocturnal New World monkey *Aotes* (douroucouli, the owl monkey), *Callithrix* (the marmoset), and finally, *Saimiri* (the squirrel monkey), also a New World species. Earlier we discussed the situation in their cortical areas; we now discuss the thalamic systems that supply them and that also receive corticofugal projections from them (figure 5.45; see Glendenning et al. 1975).

Note first of all the evolution of the structure PUL (Harting et al. 1972), In *Tupaia*, a sort of prototype, the PUL is not yet an "intrinsic" nucleus, since it receives inputs from the (superficial) SC. However, these inputs, unlike in more developed species, project to all of the nucleus, which thus can be regarded as homogeneous structure. It projects in turn to areas 18 and 19, which because of this can likewise not be regarded as "association" areas. The VM is represented at the 17/18 boundary while area 18 receives projections from the PUL alone. There is thus contiguity at the 17/18 border just as there is contiguity at the thalamic level.

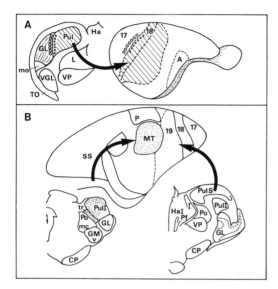

Figure 5.45
Two examples illustrating the evolution of the pulvinar: *Tupaia* (insectivore) and *Galago* (prosimian). *A, Tupaia,* the entire pulvinar receives projections from the superior colliculus and projects to a large area of the temporal cortex (areas 18 and 19). *B, Galago,* the tectorecipient part of the inferior pulvinar (Pul I, dotted shading) is what projects to the MT area, whereas the nontectorecipient part (Pul S) projects to areas 18 and 19. In both species the LGB (GL) projects to area 17. (From Glendenning et al. 1975)

In *Galago*, a distinction must be made between an "inferior" and a "superior" pulvinar (PI and PS). In this species, the projections from the SC go to the caudal PI. The rostral PI and the PS contain no such projections, marking an evolutionary change from *Tupaia* to *Galago*. In addition, in *Galago*, the tectorecipient zone essentially projects to MT (i.e., remote from area 17 and not affecting 18 and 19). These latter areas receive their visual inputs from both the nontectorecipient zones of PUL and also from corticocortical connections from 17.

In the owl monkey, the organization is essentially analogous to that in *Galago*, except that only part of PI projects to MT (Lin et al. 1974). There are other nontectorecipient regions of PUL that project to 18 and 19 (Allman et al. 1972).

In the *Saimiri* also, the PI is divided into a tectorecipient and nontectorecipient zones: The SC only projects to the ventromedial two thirds of PI (as well as to another nucleus that we have scarcely mentioned here, the posterior nucleus PO). But here the tectorecipient zone projects to areas 18, 19, 20, and 21, unlike species such as *Galago* and *Aotes*.

In conclusion, it is now well accepted that in the primate pathway and funcitonal organization there are at least two systems that channel visual messages to the cortex, one being the retinogeniculostriate pathway, and the second the retinotectopulvinoprestriate (including the area MT/STS in the prestriate bands). [To which one should also add the extrageniculostriate and the retinocolliculogeniculoprestriate path.] These thalamocortical connections are to some extent duplicated by corticocortical connections, which, on the one hand, combine the two systems at the cortical level and, on the other hand, join them at the inferotemporal region (IT), which itself also enjoys projections from the nontectorecipient part of PUL.

The simplistic idea that cortical operations are elaborated from 17 to 18 then to 19 is no longer acceptable to the extent that, even if we agree that IT remains an "association" area not receiving inputs from peripheral afferents, this certainly does not apply to those other areas, since all of them receive such inputs: area 17 from LGB, areas 18 and 19 from the tectopulvinar system and likewise for other areas such as MT (or some such as DL or DM that are seen in the squirrel monkey but not yet recognized in macaque and probably others also that are yet to be discovered).

The possible importance of these diverse circuits that carry visual information to different places continue to be debated, as for example the reasons for the duplication of thalamocortical connections with corticocortical connections. An observation by Bender (1983) established that the visual responses of pulvinar cells (PI) depend almost exclusively on the integrity of area 17: Ablation of 17 suppresses these responses in spite of the integrity of SC. In these conditions, the passage of these signals from 17 to 18 and 19 implies an obligatory transfer via PI: (17 $\rightarrow$ PI $\rightarrow$ 18 $\rightarrow$ 19). Recall the recent evidence derived from double cellular marking by Kennedy and Bullier (1985) that there are neurons at subcortical levels (including LGB and pulvinar) that innervate *both* area V1 and area V2, by axonal bifurcation. Finally, here as in other thalamocortical systems, the functional significance of the bidirectional ascending thalamocortical and descending corticothalamic projections remains to be determined. New research and above all new and original ideas are very likely to oblige a revision of the answers that have been given to these basic questions.

3.3 CORTICAL FUNCTIONAL ORGANIZATION AND RESPONSE CHARACTERISTICS

The response properties of cortical cells prove to be much more complex than those of LGB or SC. Before going on to describe these response types, we first need to specify the various stimulus configurations that are most used (figure 5.46) in cat and other species:

• Stationary spots of a given angular diameter turned on (ON) or off (OFF) on a dark background.

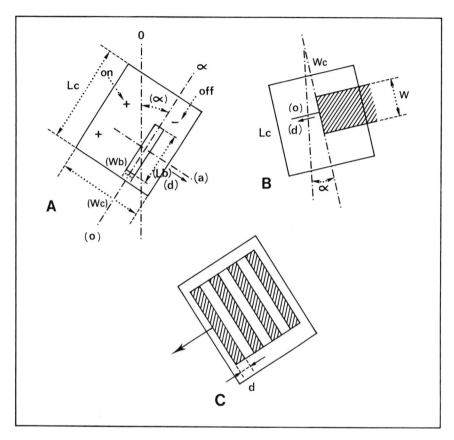

Figure 5.46
Methods of analyzing a receptive field. *A*, Geometrical variables: Lc, Wc, length and
width of the receptive field; Lb and Wb, length and width of the stimulus bar; o, bar
orientation at $\alpha°$ to the 0 orientation axis; d, direction of displacement here perpendicular to o. *B*, A dark area of width W enters a field of length Lc and width Wc. The
stimulus is displaced in the direction d. *C*, Case of a square wave grating of period
expressed in cycles/deg if it is stationary. If it is displaced the measure used is
cycles/s = cycles/deg × deg/s (deg/s being the drift velocity).

• Stationary illuminated bars of given length (Lb), width (Wb), and orientation (o)—angle α—with respect to a fixed reference (usually the principal axes of the visual field).
• Moving spots displaced at a given angular velocity (deg/sec) along a given axis (a) in a given direction (d).
• Moving bars, with the parameters (Lb), (Wb), and (o) defined, which are displaced along an axis (a), which as a general rule is perpendicular to (o), in a given direction (d) and at angular velocity (v) (deg/sec).
• Stationary or moving edges of known width (W) and orientation (o), fixed or moving perpendicularly to (o).
• According to circumstances, the above stimuli might be given the opposite contrast, for instance, dark stimulus on a bright ground rather than bright stimulus on a dark ground.

The exploitation of fixed or moving stimuli of a certain length has proved to be particularly interesting. Much has been learned from the variation of a standard response (R) as a function of one of the numerous possible variables, with the others serving as parameter [first changing (o), (Lb), and (v) but then also others such as displacement amplitude, or the stimulus' direction with respect to (o), etc.]. Plotting curves of the changes in (R) with changes in a chosen variable can yield a "tuning curve" for that variable. It has become usual also to describe cell responses in terms of *orientation selectivity* (o) or *direction selectivity* (d). These two properties are defiend operationally and specified in different ways that should not be confused. By orientation selectivity (o) we mean that a cell preferentially responds either to a given orientation (o) of a stationary bar or edge or to the displacement of such a bar or edge along an axis perpendicular to (o) whatever the direction of the displacement along that axis. By directional selectivity (d) we mean that the cell preferentially responds when the stimulus (bar or spot) is displaced in a given direction and does not respond or responds less well when the displacement occurs in the opposite direction along the same axis.

"Gratings" are also used, which are images of alternatively light and dark bars, whose contrast follows a given spatial function (e.g., rectangular as in figure 5.46, or sinusoidal) with its spatial frequency defined in cycles/degree. If the grating is moved at a given speed (in deg/s) the variation of the luminance at a fixed point is expressed in cycles/second = cycles/degree × degree/second.

With these varied types of stimulus it has been possible to recognize many types of cortical response characteristics; the detail in the classifications has been considerably elaborated since the first classification was proposed by Hubel and Wiesel (1962).

RESPONSE CHARACTERISTICS FOR STATIONARY STIMULI IN SIMPLE CELLS AND COMPLEX CELLS

By using essentially stationary stimuli (spots, bars, or edges) Hubel and Wiesel (1959, 1962, 1965) were able to distinguish two main types of receptive fields in the visual cortex (17, 18, 19) of the cat. These were simple cells (S) and complex cells (C). Table 5.6 summarizes the essential properties of these rather well codified types of cell.

Table 5.6. Comparison of response properties of simple and complex cells to stationary stimuli

Stimulus	Simple Cells	Complex Cells
Spot	Nonconcentric ON and OFF fields; possible intermediate ON/OFF zone; place of maximal response in each zone	Homogeneous ON/OFF response; identical response throughout field; (rarely) a nonhomogeneous field with one ON and one OFF region with not always a response to a fixed spot
Bar or contrast edge	Optimal oreientation ("field orientation")	Optimal orientation
At optimal orientation	Response type depends on position in field	Response type does not depend on position in field
Summation with Wb increasing	Increasing R with increasing Wb	Response max. for $Wb << Wc$; in some cases decreasing R for $Wb \rightarrow Wc$
Antagonism	Between ON and OFF fields	Nonantagonistic
Field size	small, cat 1°–3°	Usually wider (6°)
Summation for Lb increasing	Summation up to $Lb = Lc$	Standard complex summation up to $LB = Lc$ Special complex response max. for $Lb < Lc$
Spontaneous activity	Weak or zero	High

Wb, width of bar; Wc, width of receptive field; Lb, length of bar; Lc, length of receptive field; R, standard response.

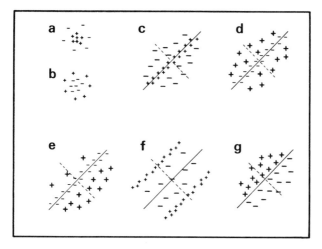

Figure 5.47
Examples of simple concentric receptive fields in the cat cerebral cortex. The concentric ON-center (*a*) and OFF-center (*b*) fields are typical of simple receptive fields in LGB but are also found in area 17 of cat and monkey. (*c*) to (*g*), Simple fields but with a specific preferred orientation axis. Cell (*c*) responds preferentially to a bright bar in the center and fields (*d*), (*e*), and (*f*) to a dark bar. Field (*g*) is asymmetrical, as is (*e*) also. These fields (*c*) to (*g*) respond best to a displacement of the bar in the direction of the dotted line. (+) signifies excitation and (−) inhibition in response to a bright bar (or excitation by a dark bar). (From Brooks & Jung 1973)

Remember from now on that, whatever their type, these receptive fields have a roughly rectangular outline with a major axis (length, *Lc*) and a certain width (*Wc*).

Using fixed spots or slits, it is found that S fields have an ON/OFF organization but show nonconcentric arrangements, as opposed to LGB cell fields. Thus an ON-response flanked by an OFF-response on one side exists and alternatively an ON-response flanked by OFF-responses on both sides of it. Most C cells show a homogeneous ON/OFF arrangement. However, this rule is not universal; some cells that show other C characteristics have a zoned ON/OFF organization (figure 5.47 and 5.48).

The S cells, just like the C cells, show a preferred orientation when stimulated by stationary rectilinear bars. The corresponding tuning curve, *R* = *F(o)*, is narrow for S cells and wide for C. Apart from that, for a stimulus with optimal orientation, the response depends on the position of the bar or edge in type S fields, whereas it does not if the field is a homogeneous ON/OFF type C.

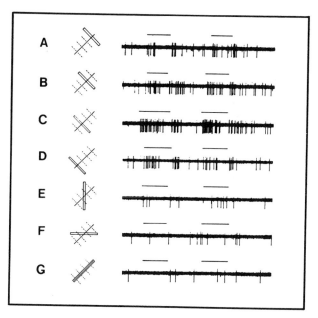

Figure 5.48
Responses of a cortical complex cell in the right visual area 18 of the cat. Left eye stimulation by a slit 1/8° × 2.5°. The field is in the area centralis and is 2° × 3° in extent. The stimulus is stationary and is switched on and off. A to D, slit oriented parallel to the preferred direction of the field and is projected to different places in the field. Stimulation marked by the horizontal bar above each trace. E to G, The slit is oriented at 45° or 90° to the preferred orientation. (From Hubel & Wiesel 1962)

One of the (perhaps most universal) differences between S and C cells appears when a bar of optimal orientation is used but its width (Wb) is modified. In S cells it generates a summation in the interior of each homogeneous part of the field (whether ON or OFF). In C cells, however, the results are more complicated. For example, the optimal bar width (Wb) can be considerably less than the cell's field width (Wc) whatever the organization of the C cell, whether homogeneous ON/OFF or, in the more frequent case, ON or OFF.

Another distinction arises from what happens to a response when the length (Lb) lying along the optimal axis (o) is increased. S cells and also a subgroup of the C cells (called *standard* C) show a regular summation, with the response increasing as Lb increases up to the length (Lc) of the field. In contrast, other C cells (called *special* C) show a response that is in practice maximal for a length (Lb) <

(Lc). Beyond that the response stays more or less the same until (LB) = (Lc).

In their original definitions, Hubel and Wiesel extracted a third cell category called *hypercomplex cells* (HC). These have a peripheral inhibitory region as a fundamental characteristic. Their work also led them to distinguish two subgroups of HC. Some cells (called *lower-order HC*) respond to a bar or a rectilinear contrast edge, stationary or moving, in an optimal orientation, but only on condition that the length (Lb) does not exceed a certain value. If (Lb) > (Lc) the response decreases, which proves the existence of peripheral inhibition. Other cells (*higher-order* HC) only generate responses under the influence of more comlex stimuli, such as a bright corner defined by two perpendicular dark boundaries (figure 5.49).

We have seen how the terminations of X, Y, and possibly W cell types are arranged with respect to the various cortical layers of area 17. Here we study the laminar arrangements of these types of cells with simple or complex response characteristics. Experiments show that simple cells are concentrated at two levels, the superficial parts of layer VI and all layer IV. Standard complex cells, in contrast, occupy either the deep layers V and VI or the superficial layers II-III (Gilbert 1977, 1983; cf. Wiesel & Gilbert 1983).

COMMUNAL ORGANIZATION OF S, C, AND HC CELLS

Once again we will begin with the original scheme of Hubel and Wiesel (1962) that proposed a "hierarchic" elaboration of the re-

---

Figure 5.49
Examples of the behavior of a hypercomplex cortical cell in cat area 18. Stimulation of the right eye, which is in this case dominant. Receptive field 2° × 4° in extent with an inhibitory zone in its right half (see dotted contours). *A*, The stimulus is a band of light oriented to 2 o'clock, dark below and dark also to its full width at its (90°) right boundary. Luminance in the bright region 1.3 log cd/m² and in the dark region 0.0 log · cd/m². From above to below (1 to 5): advance and return of the luminous stimulus (along the arrows). From 1 to 3: the area of the field illuminated increases and the response also. In 4 to 5: the illuminated stimulus bites more and more into the inhibitory zone of the field, decreasing and even suppressing the response. Each stimulus sweep lasts 2 s. *B*, Displacement always in the same direction, upward only, of an increasingly (1 to 6) obtuse angled stimulus. The inhibition is maximal when the angle is flat (6). *C*, Same type of (2 deg/s) displacement of a bright right angled stimulus accompanied by a second one that is closer or further away from the first and therefore biting more or less into the inhibitory zone. *D*, Displacement of two bright edges of the same orientation but which have different separations. Here again the response decreases for a given illumination of the excitatory region in proportion to the amount of the inhibitory region that is encroached upon. (From Hubel & Wiesel 1965)

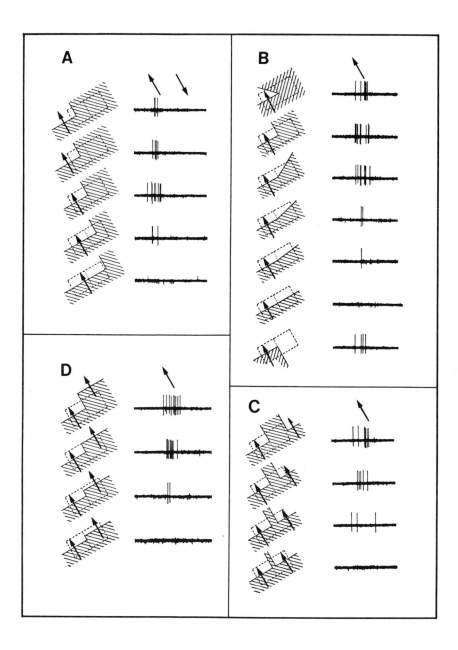

ceptive fields (figure 5.50). They posited that S cells receive their inputs from a given number of geniculate cells, either ON-center or OFF-center; the ordered juxtaposition of each can explain the elongated, rather than concentric, nature of the field.

The more complicated nature of the C cells would be due to a convergence from several simple cells, and this could explain the uniform ON/OFF configuration by exploiting short intracortical connections. Similarly, a corresponding extension of this arrangement would explain the hypercomplex nature of HC cells, several C cells converging on an HC unit with the appropriate combination of these fields determining the particular peripheral inhibitions. According to the original hypothesis, S cells are localized chiefly in area 17, whereas C cells predominate in 18 and 19. The HC cells are found only in areas 18 and 19. What is seen therefore is a hierarchical "cascade" arrangement from simple to more complex from 17 to 19, which at the time was strictly in line with traditional notions of brain behavior.

The hierarchical arrangement was disputed by a good deal of experimentation that led, one way or the other, to contradictory results and stimulated the proposal of a new concept, that of the visual information being treated by geniculocortical paths that are arranged *in parallel.*

The classification of cortical cells has been reviewed by various researchers (Henry et al. 1973, 1974; Rose & Blakemore 1974; Goodwin & Henry 1975; Henry 1977; Rose 1977; Orban & Kennedy 1981; Payne & Berman 1983; cf., for the monkey, Schiller et al. 1976a,b,c; De Valois et al. 1979, 1982) and here we summarize two aspects.

The hypercomplex categorization (i.e., the existence of an inhibitory zone at the extremities of the field which is not by itself responsive) has also been shown in some simple cells (since referred to as S_H or as *hypercomplex type I*) and has equally been found in complex cells (referred to as C_H or as *hypercomplex type II*). The hypercomplex character thus ceases to be a unique entity.

The types of cell in area 17 have thus become more numerous than Hubel and Wiesel envisaged. Effectively, we see there: S cells, S_H cells, C cells (complex wide field), B cells (complex narrow field), A cells (wide field complex with separate ON and OFF regions), and finally, cells with concentric field arrangements ("geniculate fields"). Numerous simple cell types have been found in area 18 since the original scheme was conceived. We will return to this when dis-

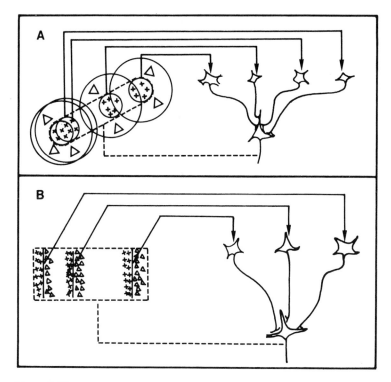

Figure 5.50
Diagrams to illustrate the hierarchical organization of simple (A) and complex (B)
receptive fields. A, A limited number of LGB cells (of which four are shown above
right) have ON-center receptive fields arranged along a straight line on the retina. All
project to the same cortical cell with excitatory synaptic contacts. The receptive field
of the cortical cell becomes an elongated ON-center cell as shown at the left hand side
by dashed lines. B, A given number of simple cortical cells, three of which are shown
in the diagram, are assumed to project to a single cortical cell at a higher hierarchical
level. Each afferent neuron has a receptive field arranged as shown to the left with an
excitatory zone (+) and an inhibitory zone (−) to either side of a central straight line
boundary. The boundaries of these fields are thus distributed inside the rectangular
area shown by the dashed lines. Any edge crossing this field horizontally, whatever
its position, will generate an excitation of this higher order cell for stimulus ON and
an inhibition for stimulus OFF. (From Hubel & Wiesel 1962)

cussing movement sensitivity. Finally and notably, it has been shown by several researchers (e.g., Bullier & Henry 1979a,b) that the C elements of area 17 can, quite as much as the S, receive a direct *input* from the geniculate.

It now becomes necessary to postulate the existence within cortical systems, whether simple or complex, of *inhibitory interactions* according to an organization that continues the arrangements postulated for the LGB level (see section 2.2 above). Thus a cortical cell may be excited by a small number of geniculate afferents (one in the limit) but also receive other inhibitory influences from nearby cells. This idea rests on the demonstration of IPSPs in visual cortical cells that are generated particularly by moving stimuli (Creutzfeldt et al. 1974) and supported by neurochemical results in favor of intracortical inhibitory interactions. We will discuss these briefly below.

NEUROCHEMICAL MEDIATORS OF THE SPATIAL SELECTIVITIES IN CORTICAL CELLS

We now describe the results that demonstrate the important role of cortical inhibitory interactions, all the geniculocortical fibers providing excitatory input and the inhibitions being effected by local cortical interneurons. Recent neurochemical research supports this hypothesis particularly for orientation (o) or directional (d) selectivity of cortical cells, these characteristics being linked to cortical lateral inhibition operating via GABAergic interneurons.

Physiologically, the proof of this type of inhibition rests, rather than on intracellular investigations, on the iontophoretic administration of bicuculline (antagonist of GABAergic receptors) to pyramidal-type cortical cells, that is those that have previously been identified as possessing S or C responses (Rose & Blakemore 1974b).

In this way it has been shown that an S cell's (o) selectivity was maintained under GABA antagonists but its (d) selectivity was suppressed, and from then on the cell responds in both directions of movement of a stimulus among a given axis while still preserving a certain orientation preference (Sillito 1975a,b; see also (Trans.) Sillito 1977, Sillito et al. 1980). This persistence of the (o) selectivity has more recently been attributed to an incomplete inhibitory block. When the action of bicuculline is coupled with that of 3-mercaptopropionic acid (3-MP), a GAD inhibitor (i.e., inhibiting the enzyme synthesizing GABA from glutamate), then in those conditions both the (d) and the (o) selectivity are suppressed (Tsumoto et al. 1982; figure 5.51).

The case of complex cells proves to be equally interesting. Applica-

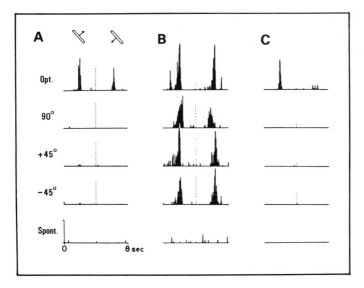

Figure 5.51
Effects of 3-MP and of bicuculline on the orientational and directional sensitivities
of a visual cortical cell. *C*, Control response showing that the cell is both orientation
and direction sensitive; movements according to the inset diagrams above column A.
A, Responses obtained during intravenous injection of 3-MP, measured after 20 to 25
min. Abolition of the directional sensitivity but maintenance of the orientation sensitivity. *B*, Simultaneous injection of 3-MP and administration of bicuculline. In this case
there is abolition of both directional and orientation sensitivity. (From Tsumoto et al.
1982)

tions of both GABA antagonists produces analogous effects, suppressing both the (d) and even (o) sensitivities, that is, the orientational selectivity properties of these cells are also dictated at least in
part by a process of cortical inhibition. This means that the original
model of intracortical hierarchical organization by Hubel and Wiesel,
in which the C cells only receive inputs from S cells, all of them
excitatory, proves once more to be inadequate. Like the S cells, the
C cells must receive a direct input from the geniculocortical pathway.

Histologically and *histochemically*, many efforts have been made to
specify the presumed inhibitory interneurons and the involvement of
GABA as a transmitter. As we have seen, histology has demonstrated
several intracortical interneurons, stellate units with smooth dendrites, different pyramidal units, and other cells with spiny dendrites
that have basket terminals in the cell body region of pyramidal cells
(which suggests a powerful inhibitory influence from the latter). After

injecting it into the visual cortex, the spread of ^{3}H-GABA into interneurons can be measured and this also corresponds effectively
with the histological "stellate/smooth dendrite" classification above.
It is also known that GABA is "pumped" at GABAergic terminals
and accumulated by the perikaryon. When ^{3}H-GABA is injected into
layers V and VI, it is seen in neurons in layer II in which there has
been retrograde transport, and these seem to be cells with double
dendritic trees.

Immunohistological characterization by GAD, the enzyme for
GABA synthesis from glutamic acid, has enabled even more specific
characterization. GAD-positive terminals have been localized to the
somas, the proximal dendrites, and axon terminals. These terminals
make *reciprocal* synapses with the dendrites of pyramidal and stellate
cells. The somas of these GAD$^+$ neurons receive both reciprocal and
nonreciprocal synapses. Finally, stellate cells with smooth dendrites
are involved as inhibitory interneurons in the cortex (Ribak 1978).

TONIC AND PHASIC CORTICAL CELLS: X AND Y TYPES

We saw above how the response properties of X, Y, and possibly W
retinal cells are replicated in the thalamocortical units in LGB (Ikeda
& Wright 1975a,b). The further elaboration of these signals needs to
be undertaken remembering that, as we have seen, cortical cells present two other basic types of response, simple (S) and complex (C).
The X and Y afferents (considered alone) project to different cortical
levels (in particular in layer IV), which encourages the speculation
that four independent combinations ought to be possible: S-X, S-Y,
C-X, C-Y.

In other words, it is necessary to discover the extent of S and C
cell distributions with either good temporal resolution but bad spatial
resolution (Y-type) or with good spatial resolution and bad temporal
resolution (X-type). At present, this apparently has only been
achieved for cat S cells in area 17 (Mullikin et al. 1984a,b). By using
some well-established techniques and criteria (tonic or phasic nature
of the response to a contrast step stimulus, extent of the excitatory
field, movement sensitivity, spatial homogeneity or heterogeneity of
field characteristics; see chapter 4, section 5.3), it has been shown
that S cells comprise two subassemblies, one with X, the other with
Y characteristics, with their levels of cortical localization essentially
corresponding with the known terminations of X and Y inputs from
the thalamus (see section 3.2 above).

No doubt data for the other cell types will soon become available. Maybe the general idea will be confirmed that channels for X, Y, and even W types of information constitute independent channels all the way up to their cortical level.

MOVEMENT SENSITIVITY

[The terms orientation and direction sensitivity will be used as defined in section 3.3 above.] Up to the present we have only considered cortical cell responses to stationary stimuli. At subcortical levels it has been established that there are cells sensitive to *movement* in both SC and LGB and even in the retina. In some cases, the sensitivity arises as an intrinsic property of the local cell network and is unpredictable from responses to fixed stimuli (as in the case of the rabbit retina, as we have seen, and of the SC in a variety of species and also to some extent in LGB). For other cases, as in the cat retina and often in LGB, the response to a moving stimulus is the predictable response to a stimulus moving across ON and OFF areas and thus is only a simple consequence of the response characteristics found in the spatiotemporal domain for stationary stimuli.

Our discussion of movement sensitivity in cortical cells will benefit from a few preliminary remarks.

Most studies have been made keeping the fundamental division of cell types into S and C, with a possible inhibitory fringe H and in some cases, adopting subdivisions within class C into A and B cells as proposed by Henry (1977), as well as taking into account the more recent criteria separating X-type from Y-type cells. As in the retina, and later in SC and LGB, consideration is made as to whether or not movement sensitivities are predictable from static measurements of field geometry.

As in comparing LGB responses with retinal, it is important to distinguish between those cortical properties that have arisen from local interactive mechanisms and those that are merely the effect of what is in the signal input from lower centers.

Differential Behaviors of S and C Cells

Let us first examine the behavior of S and C cells to moving stimuli without, for the moment, considering changes in speed (figure 5.52; see, e.g., Goodwin & Henry 1978). Most S cells are (d)-selective, whereas many C are not. For movement in the optimal direction, the response of an S cell to a light (L) or dark (D) bar crossing the re-

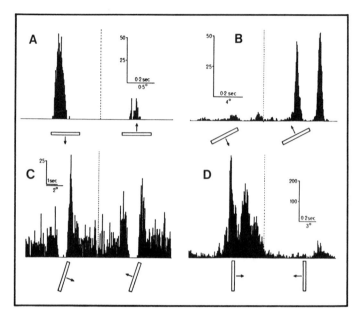

Figure 5.52
Sensitivity of cortical cells to stimulus movement. Discharge frequencies as a function of time for a repetitive displacement of a slit that is optimally oriented to the receptive field in four types of area 17 cortical cells in the cat; responses to stimulating the dominant eye in each case. Responses in spikes/s against displacement of the slit with respect to the mean position in degrees of arc and seconds (see scales). For each cell, responses to two opposite directions of movement. *A*, Simple cell, unimodal, d-selective (stimulus slit 1.5° × 0.2°: 20 deg/s). *B*, Simple cell, bimodal, d-selective (3° × 0.2°: 20 deg/s). *C*, Simple cell with central inhibition (3° × 0.2°: 1.3 deg/s). *D*, Complex cell (4° × 0.5°: 15 deg/s). (From Pettigrew et al. 1968a)

ceptive field (as defined by static stimuli) consists in one or two abrupt discharge peaks, called respectivley *unimodal* or *bimodal* responses. The spatial extent of the peak or peaks is smaller than that of the static receptive field. In contrast, for C cells the discharge is maintained throughout the whole field with a maximal response near the center. (Pettigrew et al. 1968a,b).

When a bar, or even more so an edge, moves in the field of an S cell, the excitation is preceded by an inhibition of the spontaneous activity of the cell. This inhibition, unlike the excitatory peak, is not (d)-selective. No inhibition of this sort has been described for C cells.

When an S cell is subjected to stimulation by a moving grating (alternate bright and dark bands), the S cells respond well but the C cells' responses merge into each other quite quickly. Conversely, when presented with a bar stimulus constructed of random dots moving with respect to a background of the same sort of random structure, the S cells do not respond, whereas the C cells do (camouflage perception).

A whole series of experiments (Bishop et al. 1973, Goodwin et al. 1975) that we can only summarize, have been aimed at understanding the mechanisms for directional sensitivity, particularly for the S cells, which show this effect most clearly (figure 5.53).

[In no case is the (d)-selectivity tightly linked to any spatial organization of ON and OFF subregions established for the cells by static stimuli; in other words, directional sensitivity is not predictable from that organization.

Using simple edges representing a passage from dark (D) → light (L) or the opposite, it is possible to show in an S-cell field that there are two zones of maximal response, one for the light edge L ("center" of ON-discharge) and the other for the dark edge D ("center" of OFF-discharge). In a given S cell these two are spatially separated to a greater or lesser extent, giving rise to the complexity of the responses of such cells to a bar, which is in effect a succession of two edges, one L and the other D. In C cells these two "centers" are always essentially overlapping. Furthermore, the existence of these two "centers," one for D, the other for L, explains why the (d)-selectivity is practically the same whether the bar stimulus contrast is positive (bright bar on dark ground) or negative (dark bar on bright ground).

Finally, there is a selectivity even *within* a zone of homogeneous response to a static stimulus (either ON or OFF). In other words, this (d)-selectivity is in no case linked to an antagonistic interaction between (static) ON and OFF zones: to the contrary, it must be due to the existence of *local inhibitory interconnections* (as already described for the rabbit retina) arranged so that movement in the nonpreferred direction unlocks intracortical inhibitory mechanisms that are particularly sensitive to movement and are not detectable with stationary spot or bar stimuli (Barlow & Levick 1965).]

Note at this point that these properties allow the introduction of new distinctions betwen S and C cell types that have led, as we shall see, to the specification of a large number of cells as S in area 18, unlike the original conclusions of Hubel and Wiesel.

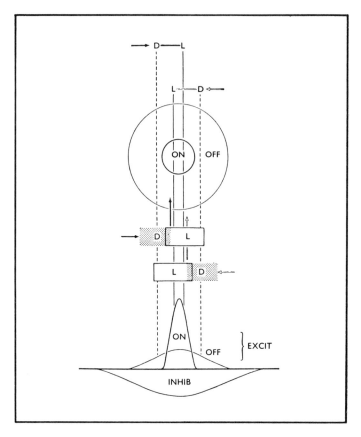

Figure 5.53
Response of a simple cell to a moving stimulus. Diagram showing the relationships between the excitatory (EXCIT ON and OFF) and inhibitory (INHIB) components of the receptive field of a simple cortical cell together with the ON- and OFF-regions of a geniculate cell. The vertical lines represent the positions where maximal discharge is obtained for the displacement of a light edge (continuous lines L) or a dark edge (dashed vertical lines D) in a right-left direction, or in the opposite left-right direction. The rectangles L and D mark the discharge centers for the cases of the light and dark edges respectively. The solid vertical arrowhead shows the maximal discharge position for a slit moving left → right across the field and the open arrowhead is for a right → left movement. The diagram aims at explaining the discharges observed when an edge or bar crosses the receptive field of a simple cortical cell. (From Bishop et al. 1973)

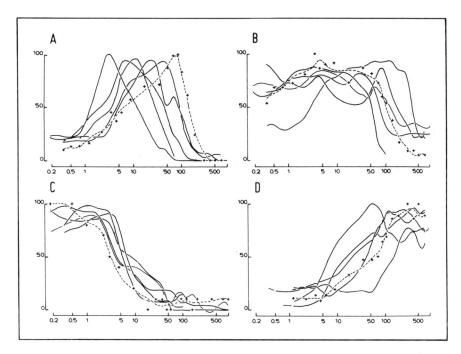

Figure 5.54
Characteristic responses (as % maximal response) to stimulus speed (deg/s) for the four different cell types. *A*, Cells sharply tuned to stimulus speed. *B*, Broadly tuned. *C*, Low-pass tuned. *D*, High-pass tuned. In each collection of curves one dotted curve shows both the curve and the experimental points from which it was obtained. (From Orban et al. 1981)

Differential Responses to Stimulus Speed

Let us now approach one of the interesting points concerned with movement, namely, the responses of S and C cells to the speed of a moving stimulus. Four different modes of response can be distinguished, sometimes in area 17 and sometimes in 18 (figure 5.54; see Orban et al. 1981):

• Cells sharply tuned to speed, *velocity tuned* (VT). These respond optimally at a given speed (generally between 2 and 100 deg/s) and their response decreases at both higher and lower speeds.
• Cells responding for a broad band of speeds, *broad-band velocity* (VBB), consequently not very speed sensitive.
• *Low-pass* cells (VLP), only responding for low stimulus speeds (<5 deg/s, to give an impression of the range in question).

• *High pass* cells (VHP), only responding at high speeds which can exceed 500 deg/s.

In actually attributing properties such as these to one or the other of the classes S or C, authors' practices vary subtly, since in some cases different subclasses are introduced within category C and in other instances the situation in area 17 is dissociated from that in 18. But essentially we have the following:

In 17, the VT and VLP categories are S cells or B cells (i.e., C cells with restricted receptive field; see section 3.2 above), whereas the VBB cells are of type C and A ("special" C cells with separate ON- and OFF-zones; see section 3.2). In 18 the S cells are often type VBB and the C and A cells often type VHP. Correspondingly, most cells in 17 are sensitive to slow movements, whereas 18 is rich in cells responding to rapid movements. Apart from that, the movement sensitivities increase with target eccentricity both in 17 and particularly in 18 (figure 5.55). Finally, we cannot fail to associate these differences with the modes of innervation in 17 and 18, knowing that 17 receives inputs from X and Y mechanisms, whereas 18 only enjoys phasic Y inputs.

Two noteworthy conclusions can be drawn from this: (1) as noted above, area 18 contains, like 17, a good proportion of S cells in contradiction to the conclusions arrived at from only static stimulus tests. (2) Area 18 appears to be specialized for the perception of rapid target movements (up to at least 700 deg/s), whereas area 17 is particularly sensitive for slow or very slow movements (0.5 deg/s; see Orban et al. 1975; Orban & Callens 1977).

A Specific Role for Area MT-V5 in Macaque
There have been several studies on the macaque MT area (Maunsell & van Essen 1983d, Mikami et al. 1986a,b, Newsome et al. 1986). The sensitivity of these cells to direction of movement and to the speed of the target are particularly well marked, with inhibitory mechanisms controlling both the directional properties and the preferred speed range. One of the factors facilitating these types of sensitivity is the existence of much wider receptive fields in MT than in V1, so that a cell in MT can respond to a notably wider angle of movement and to higher speeds than would be possible in V1. A basic complementary piece of evidence for this concerns the effects of applying stroboscopic stimuli. In humans these can create the classic perception of apparent movement. By manipulating the spatial and

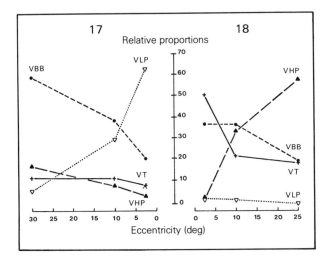

Figure 5.55
Proportions of the four types of speed sensitive cells in area 17 (left) and 18 (right) as a function of stimulus eccentricity. VT, sharply velocity tuned cells; VBB, broad band tuning; VLP, low-pass tuning; VHP, high-pass tuning. (From Orban et al. 1981)

temporal characteristics of this sort of stimulation, the results of psychophysical experiments in human subjects has been compared with the relative cell responses in V1 and V5 in the macaque. Here again the comparison favors V5 over V1, which strongly suggests a special function of MT for processing not only real but also apparent movement.

Having just suggested that a single set of mechanisms can deal with both the real and apparent movement of light sources over a limited angular distance, we are hypothetically postulating that cells sensitive to (d)-selective movement possess some very well-dedicated functional properties that are capable of integrating along a target's trajectory as a function of time and of space simultaneously.

From this, to the extent that the visual system can effect an interpolation between the positions of static images and thus perceive image positions (even if they do not exist) *between* these places in the same way that it does when confronted with a real movement, then these mechanisms can generate perceptions that do not differ at all from one another. Such integrators in space-time would not be able to distinguish real from apparent movements.

Note also that most area MT cells are binocular and very sensitive to disparities, which might well suggest their particular suitability for contributing to the perception of movement in three-dimensional space (Maunsell & van Essen 1983b).

Another study has been devoted to the area that is immediately adjacent to MT and is situated in the dorsal part of the median superior temporal sulcus, area *MST* (Saito et al. 1986). Direction-sensitive cells are found there with a variety of behaviors, some sensitive to rectilinear movement in the frontoparallel plane ("D"), some to change in size of a stimulus ("S"), and still others to the rotation of a shape ("R"). The hypothesis proposed is that this region, called "DSR" carries out these operations by effecting a serial integration beyond MT.

ACUITY AND SPATIAL SELECTIVITY OF VISUAL CELLS

We have already discussed how visual psychophysics has exploited the use of stationary and moving gratings. These stimuli have facilitated similar animal research in various levels of the nervous system (retina, LGB, and cortex) measuring the spatial selectivity and its relationship with contrast in the cat and occasionally in the monkey. [However, this experimentation sometimes exploits a drifting grating image presented to the animal and sometimes uses a stationary grating with an alternation of the contrast between the fixed stripes. The two viewpoints, sensitivity to spatial contrast and sensitivity to movement, are not always as clearly separated as in human experiments.] Thus animal experiments manipulate two variables, the grating spatial frequency and the contrast between the bright and dark bands, and proceed either by determining thresholds or by measuring supraliminal changes (figure 5.56).

General Measurements
The acuity at a cellular level, at a given contrast, may be measured by finding the *highest spatial frequency* in an alternating grating that can generate a detectable response. The cell continues to respond as the spatial frequency increases but only up to a certain maximal spatial frequency for that cell, at which the response is no longer detectably different from the cell's spontaneous activity. This allows a general estimate of acuity and shows that it is maximal for cells serving the area centralis and decreases for those registering images situated toward the periphery of the retina. In the cat, the mean value for this type of experimental estimate of the acuity threshold is around 6 cycles/deg. Behavioral measurements, of which some are of long

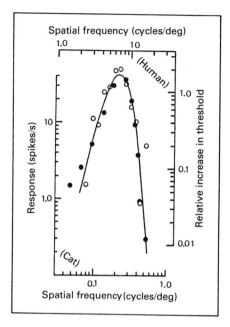

Figure 5.56
Response of a simple cell in cat visual cortex to a sinusoidal grating. Comparison with the adaptation of detection sensitivity generated by a similar stimulus in humans. Black circles, response of the cat cell as a function of grating spatial frequency for a grating of contrast 0.5 displaced in the preferred direction for the cell at a speed of one bar/s. Open circles, human response adaptation after prior exposure to a grating of contrast 0.7 and a spatial frequency of 7 cycles/deg as a function of the spatial frequency of the test grating. The scales have been manipulated so as to superimpose the two sets of observations, human and cat, over each other. Note that the curve for cat is narrower in absolute spatial frequency spread. (From Brooks & Jung 1973)

standing, showed results of the same order (5.5 cycles/deg). Human psychophysical tests generally show much higher acuity values (50 cycles/deg; see Brooks & Jung 1973).

Then there is the determination of the variation of cell discharge rate with spatial frequency toward the low spatial frequency side. There, depending on the case, the curve might be flat or might show a maximum at a certain spatial frequency of the grating, (Bishop et al. 1971a,b) just like the results obtained from human psychophysics.

There is also the study of how cell discharge varies, at a given spatial frequency, as a function of the grating contrast. As in the results above (from both human psychophysics and the amplitude of visual evoked potentials), there is a linear increase (in this case in response discharge rate) as a function of the log of the contrast, at least for one category of cells, the cortical S cells.

Once again, threshold contrast values can be measured, that is, the contrast magnitude for a given grating spatial frequency at which a cell first shows a detectable change in its activity can be compared with the spontaneous discharge. In practice, the reciprocal of the threshold value is usually specified. This is the *contrast sensitivity*. The curve obtained with the spatial frequency of the grating as independent variable is very like that in the previous paragraphs with a maximal sensitivity at a particular spatial frequency.

Finally, using either visual function, the attenuation of response toward high spatial frequencies can be measured, namely, the spatial frequency at which the response or the sensitivity has decreased by 1 log unit with respect to the response at "zero spatial frequency" (in the absence of any succession of stripes). This level of attenuation varies with cell type, reinforcing the hypothesis of the researchers (already obtained from other data) suggesting the existence of separate channels for the discrimination of spatial frequencies (Campbell et al. 1969a, Jacobson 1976).

Cell Categories at Different Levels of the Visual System
Given such results, the question clearly arises as to which types of retinal, geniculate, or cortical mechanisms (to consider the principal pathway only) are likely to elaborate the particular characteristics seen in sensitivity to spatial frequency. Essentially, conclusions are referred to the distinctly different systems that have been discovered by the use of other types of stimuli, that is, X and Y types throughout the visual system and S and C types in the cortex.

We have seen, from studying their general properties, that the retinal X and Y cells have different spatial frequency sensitivities: Tonic X cells are highly sensitive to spatial frequency and are poorly sensitive to temporal contrast; Y cells have a good temporal resolution and a poor spatial resolution. But this proposition needs to be considered carefully, because when using gratings of a given contrast as stimuli with a given speed of drift across the visual field but with a variable spatial frequency f, it is found that at the retinal level X cells show a higher spatial frequency cut-off than y, and at the low spatial frequency side the X cells tend to show a reduction in response that is much more marked than in Y cells.

At the LGB level these differences are quantitatively even more accentuated. The two geniculate operational mechanisms, one with X and the other with Y inputs, each tend here to show the existence of an optimal "f," but it is nevertheless clear that the Y cells remain more sensitive to very low spatial frequencies than the X, whereas the X are more sensitive to high spatial frequencies. Researchers suggest (e.g., Lehmküle et al. 1980) that, to the extent that LGB can be considered to be responsible for some of the mechanisms subserving form vision, or at least be involved as a relay for that sort of function, then it is the Y cells that comprise the basic substrate for shape recognition (which essentially requires good visual spatial frequency sensitivity at low spatial frequencies), whereas the X cells, being better analyzers of high spatial frequencies, are the complementary units for the vision of detail and texture.

Similarly there are some observations to make on the situation in the cortex. In line with the results above, behavioral observations in the cat also seem to confirm the importance of X cells for high spatial frequency vision and spatial acuity and of the Y cells for the perception of low spatial frequency contrasts. After surgical elimination of area 17 (which is the cortical region that chiefly benefits from a large projection from X type mechanisms, as we have seen), the animals lose all sensitivity to high spatial frequency contrast while preserving a good discrimination of low spatial frequencies (Lehmkühle et al. 1982). This point may well be important in that even a rough recognition of shapes requires a good resolution of low spatial frequencies (Kabrisky et al. 1970, Hess & Woo 1978) from the Y cells and not the X, which were originally considered to be responsible for all spatial vision. It is this coarse shape discrimination that is retained after lesion of the geniculostriate system, that is, after the elimination of the basic X system while retaining the Y system; the latter has a much wider input to the cortex.

Electrophysiological exploration of the cat cortex (Hammond & MacKay 1975, 1977; Maffei 1978; Maffei & Fiorentini 1973, 1977) also points to differences in mechanisms. However, the dividing line in this case does not seem to be between X and Y but between simple and complex cells. The distinction arises in a different way: S cells show a spatial frequency *tuning curve* with a very well-peaked maximum and a tuning width for "f" that is narrow. In contrast, cells classified as C from other data have a much flatter curve. In these respects, therefore, it is the S cells, as opposed to the C (and not the X as opposed to Y) that correspond with the spatial frequency tuning systems proposed from psychophysics (see chapter 3, section 3.3). However, not everything is fully explained by that hypothesis; we will return to the question below when discussing amblyopia.

In areas 17 and 18 of the cat the cortical localization of cells has been studied according to their optimal spatial frequency (whatever their response type). It appears that cells of the same spatial resolving power (in other words, with the same optimal spatial frequency) are aligned in directions at right angles to the alignment of cells with identical orientation preference. Therefore, while the latter are grouped in vertical orientation columns, cells with the same spatial resolving power are found along tangential electrode penetrations, that is, along lines parallel with the cortical surface (Berardi et al. 1982).

Following Schiller et al. (1976a,c), De Valois et al. (1982) studied the spatial selectivity of cells in the macaque, and Foster et al. (1985) compared the spatial and temporal selectivity between areas V1 and V2 in the same species. They found that most cells in V1 and V2 have a good spatial selectivity but with some bandwidth differences (0.2 to 2.1 cycles/deg in V1 and 0.5 to 8.0 cycles/deg in V2), whereas the temporal selectivities in these areas differ more markedly. Most cells in V1 respond up to 5 to 8 Hz spatial frequency but are low-pass types (with no real temporal selectivity), whereas most V2 cells show a peak in selectivity around 4 Hz spatial frequency.

In the macaque, Hawken and Parker (1984), studying spatial contrast sensitivity of cells in layer IV, showed a difference between parts that are superficial and deep with respect to layer IVC: in layer IVCα, sensitivity is as high as it is in the magnocellular layers of LGB; in layer IVCβ, it is weaker and like parvocellular units. Taking into account the remarks already made with respect to LGB units (see section 2.2, above) little correlation between these response properties and the X/Y classification is as yet evident (De Valois et al. 1979).

ADDENDUM

Attempts to Model Contrast and Movement Detectors
We find ourselves unable to omit, in this context of physiological analysis, some interesting attempts to devise a model that can simultaneously explain the mechanisms that detect a contrast edge and also the movement of a bar. During our discussions we have encountered, more or less explicitly, two somewhat different ways of approaching explanations for the different stages of treating the information relating to form and to spatial contrasts in the visual system. Schematically we may sometimes

consider, as did Hubel and Wiesel, that there exist populations of specialized detecting units dedicated in a well-defined way to the widths and orientations of bars or contrast edges. Alternatively, the processes are sometimes viewed, as by Campbell and Robson (1968) and others, as treating information in parallel visual paths via channels dedicated to orientation and to spatial frequency (which can in the limit operate as Fourier analyzers).

These two viewpoints give rise to a certain number of difficulties that we will not detail here. They have, however, inspired the creation of a formal model of visual image processing that, as we shall see, is strictly governed by certain physiological data, in particular those concerned with the existence of X and Y channels (Marr & Ullman 1981, Marr & Hildreth 1980).

Operators Detecting a Bright/Dark Edge

First, an algorithm is suggested for detecting contrast edges and it is suggested that this takes place in several stages (in principal, successive ones).

Optimal image-filtering. Before being processed further, the original image first needs to be filtered optimally. Filtering is needed because it is hardly conceivable that a single mechanism could deal with all contrast profiles from the most gentle to the very steep. This filtering dictates two sorts of constraint: One is in the spatial frequency domain, that is, at the edges of a contrast variation, where it is conceivable that a given detector can only operate over a certain limited bandwidth of spatial frequency (say with a variance δw). The other is a constraint upon spatial localization, which needs to be as acute as possible (say a variance in the spatial domain of δx that needs to be as small as possible).

Intuitively, these two constraints must be to some extent antagonistic, since the product $\delta w \cdot \delta x$ cannot be less than a certain magnitude (that has been shown to be $\pi/4$; thus $\delta x \cdot \delta w \geq \pi/4$). From this there arises a first element of the proposed theory. It has been demonstrated that one distribution optimizes such an operation, that is, simultaneously reduces to a minimum the values of δx and δw. This is the Gaussian distribution:

$$G(x) = \sigma^{-1} (2\pi)^{-1/2} \exp(-x^2/2\sigma^2),$$

for which the Fourier transform is:

$$\hat{G}(w) = \exp(-\tfrac{1}{2}\sigma^2 w^2).$$

In this expression the spatial resolution of the image is higher and narrower the smaller the parameter σ (space constant); this is referred to as a "pixel," or a "picture element." In a two-dimensional system we have:

$$G(r) = (\tfrac{1}{2}\pi\sigma^2) \exp(-r^2/2\sigma^2).$$

For the moment we can imagine the image to be treated in this way by a whole series of filters operating in parallel and having different spatial resolutions.

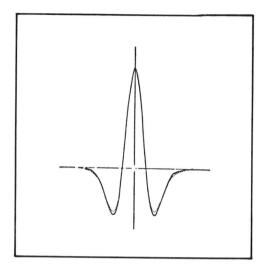

Figure 5.57
The difference of Gaussians (DOG) operator. The "Mexican hat" shaped DOG operator is the contour of the difference of two Gaussian curves of space constants σ1 and
σ2 (here σ1/σ2 = 1.6). This curve is closely approximated by the second derivative G″
(x), (dashed lines), or by the Laplacian operator (∇² G) (solid line) obtained with an
appropriate σ. (From Marr & Ullman 1981)

Detection of intensity variations. The next stage is to examine the location
of intensity changes. To do this, imagine that a first derivative of intensity is taken and this is inspected for maxima. In fact this procedure
would be somewhat lacking in sensitivity and another mechanism is to
be preferred: a search for places where the second derivative of intensity
D^2 passes through zero (zero-crossings, ZC). Thus it is found that this
operation consists in determining the ZCs of the function:

$$f(x,y) = D^2 [G(r)*I(x,y)]$$

where $I(x,y)$, the intensity of the image at a point x,y in appropriate
units, represents the image and (*) is the convolution operator. The derivative $D^2 [G(r)*(Ix,y)]$, because of the properties of the convolution, can
also be written $D^2G*I(x,y)$. Writing $D^2G = G″$, then in the (x) dimension
$G″$ can be written:

$$G″(x) = [-σ^{-3}(2π)^{1/2}] [1 - (x^2/σ^2)] \exp[-(x^2/2σ^2)].$$

This second derivative plots as a "Mexican hat"-shaped operator that
is in practice very like the function that is obtained from the difference
of two antagonistic Gaussians (DOG curves) of space constants $σ_1$ and
$σ_2$ (figure 5.57).

Thus at this stage the contrast characteristics of the image can be determined (1) by convolution of the image by the operator D^2G, and (2) by
looking for the ZCs. But there is another necessary constraint also, the

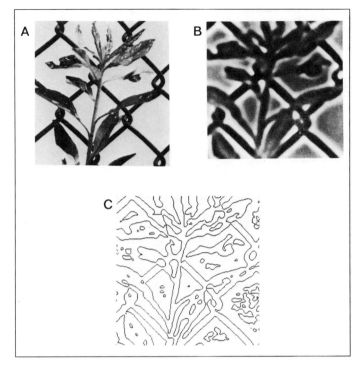

Figure 5.58
Treatment of the image by a DOG operator. Image (*A*) when subjected to a convolution by a center/surround organization of the DOG type ($\nabla^2 G$) results in (*B*) with the positive resultant values represented in white and the negative ones in black. These black and white values might represent the ganglion cell activity of respectively ON-center and OFF-center cell types "inspecting" the image. From (*B*) can be deduced a map of zero-crossings (*C*). Similar filterings for different given spatial frequencies can, combined together, embrace the total information contained in (*A*). (From Marr & Hildreth 1980)

need to recognize the direction (with respect to the x,y image plane) in which the two above operations need to be carried out. To break free from that restriction, an operator that is independent of direction is introduced. This is the Laplacian $\nabla^2 G$. It may be shown that this function ($\nabla^2 G = \partial^2/\partial x^2 + \partial^2/\partial y^2 + \partial^2/\partial z^2$) in the limit is very close to a DOG function when the ratio σ_1/σ_2 of the two Gaussian functions tends to unity.

Finally, this operation reduces to finding the zero-crossings of the convolution $\nabla^2 G * I$.

The result of such a Gaussian filtering is a representation of the image in terms of oriented segments near zero-crossing. The accuracy of this image representation will be better the smaller the σ of the Gaussian function (figure 5.58).

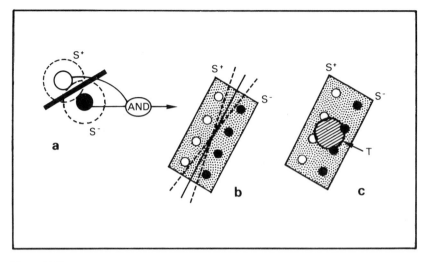

Figure 5.59
Models of zero-crossing detectors. *a*, Two S− and S+ units are associated with an AND logical operator. This arrangement can detect the zero crossing between the two subunits. *b*, A rank of such units could detect the zero-crossing of an oriented contrast edge, roughly as being between the two dashed lines. *c*, A "T" unit is added to detector *b*. If it is a T+ unit the operator STS will respond when the light border moves from S+ to S−. If the unit is T− there will be a response to movement in the opposite direction. (From Marr & Ullman 1981)

In what way can all this information be compiled to really represent the image? Marr and colleagues postulate a further necessary accompaniment, that of *coincidence:* if a ZC segment shows up in a set of independent channels (in the minimum two) for which σ is different, with the same orientation and the same position, then it should be taken into consideration in reconstructing the real image.

Application of the model. We must now examine the physiological data on which this formal modeling of the image must rely. First, note that the X retinal ganglion cells have a field arrangement which closely resembles a DOG curve (see chapter 4, section 5.3). Notice also that in the LGB, the cells in the X channel only receive a small number of ganglion cell inputs (in the limit one only). It is thus proposed that in the LGB the X channels have effected a convolution operation.

Finally, it is the field structure of the simple cell type that will be most relevant, since this sort can facilitate the detection of ZCs. First consider the case of two geniculocortical cells assumed to be side by side, one having an ON-center X field and the other an OFF-center. In this system (figure 5.59), the zero-crossing will be effected half way between the two fields. If these two are connected to an AND logic gate, the system could detect an edge but not necessarily its orientation. However, this parameter could be detected by a spatially organized range of such X^+ and X^- detectors (staying with a spatial Hubel and Wiesel type model). Thus, the orientation can be computed by this type of arrangement following a series of convolutions and the determination of the ZCs. And, very much simplified of course, that is the essential basis of this sort of modeling.

Modeling a Mechanism Sensitive to Direction of Movement

Another stage concerns the modeling of a system that is sensitive to the direction of movement. We have already seen one solution of this problem, suggested by Barlow and Levick, that involves the existence of unidirectional inhibitory connections (arranged as a NAND gate) between two receptors that are stimulated successively by a target.

Marr proposed another arrangement based on a model derived from the one above. He showed (and we will not go into the details of his argument) that to detect a movement's direction it is sufficient to carry out the following operations:

1. First, to calculate the convolution operation $(\nabla^2 G)$ with the image $G(x,y)$, this being a Gaussian distribution (exactly as above) where $\nabla^2 G * I$ can be written as $S(x,y,t)$.
2. To locate the ZCs (exactly as above).
3. To calculate (and this is the new process that is introduced) the derivative of the previous function with respect to time at the point of ZC:

$$T = \partial(\nabla^2 G * I)/\partial t = \partial[S(x,y,t)]/\partial t$$

Marr proposed that the basic unit capable of evaluating the direction of movement by means of this algorithm will consist of two units called S, one being S^+ and the other S^- (as above for the detection of an edge), to which there is added a new element situated between the two, called $T(+$ or $-)$, and which carries out the differentiation proposed in step (3). According to Marr, an element of the type $[S^+ \ T^+ \ S^-]$ would be capable of detecting the direction of a movement without it being necessary to postulate the existence of any more remote interconnections or a delay line between receptors that are some distance from each other in order to measure the movement by logical comparison mechanisms (figure 5.59).

The physiological equivalent of this model once more requires the aid of X channels but this time incorporates Y channels also. The sketch plan of such a model for movement detection would comprise two X cells (effecting the operations as above) with a Y channel element between them, that effects the differentiation $[X^+ \ Y \ X^-]$ by its phasic nature.

COLUMNAR ORGANIZATION OF THE GENICULOSTRIATE PROJECTIONS

One of the most interesting facts emerging from a study of the geniculostriate cortical projections is their *columnar organization* in the visual cortex. Two specific questions arise when considering the significance of the existence in the cat, monkey, and many other species of an organization of afferents from a given zone of the visual field being all arranged in a vertical column normal to the surface of the cortex.

The visual cortex comprises, as we know, the essential region of convergence of afferents from the two eyes (any convergence observed at the LGB level being negligible in comparison). Furthermore, physiological studies have shown clearly, in both cat and monkey, that the convergence of inputs from the right and left eyes on a given cortical cell remains a limited one and also confers on each cell a certain *ocular dominance*. In addition, and this is important, it has been demonstrated that successive cells encountered along a given intracortical electrode track normal to the cortical surface possess the same ocular dominance. Thus there are ocular dominance columns (Hubel & Freeman 1977).

This cortical organization shows that geniculate afferents from the contralateral eye (arising in the cat from layers A, C, and C2; in the monkey from 1, 4, and 6) and those from the ipsilateral eye (in the cat from A1 and C1, in the monkey from layers 2, 3, and 5), each concerned with the same point in space, are contiguous yet separated in layer IV, where they first arrive. The fact that thereafter a given ocular dominance is maintained in the layers above and below IV shows that in spite of convergence of the signals from the two eyes (a necessary condition for binocular vision), nevertheless this is not random but is organized so that there exists an ocular dominance proper to each column.

A similar question arises in respect to orientation specificity. Here also, provided an electrode penetration is normal to the cortical surface, it has been shown (particularly in the monkey) that the same preferred orientation exists in cells arranged in the column (figure 5.60; see Hubel & Wiesel 1962).

From this we can understand why, since most cortical penetrations in the macaque may be more or less oblique or even tangential, cells are experimentally successively encountered with first one ocular dominance, then another, and likewise cells with one preferred orientation and then another. Thus the question arises as to what spatial relationship might exist between these two organizations. The important fact that emerges experimentally is that the ocular dominance columns and the preferred orientation columns are separate and do not coincide. Hubel and Wiesel's (1968, 1972) work clearly shows that successive orientation columns are arranged perpendicularly to the

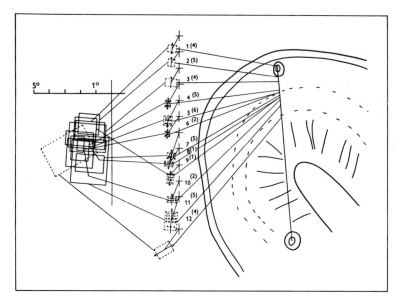

Figure 5.60
Example of a columnar arrangement of receptive fields in the visual area 17 of the cat. *Right*, Reconstruction, achieved via two small marking lesions (shown) at the ends of a microelectrode track across the cortex. Thirteen cells are recorded in the upper third of its descent. The first twelve cells are shown. The dashed lines mark the boundaries of layer IV. *Center*, Position of each field with respect to the area centralis (crosses) numbered 1 to 12, with the numbers in parenthesis relating to the category of lateralization (1 to 6 in figure 5.64) to which the cell belongs. The preferential orientation (arrows) of each of the fields except the last is practically the same. *Left*, The fields are drawn superimposed. Note the variation in their sizes and positions. (From Hubel & Wiesel 1962)

succession of ocular dominace (right and left) columns, both of them also being orthogonal to the cortical layering, of course. Their research data shows that a whole cycle of orientation columns (from 0° to 180°) is completed, then repeats approximately every 600 μm and that 800 μm is needed to go from completely right ocular dominance to completely left. Figure 5.61 shows how the researchers were also able to define a vertical cortical "hypercolumn" with right dominance columns changing to left dominance columns in one direction, accompanied by successive preferred orientation columns in the perpendicular direction going through 0°, 45°, 90°, 135° to 180°. A hypercolumn thus embraces all preferred orientations for signals from the two eyes.

The above physiological data have more recently been clearly and

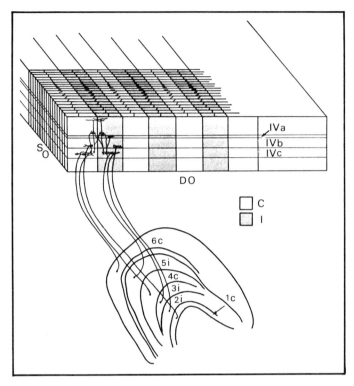

Figure 5.61
Diagram of relationships (in principle) between the ocular dominance columns (DO)
and the specific orientation columns (SO) in the macaque. Both are normal to the
cortical surface, viewed as a plane. In this figure the contralateral (c) and ipsilateral (i)
ocular dominance columns are ranged from left to right with projections from a column
of LGB cells (c, contralateral layers 6, 4, and 1; i, ipsilateral layers 5, 3 and 2). The
orientation columns are organized perpendicular to these, their preferred orientations
being indicated by the short bars on the surface. (From Hubel & Wiesel 1972)

carefully confirmed by histological and histochemical marking techniques (Hubel et al. 1978, Levay et al. 1975; figure 5.62). These results
essentially arise from the use of 2-DG as a marker for cell metabolism
on two types of preparations that have been subjected to two experimental environments: either prolonged stimulation of one eye (using
monocular occultation) or, alternatively, prolonged stimulation of
one or both eyes by bars of a fixed orientation (e.g., vertical). These
procedures reveal, depending on the method chosen, either ocular
dominance columns or orientation columns. Note that ocular dominance columns can also be studied by another autoradiographic

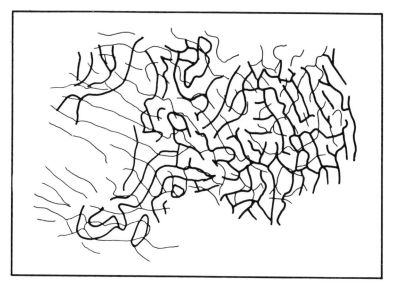

Figure 5.62
Columnar organization in the monkey: a 2-DG study. Arrangements of the orientation columns for vertical orientations and also of the ocular dominance columns, from work on monkeys either with vision limited to vertical stripes (thick lines) or confined to monocular vision (thin lines). The average distance between successive orientation columns (for the same orientation) is about 570 μm and between columns of the same ocular dominance is 770 μm. (From Hubel et al. 1978)

method (the monocular injection of ^{3}H-proline into the posterior chamber of the eye) because after a sufficiently long delay and an adequate quantity of marker being injected, a transneuronal transfer of the substance takes place in the LGB and allows identification of the cortical cells supplied from a given eye (Wiesel et al. 1974).

The following results on the situation in area 17 (V1) have emerged from the application of such methods as these in the macaque: The presence of preferred orientation columns is confirmed. The periodicity observed in the bands of marked cells after prolonged exposure to vertical bars is about 600 μm, in agreement with the physiological evidence.

This columnar arrangement of preferred orientations persists in practically all cortical layers from II to IV, with the exception of layer IVC (the principal input area for geniculate afferents), since the latter do not show orientation preference in this species. [It seems that this conclusion will need to be revised since more recently Hawken &

Parker (1981) have observed cells with orientation selectivity even in the geniculorecipient layers IVA and IVC.]

The existence of a distinct columnar arrangement for ocular dominance is also confirmed, the width of a column being 400 μm and therefore its periodicity around 800 μm.

Ocular dominance columns, unlike those for orientation, are present in all cortical layers including layer IVC.

One prediction from physiology is, in contrast, not clearly confirmed. A reciprocally orthogonal arrangement of the two types of column is not very evident. The dominance columns in reality look more like sheets or slabs with sinuous loci. In each slab is included a complete series of ocular dominances, the whole of this basic functional module spreading over about 4 mm². Figure 5.62 and its legend helps to illustrate this data.

As for other species or groups of animals, ocular dominance columns have not yet been found in the New World monkeys, *Ateles* (spider monkey) and *Saimiri* (Hendrickson et al. 1978).

In the adult cat, ^{3}H-proline has been used to research ocular dominance columnar arrangements also, particularly in layer IV. Here the results in adult animals show a clear segregation of ipsilateral and contralateral afferent inputs that have arisen in layers A1 and A of the LGB, respectively. However, unlike the case in the rhesus monkey, overlaps exist with regions of completely binocular recipient cells, both at the thalamic level and at the cortical (LeVay et al. 1978). Organization into orientation columns has also been shown in this animal (Singer 1981) and also in *Tupaia* (Humphrey et al. 1980). In the cat this is seen in both areas 17 and 18, and the bands of columns are orthogonal to the representation of the vertical meridian. What is more, this organization is resistant to changes that might have been expected to be consequent upon manipulating early visual experience. It thus seems to constitute an intrinsic property of the system (figure 5.63).

A new line of study was initiated by exploiting another marking technique employing cytochrome oxidase, which is a mitochondrial enzyme that indicates high cellular metabolism (Livingstone & Hubel 1982, 1984a,b). This marking has shown staining of "blobs" in areas V1 and V2 of the macaque. These are particularly clearly seen in layers II and III. Thus, in addition to the sheets of ocular dominance and to the preferred orientation columns there must be added this

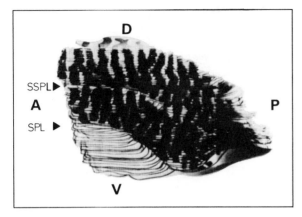

Figure 5.63
Orientation columns in the cat. View to the median face (cf. figure 5.39) of a three-dimensional reconstruction of the cortical visual area 17 in the cat. The animal had been stimulated for 50 min by vertical stripes before sacrifice and the administration of 2-DG marker. Notice the regular arrangement of the columns that show increased optical density. D, V, A, P, the dorsal, ventral, anterior, posterior boundaries of area 17, respectively. Horizontal and vertical scale: 2 mm. The two triangles to the left show the suprasplenial sulcus (SSPL) and the splenial sulcus (SPL). (From Singer 1981)

series of accumulations of cytochrome oxidase. They appear to be regularly spaced.

Using this technique, Hawken and Parker (1984) have been able clearly to distinguish subdivisions of the principal receptive layer in V1. Layer IVA, receiving from the parvocellular LGB layers, is well labeled; IVB is less heavily marked. The IVC regions that receive most of the fibers from the LGB magnocellular region and also the IVC regions receiving from the LGB parvocellular region are only feebly marked. But more important, the technique has been able to reveal very important functional distinctions, since well-controlled functional physiological experimentation (Zeki & Shipp 1988) has shown that cells in the "blobs" mostly show no orientation selectivity but are selective for light wavelength, whereas the cells outside the blobs are orientation selective but nonchromatic. So that it can now be said that within V1 there exists a segregation between regions specialized for form or shape detection, regions specialized for movement, and regions specialized for color.

The same sort of study in V2 reveals a more complex organization with alternating "thick stripes," "thin stripes," and "interstripes."

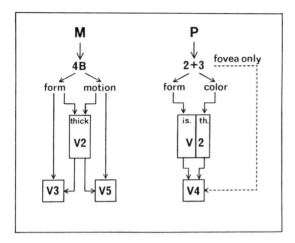

Figure 5.64
Summary diagram of the connections of the M system and the P system. is, interstripe; th, thin stripe; thick, thick stripe. (From Zeki 1990)

Electrophysiology shows that the thin stripes contain color cells and receive their input from the V1 blobs. The thick stripes contain direction-sensitive cells and receive their input from the deep layers in V1. The afferents to the interstripes come from the interblob regions of V1 and are rich in orientation-selective cells.

Having taken into account the known differences in response types in geniculate outputs and their projections to V1 and V2 as well as their continuing projection onward to the more specialized areas V3, V4, and V5 (see section 3.1), Zeki and Shipp (1988) have proposed two afferent systems serving the V1 cortex from the retina via LGB (figure 5.64). A system they call "M" comes from the magnocellular layers of LGB and essentially terminates in the middle and deep regions of layer IV at the level of the interblobs. From there the projection continues either directly or via the thick stripes of V2 toward V3 and V5. This system is specialized for orientation and directional sensitivities, in other words, for form and movement ("dynamic form").

The "P" system, originating in the parvocellular layers of LGB and terminating in the more superficial regions of V1 and uniquely in the region of the foveal representation, then projects via the thin stripes and interstripes of V2 toward area V4. This system is specialized for color and has a certain specialization for "static form."

These proposed systems thus comprise connections that treat the different attributes of visual images in *parallel pathways*. These two systems continue onward in the cortex. The "form/ color" V1-V4 system continues forward to the inferotemporal region, where form recognition occurs. The "form/movement" system involves area V5-MT, then MTS (DSR zone) on its way to the posterior parietal cortex, area 7. We have already studied some of the properties of V5-MT and of DSR; those for V4 will be outlined immediately below. A study of the integrative regions of the inferior temporal and posterior parietal regions would exceed the intended scope of this book.

THE CORTEX AND COLOR VISION

A very detailed body of data for the monkey exists that specifies the types of responses to chromatic stimulation (e.g., De Valois 1973, De Valois et al. 1974). This has been collected to address the problems of how cortical responses relate to LGB and how these responses are combined with the traditional classifications based on luminous contrast (B/W) in simple complex and hypercomplex units.

Area V1 of the Macaque
A whole series of response properties is found for V1 cortex of the macaque following the application of either achromatic stimuli using gratings with black and white (positive [W] and negative [B]) luminance contrast or, alternatively, colored stimuli (red [R], green [G], yellow [Y], or blue [B]). The following are sought as functional elements in these systems (Gouras & Krüger 1979, Michael 1981): (1) Units responding well to both B/W and to colored stimuli. Most likely, these are essentially concerned with achromatic aspects of perception. (2) Units responding differently to different colors. These, presumably concerned with color vision, comprise four distinct sub groups:

• *Cells with concentric receptive fields showing double-color antagonisms.* The center is either R^+/G^- or R^-/G^+ with the surround organized in the opposite sense, respectively R^-/G^+ and R^+/G^-. These cells are always monocular, never respond to a monochromatic diffuse stimulus (because of the center/surround antagonism), nor do they respond to an achromatic contrast. Their cell bodies are located in layer IVC. These cells constitute a first step in the treatment of color information. They receive a combination of direct inputs from LGB, either from two categories of type II fibers (in Hubel & Wiesel's classification, see section 2.2 above), that is, either from R^+/G^- and R^-/G^+ homogeneous units, or from type III fibers, namely, chromatically homogeneous units, some R^+/R^-, the others G^+/G^-.

• *Simple cells with double-color contrast.* These may comprise a central field of the R^+/G^- (or inverse) with adjacent peripheral fields of the opposite contrast. Others may be less complicated, operating as only two adjacent antagonistic fields. It will be remembered that most of these have an orientation selectivity that does not depend on the color of the stimulus (provided the light is an adequate stimulus), that most of them are monocular, that their cell bodies are ranged among the collection of layers IV and, according to some authorities, they receive their input not directly from LGB but from concentric, double-color contrast elements of the first type above.

• *Complex cells with color properties.* These cells have rectangular or square fields. They respond very poorly to stationary stimuli in general but respond very well to stripe or edge contrasts and sometimes only to the boundaries between two different colors. They may respond best to R or best to G. Most of these cells have a directional sensitivity. Most of them are found to be binocular. Their cell bodies are found in layers II, III, V, and VI. In the hierarchical view of the pathway proposed by Hubel and Wiesel, these cells receive their input from several simple cells.

• *Hypercomplex cells.* Essentially, the differences from complex cells are those usually recognized: responses to moving stimuli with their preferred orientation and direction of movement being well determined but with some color characteristic added. In the typical case, they need an optimal length and, as in achromatic hypercomplex cells, they have inhibitory flanking fields. The central and flanking inhibitory regions always have the same spectral sensitivities. These cells receive their inputs from several complex cells according to the proposed hierarchical intracortical scheme of response elaboration and from that perspective these units may be regarded as the final stage (in area 17) of an integration that has simultaneously taken into account both the spatial and chromatic qualities of the stimulus.

There is one final point to be made concerning the cortical distribution of these cells as determined from systematic vertical and inclined electrode penetrations of the cortex. Michael (1978a,b, 1979a,b, 1981) proposes the existence of "color columns" within which all the cells need colored light and do not respond to white. In such a column the concentric and simple (see above) units always show the same double-opponent color antagonisms and that the hypercomplex types (see above) in general react best to the central color of the other concentric and simple cells. Other "achromatic" columns contain cells that respond both to color and to black/white. The color columns are geometrically separate from the ocular dominance columns and from the preferred orientation columns.

Cortical Color Sensitivity and the Perception of Color Constancy
We have mentioned already how the problem of color constancy arises. The impression of the color of a reflecting surface or other object remains fairly constant in spite of changes in the light source that illuminates it (daylight, artificial light, etc.). In any case, it is clear that no explanation based solely on luminous energy and wavelength can account for that perceptual constancy. Early suggestions were based on the involvement of cognitive processes (constancy being seen as the result of either training, or a memory mechanism, for example, as proposed by Hering or Helmholtz). Other more recent theories depend on processing mechanisms that treat all the color information available from the total scene and then compare the data perceived simultaneously from several parts of the visual field, that is by processing in many parallel afferent channels (Land 1974, 1983; see chapter 3, section 6.2).

Whatever the process brought into play, most people judge that the cerebral cortex must be involved in it. Zeki (1980b, 1983, 1990) has systematically studied the problem from that viewpoint and, by exploring in turn the sensitivity of cells to colored stimuli from both primary sources and from colored surfaces presented in the receptive field, he has been able to establish a functional distinction between responses in V1 (area 17) and those in V4.

Studies in area V1. Studies of cell responses in the striate cortex used the following protocol: (1) Determination of the action spectrum for the cell by the usual methods. This gives an objective measure of its general color specificity, which Zeki judged to be its wavelength specificity in this measurement and not due to any subjective perception of the color. (2) Studies were then made of the cell responses to the presentation of colored fields illuminated by different continuous spectral distributions of light (in long, medium, and short light wavelengths) the chromaticities of which could be estimated by the experimenter (using the method of "Mondrian" mosaics of colors exploited by Land).

The experimental data established the following important facts for V1: A cell that demonstrates an absolutely clear wavelength specificity (say, to red) under monochromatic stimulation (as demonstrated by results from other teams of workers as well as the present) does not necessarily respond to the presentation of fields judged, for example, to be red in their environmental context when lit by stimuli of different spectral content. The cell will only respond provided that the reflected bundle of light has a given content of long wavelengths. Even if the color is red as viewed by an observer, it will not respond if there is an insufficient quantity of long wavelengths in the reflected light. Even if the color of the field is not red (green, for example), illumination with a certain abundance of long wavelengths and that in the context of the observation does not change the observer's subjective impression (of green) can nevertheless excite a response in the cell.

In summary, V1 cells code *the wavelength and not the color* as it is judged by the subjective experience of an observer who is, after all, the only person who can judge and report the color perception.

Studies in area V4.   The behavior of cells in V4 appears to be quite different and justifies the suggestion already made that V4 may be an area primarily dedicated to color analysis. When these cells are tested for their color sensitivity by the standard method (monochromatic source with calibrated energy output), the wavelength specificity is at least as clear if not better than in V1, with cells' individual sensitivity peaks being generally sited at 480, 500, and 620 nm.

But using Land's method, the response patterns of these cells are found to *parallel an observer's color perception.* Thus we find a regimen of response characteristics quite distinct from those of V1 cells. In V4, what determines the response follows closely what determines the subjective impression of color.

The question remains as to the origin of the distinctive functional differences between the cellular behaviour in V1 and V4, the one population being "wavelength detectors," the other "analyzers of color." The receptive fields of V1 are very restricted and the information they convey is in spatially narrow channels, whereas V4 cells show much wider receptive fields which perhaps satisfy the conditions needed for "subjective" color responses: a comparison between samples of the various colors in the environment of a colored field rather than only an isolated (one might say, Newtonian) specification of that small colored field is needed. The breadth of the receptive fields in area V4 may allow the comparison of inputs from various sections of the total visual field that is required by Land's theory for true color perception.

BINOCULAR INTERACTIONS

In this section we consider several problems posed by both functional data and study of the binocular visual mechanisms, which are predominantly sited in the visual cortex.

Binocular Information Convergence upon Cortical Cells
Binocularity is one of the important response characteristics of cortical cells. Among all the cortical cells that are dedicated to visual fields in the cat or monkey, effectively 95% are influenced by both eyes, by excitatory and/or inhibitory interactions. This binocularity seems to be governed by the cortical layer that a particular cell occupies.

In the *monkey*, in layer IV of area 17, which receives geniculate inputs, the cells are generally dominated by the inputs from one eye or the other. Binocularity is further elaborated to a greater or lesser extent in the most superficial (II and III) and deeper (V and VI) layers of the cortex, thanks to intracortical connections.

The classification of the extent of binocularity first introduced by Hubel and Wiesel (1962) has proved to be valuable and is still used. This consists in arranging cell types according to the relative response generated by a stimulus to each eye: (1) exclusively contralateral, (2) contralateral dominant, (4) ipsilateral dominant, (5) exclusively ipsilateral, with type (3) being activated equally via either eye. Sometimes seven classes are used, comprising intermediate degrees of contralaterality or ipsilaterality (Figure 5.65).

In the *cat*, this type of classification leads to histograms that essentially show (based on pooled data from all cortical layers) that most cells are binocular with only a small population of monocular cells (figure 5.65).

There are also species differences between simple (S) and complex (C) cells' binocularities. In the cat, 80% of either S or C cells show predominantly binocular dominance, whereas in the monkey 80% of S cells are monocular and 70% of C cells are binocular. There seem to be evolutionary differences in cell development concerned with

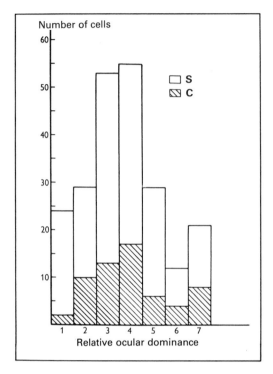

Figure 5.65
Distribution of 223 visual cortical cells according to ocular dominance. Combined histograms for the distribution of simple cells (S, open columns) and complex cells (C, hatched columns). Cells are classified according to relative dominance: (1) absolute dominance by the contralateral eye; (2) strong dominance by the contralateral eye; (3) slight dominance by the contralateral eye; (4) no marked difference in eye dominance; (5) slight dominance by the ipsilateral eye; (6) strong dominance by the ipsilateral eye; (7) absolute dominance by the ipsilateral eye. (From Hubel & Wiesel 1962)

the formation of cortical ocular dominance columns also. We shall return to this later.

A second question posed by binocular vision, concerned with the organization of the nervous projections in mammals, is that of the representation of the vertical meridian. In fact, if each hemifield were totally projected to the contralateral hemisphere and only there, then there would be no superposition of a fixation point sited on the vertical meridian and (once more, theoretically) no proper binocular vision. In reality, each region of the vertical meridian sends some fibers into both optic tracts, consequently, each central (or foveal) zone has apparently a bilateral representation (see section 3.1, above). In addition, it has been shown that many callosal connections exist between the zones of projection of the vertical meridian to each side of the brain.

Evidence for the Mechanisms Subserving Steroscopic Vision
We have laid out previously (in chapter 3, section 8.1) the general theoretical considerations concerned with binocular vision. Here we shall consider the precise neurophysiological problems that this visual processing implies. In particular, we need to discover whether psychophysical hypotheses that link the perception of the third dimension to exploitation of the disparity between retinal images are confirmed in the behavior of cortical neurons. In this respect quite a series of relevant experiments are available in both cat and monkey, carried out by investigating the anesthetized animal (notably cat and monkey) and the alert, awake monkey.

While these two types of experiment impose very different methodological constraints, their results complement each other very well in the main. In the case of the anesthetized animal, notably studied in the cat by a team led by Bishop (reviewed 1973), curarization has also been employed. As a result, the two optic axes are well fixed but are horizontally divergent (and more rarely vertically also). Because of this effect, the divergence must be determined with the greatest possible precision, using rather subtle precautions that we will not describe here, to define with minimal uncertainty the spatial relationships between the stimuli that excite a given cell via the two eyes. It is not easy to measure directly the real degree of disparity of the receptive fields viewed from each retina. Investigators must therefore make more indirect analyses (cf. Bishop 1973, Joshua & Bishop 1970), which consist in comparing the visual fields of a large series of cortical cells for stimualtion via each eye (figure 5.66).

More recently, experiments have been conducted using alert awake monkeys (Poggio & Fisher 1977, Poggio & Talbot 1981). The animal sees an illuminated source that it has been trained, by being rewarded with food, to fixate on continuously first with one, then with the other eye. Responses of a cortical cell are recorded while a moving stimulus crosses the animal's visual field. Depending on the conditions, the stimulus is a single real line or bar (1) passing through the plane of the point on which the animal is fixating, or (2) situated within this plane (generating a convergent disparity), or (3) situated beyond it (generating a divergent disparity). Alternatively, a *dichoptic* stimulus may be used, exploiting two (line or bar) stimuli, each seen

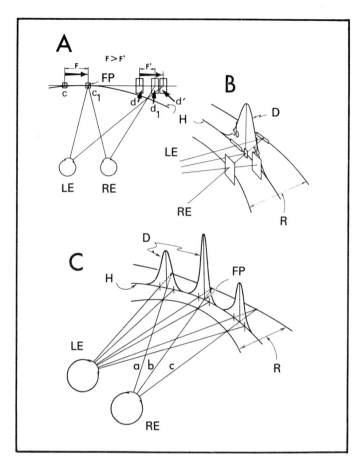

Figure 5.66
Construction of the horopter and Panum's area in the cat. (Data from a curarized animal). *A,* Principles for determining the horopter, H. Because of the paralysis the axes of the eyes are divergent and the two fields c and c_1 corresponding to the fixation point are separated by an angular disparity (F). As the line of view is moved toward the periphery, experiment shows that the distance between the fields corresponding to d and d_1 diminishes (F' <F). If c and c_1 become superimposed (i.e., assuming normal convergence between the two eyes has taken place) the field d to the left of d_1 now passes to the right (d') of d_1 since F' <F. A crossed disparity is thus established in the flat tangent plane. From this disparity, the authors construct a point on the horopter which is at the intersection of the lines from d to the right eye (RE) and from d' to the left eye (LE). This point is in front of the frontal plane FP and corresponds well with the position of the horopter. *B* shows how the authors calculate the extent of Panum's area (R) from the distribution (D) of the disparities ("F") between pairs of fields corresponding to given eccentricities. Panum's area being bounded by the disparities that can give binocular fusion, the authors consider it to be determined by the dispersion of disparities F at a given chosen eccentricity. In practice, they use the standard deviation of the distribution (D) for such an estimate. *C,* Experiment shows that (D) is a greater dispersion for lateral vision, (a) or (c), than for central vision (b); Panum's area is much reduced, relatively, toward the periphery of the visual field. (From Bishop 1973)

by only one eye, thanks to a system of screens. The stimuli are controlled so that the viewing situations are similar to those for the single image, with either the appearance of coincidence on the horopter, or of a convergent or divergent disparity.

The various responses must then be sorted out from the mass of data obtained in this way. Recall that, from the neurophysiological standpoint, it is a matter of discovering which units might be effective in making a spatial analysis, judging by their types of responses. These units need to identify corresponding parts of the binocular images as well as to measure the disparity due to binocular parallax that the stimulus images signal by their position (positional disparity) or orientation (orientation disparity) when they are displaced so that in principle a movement in depth can be created. We should not be surprised that the results at this stage are relatively complicated to unravel (see De Valois & De Valois 1980).

Positional Disparity

Geometrically static data.   Let us first of all examine how the correspondences between fields viewed by the separate eyes are presented. In this respect, two parameters in particular must be considered: the differences in shape of the two fields and the angular disparity between the right and left fields.

In many cases, the fields presented to the two eyes have the same orientation; sometimes they also have the same size (coincident fields) and sometimes different sizes, with one being more extensive than the other.

The angular differences between corresponding fields (of identical or nearly so fields, as above) have also been studied in detail. The experiments were carried out with paralyzed eye muscles in cat (i.e., in conditions where it is difficult to estimate the degree of coincidence) and have shown that for a given fixation distance, these angular disparities between corresponding fields traced on a tangent screen have notable properties: (1) The angular disparity has a tendency to decrease with increasing eccentricity, other things being equal; and (2) when measured for a large number of neighboring visual fields in visual space, these values of disparity statistically show some scatter.

On the basis of such data, Bishop's group managed to construct the horopter and define Panum's area. Because the angular disparity of the fields seen by the two eyes in a divergent setting of their optic axes diminishes with increasing eccentricity, the curve obtained in the horizontal plane, while being strictly different from the Vieth-Müller circle, differs from the tangent plane by curving inward toward the animal. In addition, when the spatial distribution of a variety of fields is examined in detail for nearby retinal positions, if one of the left fields and its corresponding right field coincide graphically, this coincidence does not necessarily transfer to a coincidence of all other fields. The resulting disparities (marked F in figure 5.66, to which refer for further geometrical explanation) of some minutes of arc at 1° have every likelihood of being real disparities. Such, in any case, is the authors' assumption; they also suggest that the dispersion of the values of F around a mean might be a way of defining Panum's area for a given distance and for given positions of the axis of gaze of course.

Dynamic data: Interocular facilitation and inhibition. Perhaps more interesting than those purely geometrical investigations are the data obtained when the anesthetized animal, in this case the cat, is stimulated with two corresponding fields simultaneously. Barlow et al. (1967), Pettigrew et al. (1968b), Nikara et al. (1968), and Nelson et al. (1977) have demonstrated that facilitatory responses occur for well-defined positions of the two stimuli, one applied to the right eye, the other to the left. These "tuning" curves of ocular correspondence are generally very peaked, the discharge of the cell diminishing very rapidly when the two stimuli are even minutely displaced from this critical optimal position (figure 5.67). Such interocular reinforcement is not necessarily obtained when the stimuli are in perfectly corresponding places in the monocular fields. In some cases, the largest response arises for a given disparity between the right and left stimuli (figure 5.68).

The situation observed is thus one of a cortical mechanism that can estimate the position of a certain stimulus with respect to the visual axes of the two eyes. This fits very well with our ideas on the nature of vision in depth. However, one difficulty does arise from this type of experiment. The angular disparity between optimal stimuli (the order of a degree) is much larger than the established values for stereoscopic acuity (the order of one minute of arc).

Experiments in the alert monkey. New and interesting data (Poggio & Poggio 1984) are now available in the unanesthetized animal (figure 5.69). It is now possible to distinguish two fundamental types of visual cortical cells, each type itself being divisible into two subgroups. Remember that in this sort of experiment the eyes are in natural fixation positions and thus are convergent on a given point in visual space.

1. *Cells "tuned" for distance.* Having first measured the responses for monocular stimulation via each eye, it can be established that these cells enjoy a considerable discharge change on binocular stimulation particularly at a point at a given well-defined distance with respect to the fixation point *F*. In most cases, this distance tuning is seen as a facilitation with respect to the monocular responses (first subgroup) or for a limited number of this sort of cell by a corresponding inhibition (second subgroup). Apart from this, the maximal effect is sometimes obtained for a zero disparity and sometimes for a disparity with respect to the horopter of a few minutes of arc, this value effectively repeating what is found from psychophysical data on stereoptic acuity and essentially corresponding well with the known extent of Panum's area.

2. *"Reciprocal" cells.* These are also called "near" or "far" cells, and they differ most from the distance-tuned cells by their reciprocal organization. Their behavior is such that they are identified by a discharge acceleration from a stimulus separated from the fixation plane in one direction and by the opposite response (i.e., an inhibition) to a stimulus separated from the fixation plane in the other direction. Two categories are thus recognizable: "near cells" that accelerate in response when the stimulus is moved from the *F* plane toward the observer (when a "crossed disparity" is established) and are slowed in response when the stimulus is further away from the *F* plane (with "direct disparity"). "Far cells" show the opposite response characteristics.

The latter results suggest that these two sorts of disparity detector provide two mechanisms that are linked with perception of the third spatial dimension, depth: (1) Cells of the second type ("near/far") are responsible for "coarse stereoscopy." They will also reflexly release a global adjustment of vergence. (2) Cells selective to disparities near the point of convergence underpin "fine stereopsis" as well as the adjustments that are necessary for maintaining an appropriate convergence. These are concerned with a perception of more detailed relief features.

Poggio and Poggio also cite some human observations in support of their conclusions (and this leads us briefly back to psychophysics).

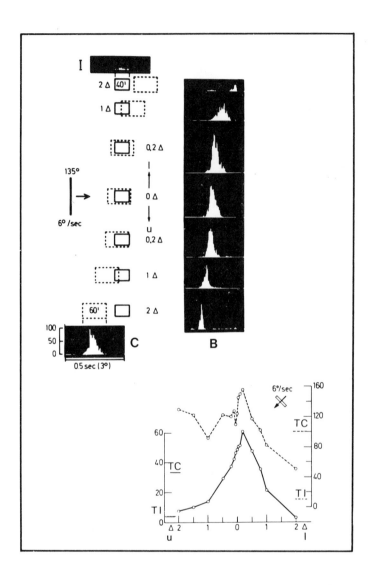

A study by Richards (1970), based on investigation of a rather wide population of subjects with different sorts of astereoscopy or with partial deficits in the perception of relief that can arise, seems to show the existence in the human of three distinct stereoscopic systems; "fine" stereoscopy, "near" stereoscopy, and "far" stereoscopy. These systems can be affected independently, thus creating partial deficits (see chapter 3).

Orientation Disparity

As we have emphasized above, positional disparity is only one possible manifestation among others related to stereoscopic vision. Another disparity is that created by binocular viewing of a receding line, which can generate an impression of depth. Optically, this disparity corresponds to two retinal images that are oriented differently on the two retinas. From this arises the neurophysiological problem: What agreements and disparities of preferred orientation can be found in the organization of corresponding receptive fields of a given cortical cell when it is stimulated through one and the other eye? Presently available results (in paralyzed cat with divergent eyes and using inde-

◄ Figure 5.67
Binocular interaction at the level of the striate cortex in the cat. Study of a cell that is optimally activated by the displacement of a slit at a speed of 6 deg/s according to a direction of movement upper right → lower left (135°, inset at lower right). The response is studied to stimulating the ipsilateral eye alone (I) or contralateral eye alone (C) or both eyes together (B), but arranging different binocular disparities between the zones stimulated ipsilaterally and contralaterally. Mean histograms are drawn. (Ordinate: number of spikes. Abscissa: time 0.5 s = 3°.) The response of the ipsilateral eye is much less than that of the contralateral. Between these two histograms for binocular stimulation, the disparity between the ipsilateral and contralateral fields are dispersed with respect to each other by a prism, maximal angular disparities being indicated for each case (varying from 40 min arc in one direction, top histogram, to 60 min arc in the other, bottom histogram. The dispersive power of the prisms used in diopters is also indicated). The histograms for binocular stimulation are shown to the right, there being an optimal response for a given disparity of images. The disparity direction for the contralateral visual field is indicated by the arrows, l being to the lower left, u being to the upper right. *Below,* Curves established for the same cell, either taking as a marker the peaks (dotted lines) or the mean values (solid lines) of the histograms. Abscissa: dispersing power of the prism in diopters, the prism being placed over the contralateral eye and sometimes displacing its field upward (u) and sometimes lower down (l); right ordinate: spikes/s for the peak responses also showing the responses for the standard discharges for ipsilateral stimulation alone (TI) and for contralateral stimulation alone (TC); left ordinate: similarly for the mean discharges in spikes/s. Note the existence of an optimal response and a clear facilitation for certain positions of relative disparity of the fields. (From Pettigrew et al. 1968)

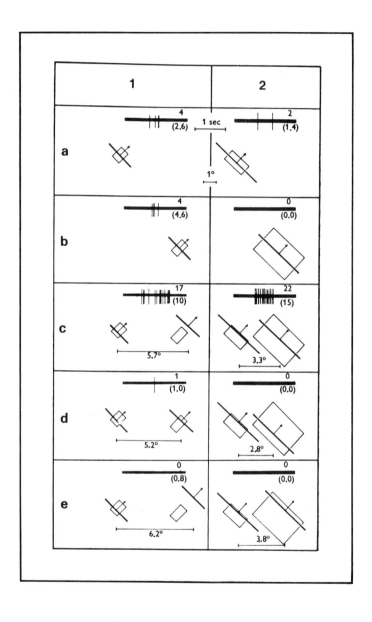

pendent stimuli) are as follows (Blakemore et al. 1972, Ferster 1981; figure 5.70). For units with orientation selectivity, the optimal orientation is not necessarily the same for the two eyes. From a rather large sample of units it is seen that disparities can attain 15° (SD 6° to 9°). However, for the majority of cells the disparity is small or zero. These disparities have been observed in all sorts of cells, whether S or C and whether or not they have an inhibitory fringe (HCI or HCII).

When the orientation of the stimulus to one eye is changed with respect to that in the other (assumed fixed), it is possible to plot orientation tuning curves (as above for positional tuning curves). It is found that the maximal response occurs when the disparity between the two stimuli corresponds to the orientations in the monocular fields (i.e., is small or zero). When the angular disparity between the stimuli increases, the cell response diminishes rather rapidly and may even turn into an inhibition (though this latter conclusion is still disputed). It seems, therefore, that there is this second neurophysiological mechanism for vision in depth provided by disparities detected by cells with orientation tuning.

Mechanisms Subserving the Perception of Dynamic Stereopsis
The term *dynamic stereopsis* implies that spatial perception is not solely related to static image disparities in position and orientation but also to movement in depth as targets approach or recede from an observer. This is, of course, related to the perception of movement in general but, unlike movement in the frontoparallel plane, movement in depth has so far been comparatively little studied even though it regulates some essential visual tasks like visuomotor control.

One set of experiments has been made in the anesthetized cat with

---

◀ **Figure 5.68**
Binocular interactions showing that facilitation of responses can occur for different disparities in the same animal. The two units, one in the left column, one in the right column, have nearby receptive fields and the same preferred orientation. For each cell, five successive stimulating arrangements are shown from monocular stimulation of each eye (left alone in *a*, right alone in *b*) then binocular stimulations (*c* to *e*). The size and position of the minimal fields on a screen to generate responses in each eye are shown. Notice the binocular facilitation in (*c*). The stimuli are at that stage separated by 5.7° for the first cell and by 3.3° for the second. When these stimuli are brought (*d*) closer together or (*e*) further apart than the optimum, there is an occlusion of the discharge. No correction has been made for the divergence of the optic axes, which in this arrangement was 6.4° between them for the area centralis. The true disparity differences for optimal response would thus be, for the first cell 0.7° and for the second 3.1°. (From Barlow et al. 1967)

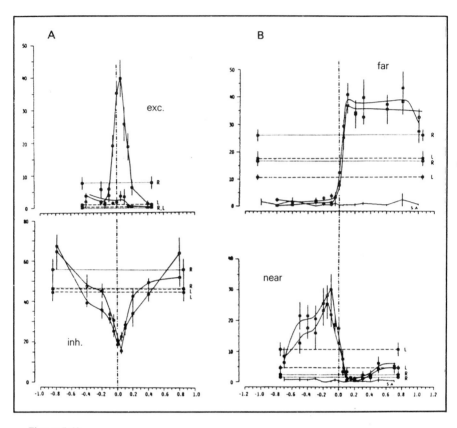

Figure 5.69
Profiles of the sensitivity to positional disparity for cortical cells in the foveal region
in the macaque. In each case an optimal bar stimulus is used presented to one or both
eyes. *Left,* Cells "tuned" to binocular disparity. *Right,* Cells with reciprocal (depth)
sensitivity. (For each cell, ordinate: mean discharge spikes/s, with 1 SE of mean shown
on the experimental points as a function of (abscissa) angular horizontal disparity in
degrees between the images to one and the other eye. The disparity is generated by
displacing the bar perpendicularly to its optimal orientation (divergent disparities
taken as +, convergent disparities taken as −). In each case, the profiles of the
responses for movements in two opposite directions of the stimulus are taken. The
responses for monocular stimulation of each eye are shown for a movement in each
direction as indicated by the dashed lines for left eye stimulation and by the dotted
lines for right eye. With respect to that response to monocular stimulation the upper
"tuned" cell shows a binocular facilitation for a certain angular disparity (exc) while
that of the lower tuned cell shows a binocular antagonism (inhib). *Upper right,* A cell
facilitated by divergent disparity and inhibited by convergent disparity ("far cell").
Lower right, A cell with the opposite behavior ("near cell"). (From Poggio & Poggio
1984)

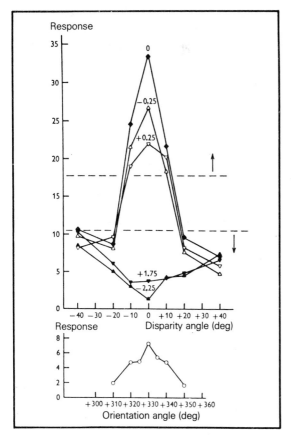

Figure 5.70
Binocular tuning with respect to the angle of presentation of an illuminated bar to each eye. For each unit, the angles for an optimal response were about 345° for the right eye and 330° for the left eye. The stimulus angle for the right eye is left constant and the angle of the stimulus to the left eye is changed. The parameter is the phase between the two moving stimuli (i.e., their mutual disparity with respect to the field boundaries: $-0°$, $-0.25°$, $+1.75°$, $-2.25°$). *Above,* Depending on the phase and on the image angle in the left eye, the combination of the two stimuli generates either a facilitation of the response (upward) or an occlusion (downward). *Below,* Orientation tuning curve for the left eye alone. (From Blakemore et al. 1972)

eyes in the paralyzed position (Blakemore et al. 1972) and another in the alert monkey. In each case, using appropriate optical arrangements, bar stimuli that can simulate approaching or receding movements of the target were applied. By this means it was possible to distinguish neurons (in cat area 18, Ferster 1981, and in areas 17 and 18 of monkey) that are indeed activated by target movements incorporating a component perpendicular to the verticofrontal plane. Activity occurs when the target appears either to approach from the front toward the head or laterally toward the side of the head, or on the contrary, to recede similarly, either frontally or obliquely. In the cat, these units can be excited monocularly. In the monkey, the situation is less simple; this type of cell is very strongly excited binocularly, over and above any varying binocular facilitation (or inhibition) that usually accompanies this type of directional spatial sensitivity. The exact listing of what directional sensitivity properties arise from these particular modes of firing is not immediately clear. However, it is certain that those cells sensitive to movements in the frontal plane itself cannot be those concerned, since the movement sensitivities are in opposite directions in the two retinas (for obvious geometrical reasons).

AMBLYOPIA

Amblyopia is basically definable as a loss of visual acuity which, under conditions that we will discuss below, can become irreversible (and this is the most frequent case). It can affect one or both eyes, and cannot be corrected by lenses. It is a deficit of complex etiology that, as we shall see, can involve several levels of the visual system. In summary, while we include this in a chapter on cortical mechanisms, this is not at all to specify a precise location for the mechanisms responsible, even though amblyopia often affects binocular vision. It is better, rather, to discuss it in terms of mechanisms that can involve any part of the total visual pathway from retina to cortex, as clearly also happens with the other functions like color vision, form vision, or the temporal perceptions that have been discussed in this section.

A Reminder of Some Clinical Data

In humans, amblyopia of an eye can be due to (1) a nonalignment of the visual axis (amblyopia of squint), (2) a difference in dioptrics between the two eyes (hypermetropia, myopia, astigmatism) that has not been corrected (nonisometric amblyopia), or (3) a pathological occlusion of one eye linked to a congenital cataract, a corneal opacity, a ptosis, and the like (deprivation amblyopia). In all cases, the child ceases to use one eye in such a way that the amblyopia brings with it a severe deficit in binocular vision and stereopsis. Uniocular amblyopia of squint is the most frequent, to such an extent that amblyopia in general is often regarded as a loss of binocular vision linked with strabismus.

Whatever the cause, human amblyopia has the following characteristics. It very specifically affects acuity in the foveal region. In the case of amblyopia of squint it is seen, by comparing the healthy eye with the other, that the deficit is indeed foveal, whereas the peripheral (>5°) acuity is scarcely different from normal. This depression of visual acuity need not arise from a total visual disuse but is concerned with foveal form vision and perhaps of binocular vision also.

Amblyopia of squint is generally agreed to be a central phenomenon, as we shall see, even though some workers invoke a retinal origin.

In general, the deficit is irreversible after the subject's age exceeds a critical period (the first few months or at most the first few years of life), during which some treatment is possible but beyond which all treatments become ineffective. The effect suggests that the lack of proper use of one fovea brings with it a permanent functional loss after the critical period and, as the data given below will prove, quite probably a degeneration of the corresponding visual pathways.

Although it is not necessary in this context to go into the precise details of the various treatments used or suggested for amblyopia, some of the essentials should be pointed out. In general the aim is to force the amblyopic eye into normal visual exposure with a well-focused image and preferably with binocular interaction being made possible. Occlusion of the normal eye forces the amblyopic eye into normal use but a snag is that the deprivation of binocular vision continues, and there is always the danger of a treatment-induced amblyopia of the originally normal eye. Optical restriction is a treatment that complements occlusion. It has been much developed since the 1960s. The principle is simple: to upset the vision of the fixating (normal) eye for a certain visual distance and thus to force the use of the amblyopic eye for that distance. Thus, it can be arranged that one of the eyes is used for certain distances and the other for others. Sometimes the restriction will be "near," with the normal eye unable to cope with close vision and the ambylopic eye suitably adjusted for that region, then at other times ("far" restriction) the normal eye is made to be useful for close vision only (by optical correction and continuous atropine application, which lead to continual loss of far vision), and thus the amblyopic eye is used alone for distant vision. For squint amblyopia, a still more serious problem can exist when there is a foveal scotoma abolishing foveal vision and thus generating an eccentric fixation outside the fovea. In this case, optic restriction alone is not enough, but it can be supplemented by using prismatic correction that invokes a displacement of the visual axis of the normal eye and forces the amblyopic eye into a foveal fixation (by conjugate eye movement).

Mechanisms in Amblyopia

Physiologists, and histologists also, have tried to unravel the mechanisms affected in amblyopia. To this effect, experimental procedures have generally consisted in reducing the vision of one eye in an animal that is young enough for possible effects to be generated during the critical "period of plasticity," the existence of which was established from other observations in both cat and monkey.

However, the possible physiopathological procedures generating amblyopia are not all identical; three different techniques have been exploited so far: (1) Stitching down an eyelid deprives that eye of all form vision and only allows a diffuse stimulation of weak luminance to reach the eye. (2) Spoiling the dioptrics of the image to one eye deprives that eye of a clear image of forms. (3) A strabismus, convergent or divergent, is generated by unilateral operation on the appropriate oculomotor muscle.

These methods, which are all meant to reproduce certain pathological conditions found in children, are not in fact equivalent. The treatment of the eye is different in each case: In the first, all the image is suppressed; in the second, a poor image remains; in the third, using squint, the situation becomes as complicated as could be imagined.

Monocular deprivation. Hubel, Wiesel, and Le Vay (1976) first exploited eyelid suture in young cats up to a few months old (i.e., during the critical period). They then demonstrated that after several months all appropriate cortical cells responded via the normal eye but none responded to stimulation of the other eye. They found no physiological deficit at the level of the LGB. In contrast, Maffei and

Fiorenti (1976) did notice a loss of acuity in LGB cells with central or paracentral (<5°) receptive fields.

In similar experiments, Lehmkühle et al. (1980; cf. Sherman 1979) also found differences in the behavior of X and Y cells in LGB. Deprivation severely affected the responses to high spatial frequencies in Y cells but only those with fields in the binocular region. Similar effects were seen in X cells from both monocular and binocular fields but were less obvious. The authors suggest that the absence of binocular competition, notably in the Y cells, was the origin of these differences in behavior in the receiving cells at LGB.

This type of experimentation was accompanied by histological control also. Hubel and Wiesel had not found functional deficits in LGB in the cat but the LGB layers appropriate for the deprived eye were abnormally narrow. In the monkey, a just postnatal monocular stitching was followed by a histological search for any effects at LGB and cortex. It was thus found that the LGB cells served by the deprived eye are smaller in size but, in contrast, there was no clear morphological change to be seen using EM. However, injections of proline in the deprived eye showed that at the cortical level the bands of monocularity, although their alternation was preserved, had become very unequal. It is clear from all of this work that the changes most easily observed are those occurring in the cortex.

In this respect, it has also been shown that these changes are reversible provided the eyelid suture is removed before the end of the critical period. What is more, suturing the opposite eye instead (reverse-suturing) is followed by a corresponding reversal of the thicknesses of the bands (again during the critical period).

The problems arising from this experimentation remain without resolution at present: How can this plasticity be explained at the neuronal level? By what process does visual deprivation diminish the volume of the corresponding projections? Is it possible that some synapses become inactive, or, conversely, is there an increase in axons during restoration?

Dioptric interference. As already mentioned, the situation is not quite the same when one developing eye is forced into poor form discrimination. The experiments have been carried out in a variety of ways. Ikeda (1979), in 3-week-old kittens, treated the eye continuously with atropine (paralysis of accommodation and of iris constriction). She later observed a loss in acuity in LGB cells, particularly affecting the

X cells. Eggars and Blakemore (1978) raised kittens with a convergent lens in front of one eye. Cortical cells served by that eye effectively showed a significant acuity loss.

Squint amblyopia.   Hubel and Wiesel (1965) studied cats raised with one squinting eye, in divergence. They discovered a loss of binocularity in visual cortical cells but did not report any notable differences concerned with acuity loss. Ikeda (1979) carried out a systematic study of the acuity of ganglion cells in eyes made to squint, convergently or divergently, by operation at 3 weeks. She demonstrated that a very clear loss of acuity occurred in X cells of the central region both in the retina itself and in the LGB. The curves she obtained resembled very closely the loss of acuity in human amblyopia (figure 5.71).

Summary.   Mechanisms operating in causing amblyopia (or amblyopias) are far from being clearly understood. In some of them the common origin can be a stimulation of the central retina by an unfocused image. Perhaps for that condition total deprivation is a limiting case of the same effect. But there remains the difficulty of amblyopia in binocular vision. Loss of binocularity is likely to be a matter affecting the central levels, but is it an entirely central process or is there also a retinal deficit? At present, Ikeda is the only researcher who has found one. This question is an important one because if amblyopia is linked to a cortical disfunction it must involve a process linked with binocularity (directly or indirectly). If there is some peripheral retinal pathology, the loss of binocularity might be only one cause among others.

3.4 ABLATIONS AND LESIONS IN THE CORTICAL AREAS OF ANIMALS AND HUMANS

Finally, let us study how the role of the cortical visual areas can be explored using the traditional method of ablations. This method has been exploited by researchers since the 1930s on a large number of mammalian species, rodents, carnivores, and primates in particular. However, since the discovery of the multiplicity of different projection regions (which has gone well beyond tracing the fewer traditional areas), a large number of those results have now only a historical interest. In addition, for the last twenty-five years investigations have necessarily been related to the existence of the *two visual systems* that we have specified and which we shall refer to again below: the *geniculostriate system* and the *extrageniculate system,* via the colliculus

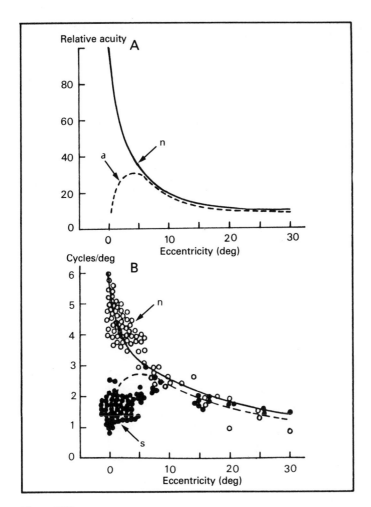

Figure 5.71
Human amblyopia and visual acuity in a cat with squint. *A,* Relative visual acuity as
a function of eccentricity in the normal (n) and amblyopic (a) human subject. *B,* Visual
acuity (in cycles/deg) in X ganglion cells for the eye of a normal cat (n) and for an eye
with a convergent squint (s) induced by surgical intervention at 3 weeks old, as a
function of eccentricity. (From Ikeda 1979)

and thalamic nuclei like the pulvinar and serving the peristriate and parietal areas.

First of all, it is notable that *partial ablations* in monkey area 17 do not reduce visual acuity to the amount that might have been predicted from electrophysiological measurements of the topological correspondences (Cowey 1967, Weiskranz & Cowey 1967). Whereas a retinal lesion brings with it an acuity loss and a scotoma that are totally predictable in conformity with the known retinal topology, the elimination of the corresponding cortical zone is accompanied by a much smaller acuity loss in the region where it ought to exist (Weiskranz 1972; figure 5.72). Cowey and Weiskranz demonstrated also that animals become able to detect stimuli in the scotoma that was initially mapped postoperatively by peripheral investigation. This improvement follows repetition of the tests. Perhaps this repetition somehow constitutes a training procedure.

In the macaque, a *total ablation of the striate area* (and probably of the circumstriate belt, which was then not well recognized) generated a deficit (Klüver 1941) that was interpreted as leaving a residual possible sensitivity of the animal to the total flux of light entering the eye. After such a deficit the visual system becomes an integrator of luminance.

Later studies elaborated and modified this conclusion. It was shown that destriate monkeys are still capable of quite a series of visual tasks, such as the localization of objects in visual space, the discrimination of targets equalized for total luminous flux but differing in luminance, a certain amount of form discrimiantion and of the spatial orientation of a grating and finally, of color. These animals were even capable of detecting transiently illuminated targets. Curiously, the absolute threshold for light detection seems to be scarcely affected. (Humphrey & Weiskranz 1967, Weiskranz et al. 1977, Dineen & Keating 1981, Schiller et al. 1972, Pasik & Pasik 1982).

One hypothesis (Humphrey 1970, Keating & Dineen 1982) proposed that the residual capacity is linked to the integrity of the second (extrageniculate) visual system.

However, to the extent that some ablations (in particular those by Klüver) had largely exceeded the limiting boundary of the striate area itself when the extrageniculate system might also be expected to have been involved, there seemed to be room for other explanations. After Pasik and Pasik (1982) found, also in the macaque, some residual vision even after elimination of the striate, peristriate, and inferior

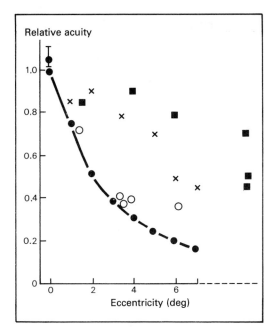

Figure 5.72
Relationships between retinal and cortical lesions and the resulting visual acuity in the monkey. Acuity expressed as relative magnitudes as a function of eccentricity. The curve shows the variation of acuity in a normal human subject as a function of eccentricity. Open circles, monkey acuity after retinal lesions (in one animal); squares and crosses, relative acuity after bilateral removal (more or less extensive depending on the animal) of the projection of the macular region on the striate cortex, the eccentricity being calculated either from the maps of Talbot & Marshall 1941 (crosses) or of Daniel & Whitteridge 1961 (filled squares). (From Weiskrantz 1972)

temporal areas, it became necessary to discover which structures are indispensable in subserving this minimal residual discrimination. It seems that neither destruction of the pulvinar nor of the colliculus nor of the pretectum, nor of all these structures combined, suppresses this elementary capacity for discrimination. However, a lesion of the accessory optical system (see section 1.3, above) decisively establishes that system as being essential for this residual vision, which might well correspond with what was described by Klüver as a detection of total luminous flux.

Some attention has also been paid to color vision. We have mentioned above that this is retained after elimination of area 17 in the macaque but that a wider cortical ablation suppresses it. This therefore excludes the colliculus as a possible site for color vision. However, in species in which the retina is essentially all-cone (squirrel and *Tupaia*), some color vision does seem to be retained after elimination of the geniculostriate system, so in this particular case there may be some possible involvement of the colliculus.

Some different experiments that are worth study involve species that are phylogenetically lower than the macaque but which nevertheless remain in the same general line of evolution that led from the insectivores to the primates via the prosimians. As we saw above, some of these species have been subjected to detailed research on their cortical visual areas and on the thalamic nuclei that serve them. The first is the insectivore *Tupaia* in which, as we have seen, the dual arrangement of the projections is relatively simple: The geniculate system projects to area 17, whereas the thalamic pulvinar projects to the peripheral temporal region. It has been established that ablation of 17 only affects the more difficult discrimination tasks; apart from that, the animal shows no obvious changes in behavior. It can avoid obstacles, discriminate simple shapes and colors, and it makes no significant errors of depth discrimination. But there does seem to be a certain deficiency in visual acuity. In contrast, the elimination of at least part of the pulvinar system generates a notable deficit in form discrimination; furthermore, the animal is unable to modify its strategies and adopt another one after a course of training. It seems that the extrageniculate system is able to support an important part of visual function including aspects exploiting temporal mnemonic cues.

At a further stage of phylogenetic evolution, the connections in *Galago* are already much more complicated. After an area 17 ablation the behavioral deficit is much greater. Behavior involving visual guidance is affected as well as vision in depth and form discrimination. After a temporal lesion, the effects differ depending on whether the lesion is ventral, temporal, or is one that specifically affects area MT. MT seems to control visuospatial recognition, whereas the ventral zone seems to exploit temporal cues. The conclusion suggested is, however, somewhat surprising compared with other conclusions that we shall be referring to below, which suggest that the striate system is predominantly visuospatial, whereas the system considered to be extrastriate shows up as being the one particularly exploited in utilizing temporal cues.

These conclusions are concerned, in our view, with an aspect other than merely examining the respective roles of area 17 and the peristriate region. What has in fact been compared is more probably the function of 17 against that of a territory, which in the macaque would be the inferotemporal area, for which a role is already well recognized, this being to control visual mechanisms on the basis of chronological temporal and mnemonic information.

There have also been systematic measurements in the cat. Certainly some of them are rather out of date. But it is very obvious that, since in the course of time a large number of different cortical visual areas have been specified (see section 3.1, above), at least part of the older work is no longer very useful.

Nowadays, results are available from exploiting a whole series of what have become standard tests comprising (1) measurement of acuity thresholds by employing as stimuli either gratings of known spatial frequency or patterns of parallel or nonparallel lines, (2) tests of form discrimination (vertical vs. horizontal bars, circles vs. other figures, polygons vs. circles, etc.), (3) receptive field estimates by perimetry, (4) measurement of flux discrimination, and (5) of visuomotor guidance.

The global conclusions from these batteries of tests are as follows: Removal of areas 17, 18, and part of 19 (roughly an ablation of the lateral gyrus) generates no deficit in form discrimination. Even preoperative training is not lost. Visuomotor guidance remains normal, as does visual field as mapped by perimetry. However, the acuity threshold seems to be reduced by about 30%.

After ablation of some other areas to which visual projections have been identified (i.e., areas 19, 20, 21, and 7, representing roughly the alteral suprasylvian region and the zones edging the sulci that are its boundaries) but leaving areas 17 and 18 are still intact, animals can still discriminate luminous fluxes normally but suffer severe loss of form discrimination and severe deficits in visuomotor guidance.

Note that, taking into account the complex connectivity of the LGB to the cortical areas, an ablation of the lateral gyrus causes the loss of about 84% from that thalamic nucleus (layers A, A1, and C in particular), whereas an ablation of the second type described above chiefly involves layers C and the MIN nucleus of LGB together with certain pulvinar regions.

Sprague et al. (1972) had shown that removal of all known visual cortical areas on one hemisphere produced a persistent contralateral neglect ("cortical blindness"). This "inattention" syndrome was largely reversible by removal of the opposite superior colliculus. The conclusion was that there is a delicate balance between (1) an excitatory descending influence from each visual cortex to its ipsilateral superior colliculus and (2) a counterbalancing inhibitory input from the contralateral to the ipsilateral colliculus via the intercollicular commissure. The contralateral neglect after a cortical unilateral ablation may thus be due (after Sprague) to the functional loss of the visual cortical facilitatory influence on the ipsilateral colliculus, which allows it to be dominated by the intercollicular inhibition (see also Stein 1988).

At this point it is worthwhile examining some clinical data for the human case, particularly from recent work. In general, an ablation in visual cortex (area 17?) brings with it a total cortical blindness in the scotoma or in the hemifield if one whole hemisphere is lesioned. In current clinical practice, testing is by perimetry with either verbal responses or manual pressing of a button when a stimulus is presented in different parts of the field. With this technique, the blind zone is usually clearly identifiable and there is no sign of any recovery (Holmes 1945).

However, some observations that are already somewhat old have shown the persistence of some elementary light perception that is limited to vast changes in stimulus luminance or to stimulus movement in the blind zone. This residual sensitivity had been attributed to the lesions probably being incomplete. But other observations caused a continued interest in this problem. For example, in 1917 Riddoch discovered from studying the effects of World War I cranial wounds that there could be a loss of foveal vision but with retention of the "detection of a movement in the blind field but without form or color." Even a certain spontaneous recovery can occur in some cases in the following order: first, luminous sensitivity, then movement sensitivity, then form, then colors.

Thereafter the data have multiplied, first suggesting, then establishing that destriation does not lead to a complete blindness. However, most of the earlier observations were not entirely definitive until the work of Pöppel et al. (1973) demonstrated a residual power of localization within the scotoma by using appropriate saccades as a measure. Quite a series of observations followed this work with the subject being submitted to forced-choice tests. The subject needed to detect and indicate, if not "see," a stimulus presented in the blind area either by occular fixation or by manually pointing to where he thought he had "seen" the stimulus. Other effects can also be detected when the scotoma is only partial: Its extent can fluctuate spontaneously depending on the time of day; it can become reduced in area (notably in testing with contrast thresholds) for stimuli applied near its border, provided the patient's attention is appropriately directed; the scotoma can be reduced in area following prolonged training sessions (Zihl 1980, 1981; Zihl & von Cramon 1982; Perenin & Jeannerod 1975, 1978a,b; figure 5.73).

This phenomenon of "blindsight" has been the object of arguments that we shall not rehearse here, particularly because it proposes a perception which, in spite of being an effectively unconscious one, can nevertheless in humans guide an appropriately oriented conscious motor action that leads to occular fixation or to a pointing action (see Campion et al. 1983). However, blindsight phenomena also open up interesting considerations of possible substitutes for the striate cortex, all of which have their own particualr difficulties associated with definitively establishing their claims. In totally hemispherectomized patients both the geniculate and the extrageniculate systems are eliminated, and the corresponding thalamic nuclei presumably have suffered retrograde degeneration. In this situation, only infrathalamic nuclei can substitute for the cortex, with the favorite candidate being the superior colliculus (Perenin & Jeannerod 1978). In contrast, in the case of patients with a more restricted lesion, particularly in area 17 and assuming that a certain amount of good anatomical control has been possible, it can sometimes be demonstrated that the residual vision can be attributed to the extrageniculate system (Weiskranz et al. 1974).

More precise observations are now available to be considered in the context of separating out the different variables of a visual scene into channels that are functionally separate. Thus, Zihl et al. (1983) describe a case of a specific deficit of movement perception together with arguments based on present evidence to suggest that such effects might be attributed to the basal occipital region (lingual and fusiform gyrus; see Zeki 1990).

THE TWO VISUAL SYSTEMS HYPOTHESIS

To complete this review of the effects of cortical ablations we must mention a set of simplifying hypotheses and synthetic views that have dominated the discussion of experimental studies in vision for the last two decades. The suggestion is that there exist *two visual systems.*

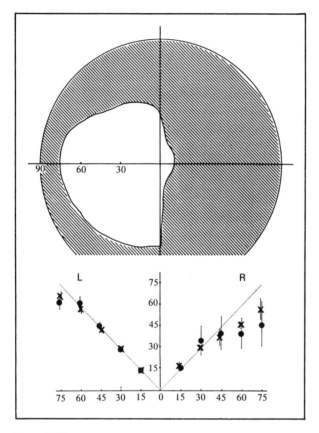

Figure 5.73
Possible visual spatial localization in a subject with a left hemisphere decortication.
The visual field was first plotted by traditional perimetry. The hatched zone shows
the region within which the subject could not "see" the test spot. The subject is
submitted to a forced-choice experiment in which he is obliged to point to the target
whether he can "see" it or not. In this typical case, the pointing was made with the
left hand and the target was a stationary grating of 8° (dots) or moving at 4 deg/s
(crosses) exposed for 500 ms. Notice that in the hemianopic field the localization, while
being defective and showing a greater dispersion than the normal side, is nevertheless
possible. It is less good the more eccentric the target. (From Perenin & Jeannerod
1978a)

Alongside the *geniculostriate* system there is another *extrageniculate* system, which involves the superior colliculus and/or the pretectum, then a group of thalamic nuclei comprising the alteral posterior nucleus and/or the pulvinar, then projecting onward to the temporal and parietal areas according to the organization that we have already to some extent detailed above.

Based on that idea of a dual connectivity is a corresponding hypothesis for duality of function which broadly is as follows: The geniculostriate system is essential for processing the detection and recognition of form, whereas the extrageniculate system has a role for localization (i.e., is dedicated to measuring the spatial parameters defining the situation of visual targets). The geniculate system comprises a wide representation of the macula (or in the primate case of the fovea) and a relatively much more restricted one of the more peripheral retina. This representation essentially involves X type ganglion cells as mechanisms for spatial resolution and to a lesser extent Y cells for temporal discriminations.

In contrast, the extrageniculate system has a wide representation of the peripheral retina (it is even "over-represented") and operates via Y and W ganglion cells with a good temporal resolution and an excellent sensitivity to the movement of a target but a poor spatial resolution. This wide peripheral representation also facilitates a good localization of targets in the visual field.

Let us examine the principal arguments used by researchers in favor of this synthesis. The first reason is the assembly of data concerned with the function of the colliculus, in particular from the effects of lesions. The lesioned animal is incapable of localizing sources and objects but can still, at best, identify them. We have already seen that it was from ablations of the colliculi or of cortical areas in the hamster that Schneider (1967, 1969) was able to propose a distinction between the systems for "what" and for "where," the first geniculocortical, the second collicular. At about the same time, other workers included the appropriate thalamic and cortical stages into the hypothesis of an extrageniculate system dedicated to visuospatial localization.

The data we have discussed above in fact only partially confirm this hypothesis, especially when the details of the deficits linked with cortical ablation are considered. It is in effect agreed that if *Tupaia* presents a clear contrast between the deficits after astriate and temporal lesions, this distinction soon becomes more blurred in the case of

Galago and even more so in macaque. It really is not possible to affirm that a peristriate elimination brings with it a purely localization deficit, whereas an area 17 lesion generates a purely identification loss. The case of the cat is not necessarily any simpler, since the pulvinar system itself seems to be concerned with a certain type of form vision.

Lesion studies by Bender (1988) in the macaque also raise problems. After lesions of the inferior and lateral pulvinar, no impairment was noticed in any of the components of visually guided behavior (eye-head coordination, visual attention, oculomotor control), in sharp contrast to most target localization tasks for which the colliculus is essential. These data indicate some independence of the tectum vs. the pulvinar and are not really compatible with the first simplified hypothesis for the "two visual systems."

In fact, the proposition appears to be more exact as soon as one no longer considers the peristriate region, or its equivalent in the cat, but rather the parietal area itself, which in the monkey is essentially represented by area 7. It is now well established that this cortical region plays an essential part in exploratory behavior and in the recognition of extracorporeal space. There is an additional argument. Representations of visual space in that area concern, principally, or perhaps exclusively, the retinal regions external to the fovea (in macaque) with a zero representation of the fovea. The proposition for a duality of systems might in reality be most valid if it is considered that the localization system comprises the tectopulvinocortical path to the parietal cortex and not the route to the peristriate regions.

Whatever validity might be attributed to the hypothesis of two visual systems as now formulated, it remains nonetheless necessary to try to understand why there is a multiplicity of projection areas for a single general sensory modality. There is no doubt that the interpretation we have arrived at for the visual system is insufficient at present. Nevertheless, this multiplicity of sensory areas is an experimentally proven fact in the case of all the three major special senses (see Buser & Imbert 1992 with respect to audition). What then is the raison d'être for this multiplicity of projections and for their underlying neuronal mechanisms?

One powerful idea suggested is that of exploiting the advantages of processing *in parallel*. We can conceive that in each sensory domain there are a number of channels operating in parallel dealing with the different parameters of a stimulus, such as are defined by psychophysics (in the case of vision, separate channels for color, form, and movement; see Zeki 1978a,b,c, 1980a,b, 1983, 1990). This rather modern concept of parallel channels to some extent contradicts the more traditional earlier views, supported by electrophysiological research methods, which led to the idea (tending to become obsolete) that cortical processing (to limit ourselves to that aspect) is arranged sequentially and hierarchically, such that a given area is the first to receive an afferent message and underpins a particular sort of signal processing. It then sends its outputs (in general by corticocortical connections) to a second area specialized for another class of processing, and so on. That view of events is thus a matter of processing *in series*, with a continual elaboration of the processing and with cells of more detailed specialization of information content appearing in this way at secondary levels, tertiary levels, and so on, constituting the detectors of particular parameters such as form recognition ("feature detectors").

To what extent are these two concepts contradictory? It must be said that they are rather less so than appears at first sight to the extent that, as we have seen, the two situations are closely combined in the geniculocortical striate system. Areas V1 and V2 act by sending outputs to different areas where different distinct parameters of the visual stimulus are processed. This operation is serial, since all signals pass via V1 and V2, but it also parallel as soon as the signals are distributed from there to new distinct cortical sites. Within these parallel systems there can, on the other hand, exist hierarchical integration as, for example, that between V5 and MST (DSR). Because of this, it is truly necessary to view these two classes of serial and parallel treatment as being complementary and not exclusive processing operations in the geniculocortical system.

4 THE DEVELOPING VISUAL SYSTEM

The various functional properties that have been examined in the preceding chapters and which characterize the adult visual system have, principally in the last decade, also been subjected to very detailed investigations of their development in the postnatal period. Thus it is inconceivable to finish a book on vision without at least introducing developmental aspects, if only briefly and as an appropriate conclusion. This is all the more necessary since the visual system, perhaps more than other systems, offers way of exploring that development and determining the different factors that control it as well as distinguishing what are the different innate or acquired effects that fill in the whole scene of development on its initially bare backdrop. Most of this work relates to the kitten, but several of its general laws and components have been discovered to be valid, even in time scale to some extent, for a variety of mammals.

Among these components we first need to specify are those which arise from endogenous processes of maturation which correspond to the expression of the genetic code ("inborn"), of which some are seen in the embryonic phase and others in the fetal and early postnatal periods. In outline, these first stages consist in a series of distinct events: cellular proliferation and migration, selective aggregation of immature cells to form the skeleton of the future nervous centers, cell differentiation in its biochemical anatomical and functional neuronal aspects, formation of the first synaptic contacts and establishment of neuronal networks, cell death.

Other factors are exogenous and are imposed by the individual history of the individual organism during the postnatal period. It is these that the experimenter is usually most able to modify or control, as the case may be. Among these are, essentially, visual experience itself, and extraretinal factors such as extraocular proprioception related to the sensitivity of the extraocular motor system.

We will show some evidence below how different techniques have led to the definition of a precise "critical period" within which the visual system can be changed by exposure to new visual environments. During this critical period the nervous system would normally progressively acquire its adult characteristics with the extraordinary precision of projections which, as we have seen, is particularly notable in the visual system.

It is relatively easy to manipulate the visual environment to which a young animal is exposed during development. Surgically, for example, an enucleation is possible or a deafferentation that denies a given cortical region access to its normal visual inputs. Alternatively a deprivation is possible, which totally or partially eliminates some particular visual characteristic normally present in the object space available to the immature animal and normally is specifically encoded by the nervous system.

Studies using sensory deprivation as a means of influencing visual development in a controlled way rely essentially upon discovering morphological and physiological changes in visual neurons and also upon observing changes in visual behavior. In order to understand the sort of results that this approach can generate let us discuss the changes consequent on monocular deprivation as a model. One of the first demonstrations of the influence of early visual experience on the development of morphological and physiological properties of neurons and its consequences for visuomotor behavior was carried out by Hubel and Wiesel in the early 1960s. If the eyelids of one eye in a kitten are stitched together from the first postnatal week for periods up to 2½ months, a reduction is seen in the size of LGB cells in the layer that receives afferent inputs from the deprived eye. In contrast, some physiological properties, notably the spatial organization of the receptive fields are little changed.

In contrast to this, anatomical changes were not observed at the cortical level but the physiological affects were very pronounced. Whereas in the normal animal most striate cortex units are activated binocularly, with a dominance of one eye or the other, in the monocularly deprived kitten they can only be activated from the eye that has had visual experience. Given that nearly all the cortical cells are active and that there is not a "silent" cortical region, we might suppose that the deprived eye has given up its territory entirely to the experienced one. Similar results have been obtained in the monkey.

The anatomical distribution of the geniculocortical afferents also shows anomalies when examined by various methods, notably by transneuronal transport of radioactive proline. Thus in the normal adult, inputs from the two eyes end in different bands identified physiologically as ocular dominance columns, but after monocular deprivation there is a marked narrowing of the ocular dominance columns appropriate to the deprived eye as well as an expansion of those for the eye that has had visual experience.

These physiological and behavioral effects are observed after quite brief deprivations. In kittens between 4 and 6 weeks of age, 7 to 8 days deprivation are enough to completely change the histogram of ocular dominance; 4 to 8 hours in a 5-week-old kitten suffice to make a noticeable change in cortical binocularity.

By studying the different stages in the visual pathway from the eye to the cortex it becomes clear that the principal site of the changes observed is at the cortical level. However, the eye itself becomes slightly lengthened, generating a myopia that is partly compensated for by a reduction in the refractive power of the dioptric system. This myopia, though feeble in the cat, can attain 13D in the monkey and itself be responsible for visual deficits.

The physiology of the retina itself, even when studied in fine detail by making very accurate measurements of resolution of the ganglion cells, seems to be practically unchanged. At the level of LGB neurons, a large reduction (around 30%) in the cellular area is observed. This effect is broadly limited to the binocular section of the nucleus. In contrast, physiological changes are relatively modest. The probability of recording from Y cells is reduced in the deprived layer and X cells show a spatial resolution that is reduced by a factor of 2. All these effects are, however, rather insignificant compared with the effects seen at the cortical level that we have already mentioned. In that region, it is possible to demonstrate that it is deprivation of clear pattern vision and not a reduction in total illumination which plays the essential role in the changes following monocular deprivation by eyelid suture.

The bilateral reduction of illumination of the retina by wearing clear neutral filters in front of the eyes is without effect on cortical cells' binocularity. In contrast, if one eye is covered by a diffusing filter and the other by a clear neutral filter to equalize the illumination of the two retinas, the latter eye becomes the only one capable of activating striate neurons. Clinically there are several conditions that can induce a degradation of the retinal image: The most common condition is anisometropia. This can be effected experimentally by giving the cat, for example, spectacles of −8 or −12 diopters. This procedure induces clear changes in binocularity, which are less marked than are found with total monocular deprivation of equal duration. However, if the eye deprived of focused vision can still activate cortical neurons, these show a considerable deficit in spatial resolution, with the signaling of high spatial frequency being more deteriorated than that of low.

If binocular vision is restored fairly soon during deprivation, the losses due to deprivation can be restored partially or even completely, and this is much influenced by forcing the animal to use the eye that was orginally deprived. But a longer deprivation cannot be reversed. There exists, then, a *critical period* within which the visual system can adapt to abnormal conditions imposed on its vision and also recover normal function when normal seeing conditions are restored.

Suturing the eyelids of one eye prevents the visual system from functioning correctly. It has been deprived of its normal capacity to observe objects and events in the visual world simultaneously with both eyes. It is in that respect that monocular deprivation is best

regarded as a model for studying other aspects of visual development. The general strategy it illustrates is to perturb in a limited way
the normal course of development and to examine with all possible
technical resources—anatomical, physiological, and behavioral—
how the animal reacts.

By assuming that the rules governing structural and functional
changes consequent on such perturbations are the same as those
governing normal development, we hope to establish the causal links
in the latter, stage by stage. In a general way, if the visual experience
of an immature animal is changed by a deprivation of contrast in
shapes, binocularly or monocularly, or by depriving it of a selective
dimension of vision such as movement or orientation, the performance of the visual system becomes limited to dealing only with
those aspects of vision that it has fully experienced in early postnatal
life. Observations like these not only illuminate the development of
vision but also of other sensory systems of the central nervous system. For a review of work on humans and other primates see Boothe
et al. 1985 (Trans.).

Appendix

Abridged Classification of Primates

At a variety of places in this book we have referred to different species of primates. It is useful to have a plan of their place in the general taxonomy of the order. This list can only be sketchy. We owe it to the kindness of Professor J.J. Petter. But the table has been simplified by sometimes including the complete hierarchy, sometimes the family or even the subfamily.

[The translator has provided the names in English common usage, where available, and for this is much indebted to some of the information in table 1.1. of *The Human Primate*, Richard Passingham, W.H. Freeman, Oxford and San Francisco, 1982. Where the Buser & Imbert original table or Passingham's also included obviously transliterated homophones from the common name in a local language, these have been retained, as have additional formal names for genera not in Passingham's table.

1 PROSIMIANS

1.1 LEMURIFORMES

Lemuridae
Microcebus (dwarf lemur), *Cheirogaleus* (mouse lemur), *Hapelemur* (gentle lemur), *Lemur* (common lemur), *Lepilemur* (sportive lemur)

Indridae
Indri (Indris), avahi, *Propithecus* (sifaka)

Daubentoniidae
Daubentonia (aye-aye)

1.2 LORISIFORMES

Lorisidae
Loris (slender loris), *Nycticebus* (slow loris), *Perodicticus* (potto), *Arctocebus*

Galagidae
Galago (bush baby)

1.3 TARSIIFORMES

Tarsiidae
Tarsius (tarsier)
This group is often separated from the prosimians to constitute an individual subgroup. The *Tupaia*, tree shrew, although recently classed among the primates, is also considered to be part of the insectivores.)

2 SIMIANS

2.1 PLATYRRHINA

CEBOIDS

Callithricidae
Callithrix (marmosets), (Wistiti), *Leontocebus* (tamarin), *Callimico*

Cebidae
Aotes (Douroucouli, night monkey, owl monkey), *Callicebus* (titi), *Pithecia (saki)*, *Chiropotes* (saki), *Cacajoa* (Oakari), *Alouatta* (howler, howling monkey), *Cebus* (capuchin, sajou or sapajou), *Saimiri* (squirrel monkey), *Ateles* (spider monkey), *Brachyteles* (woolly spider monkey), *Lagothrix* (woolly monkey)

2.2 ANTHROPOIDS

CATARRHINA

Cercopithecidae
Macaca mulatta (macaque, rhesus monkey) *Cynopithecus* (black ape), Cercocebus (mangabey), Papio (baboon, chacma, hamadryas), *Mandrillus* (drill, mandrill), *Theropithecus* (gelada), *Cercopithecus* (guenon), Miopithecus (talapoin), *Erythrocebus* (patas monkey), *Presbytis* (common langur), *Rhinopithecus* (snub-nosed langur), *Pygathrix* (douc langur), *Nasalis* (proboscis monkey), *Colobus* (Guereza)

HOMINOIDS

Pongidae
Pongo (orangutan), *Pan* (chimpanzee), gorilla

Hylobatidae
Hylobates (gibbon), *Symphalangus* (siamang)

Hominidae
Homo (man)

References

Abrahamson E & Wiesenfeld J (1972) The structure, spectra and reactivity of visual pigments (pp 69–121). In Dartnall H (Ed), Handbook of Sensory Physiology VII Vol. 1. Photochemistry of Vision. Springer-Verlag, Berlin

Aguilar M & Stiles W (1954) Saturation of the rod mechanism of the retina at high levels of stimulation. Optica Acta *1* 59–65

Allman J & Kaas J (1971a) A representation of the visual field in the caudal third of the middle temporal gyrus of the owl monkey (*Aotus trivirgatus*). Brain Res *31* 85–105

Allman J & Kaas J (1971b) Representation of the visual field in striate and adjoining cortex of the owl monkey. Brain Res *35* 89–106

Allman J & Kaas J (1974a) The organisation of the second visual area (V II) in the owl monkey: a second order transformation of the visual hemifield. Brain Res *76* 247–265

Allman J & Kaas J (1974b) A crescent shaped cortical visual area surrounding the middle temporal area (MT) in the owl monkey (*Aotus trivirgatus*). Brain Res *81* 199–213

Allman J & Kaas J (1974c) A visual area adjoining the second visual area (V II) on the wall of the parieto-occipital cortex of the owl monkey (*Aotus trivirgitus*). Anat Rec *178* 297–298

Allman J & Kaas J (1975) The dorsomedial cortical visual area: a third tier area in the occipital lobe of the owl monkey (*Aotus trivirgatus*). Brain Res *100* 473–487

Allman J & Kaas J (1976) Representation of the visual field on the medial wall of occipital-parietal cortex in the owl monkey. Science *191* 572–575

Allman J, Kaas J & Lane R (1973) The middle temporal visual area (MT) in the bush baby (*Galago senegalensis*). Brain Res *57* 197–202

Allman J, Kaas J, Lane R & Miezin F (1972) A representation of the visual field in the inferior nucleus of the pulvinar of the owl monkey. Brain Res *40* 291–302

Alpern M & Campbell F (1962) The behaviour of the pupil during dark adaptation. J Physiol *165* 5–6P

Anstis A (1978) Apparent movement (pp 655–674). In Held R, Leibovitz H &

Teuber H (Eds), Handbook of Sensory Physiology VIII. Perception. Springer-Verlag, Berlin

Apter J (1946) Eye movements following strychninization of the superior colliculus of cats. J Neurophysiol 9 73–86

Avendano C & Juretschke M (1980) The pretectal region of the cat: a structural and topographical study with stereotaxic coordinates. J Comp Neurol 193 69–88

Ayoub G & Lam D (1984) The release of gamma-aminobutyric acid from horizontal cells of the goldfish (Carassius auratus) retina. J Physiol 355 191–214

Bader C, Bertrand D & Schwartz E (1982) Voltage-activated and calcium-activated currents studied in the solitary rod inner segments from the salamander retina. J Physiol 331 253–284

Bader C, Macleish P & Schwartz E (1979) A voltage-clamp study of the light response in solitary rods of the tiger salamander. J Physiol 296 1–26

Baer W & Appleburry M (1986) Exploring visual transduction with recombinant DNA techniques. Trends Neurosci 9 198–203

Baker H (1949) The course of foveal light adaptation measured by the threshold intensity increment. J Opt Soc Am 39 172–179

Barlow H (1953) Summation and inhibition in the frog's retina. J Physiol 119 69–88

Barlow H (1956) Reliability, false positives and threshold. J Opt Soc Am 46 634

Barlow H (1972) Dark and light adaptation (pp 1–28). In Jameson D & Hurvitch L (Eds), Handbook of Sensory Physiology VII Vol. 4 Visual Psychophysics. Springer-Verlag, Berlin

Barlow H & Levick W (1965) The mechanism of directionally sensitive units in the rabbit's retina. J Physiol 178 477–504

Barlow H & Levick W (1969a) Changes in the maintained discharge with adaptation level in the cat retina. J Physiol 202 699–718

Barlow H & Levick W (1969b) Three factors limiting the reliable detection of light by retinal ganglion cells of the cat. J Physiol 200 1–24

Barlow H & Mollon J (Eds) (1982) The Senses. Cambridge University Press, Cambridge.

Barlow H & Sparrock J (1964) The role of afterimages in dark adaptation. Science 144 1309–1314

Barlow H, Hill R & Levick W (1964) Retinal ganglion cells responding selectively to direction and speed of image motion in the rabbit. J Physiol 173 377–407

Barlow H, Blakemore C & Pettigrew J (1967) The neural mechanism of binocular depth discrimination. J Physiol 193 69–88

Barlow H, Levick W & Yoon W (1971) Response of single quanta of light in retinal ganglion cells of the cat. Vision Res Suppl 3 87–101.

Bartlett N (1965) (pp 154–207). In Graham C (Ed), Vision and Visual Perception. Wiley, New York

Bartley S (1951) The Psychology of Vision. (pp 921–984) In Stevens S (Ed), Handbook of Experimental Psychology. Wiley, New York

Baumgartner G (1978) Physiologie des zentralen Sehsystems. (pp 264–348) In Gauer, Kramer, Jung (Eds), Das Sehen. Urban & Schwartzenberg, Müchen

Baylor D & Fettiplace R (1977) Kinetics of synaptic transfer from receptors to ganglion cells in turtle retina. J Physiol 271 425–448

Baylor D & Fettiplace R (1979) Synaptic drive and impulse generation in ganglion cells of turtle retina. J Physiol 288 107–127

Baylor D & Fuortes M (1970) Electrical responses in single cones of the retina of the turtle. J Physiol 207 77–92

Baylor D & Hodgkin A (1973) Detection and resolution of visual stimuli by turtle photoreceptors. J Physiol 234 163–198

Baylor D, Lamb T & Yau K (1979a) Responses of retinal rods to single photons. J Physiol 288 613–634

Baylor D, Lamb T & Yau K (1979b) The membrane current of single rod outer segment. J Physiol 288 589–611

Baylor D, Matthews G & Nunn B (1984) Location and function of voltage sensitive conductances in retinal rods of the salamander Amblystoma tigrinum. J Physiol 354 203–233

Baylor D, Matthews G & Yau K (1980) Two components of electrical dark noise in toad retinal rod outer segments. J Physiol 309 591–621

Belgum J, Dvorak D & McReynolds J (1984) Strychnine blocks transient but not sustained inhibition in mudpuppy retinal ganglion cells. J Physiol 354 273–286

Belgum J, Dvorak D & McReynolds J (1983) Sustained and transient synaptic inputs to on-off ganglion cells in the mudpuppy retina. J Physiol 340 599–610

Belgum J, Dvorak D & McReynolds J (1982) Sustained synaptic input to ganglion cells of mudpuppy retina. J Physiol 326 91–108

Bender D (1981) Retinotopic organisation of macaque pulvinar. J Neurophysiol 46 672–693

Bender D (1982) Receptive field properties of neurons in the macaque inferior pulvinar. J Neurophysiol 48 1–17

Bender D (1983) Visual interaction of neurons in the primate pulvinar depends on cortex but not colliculus. Brain Res *279* 258–261

Bender D (1988) Electrophysiological and behavioral experiments on the primate pulvinar (pp 55–65). In Hicks T & Benedek G (Eds), Vision within Extrageniculo-Striate Systems (Progress in Brain Research Series Vol 75). Elsevier, New York

Benevento L & Davis B (1977) Topographical projections of the prestriate cortex to the pulvinar nuclei in the macaque monkey: an autoradiographic study. Exp Brain Res *30* 405–424

Benevento L & Rezak M (1975) Extrageniculate projections to layers VI and I of striate cortex (area 17) in the Rhesus monkey (*Macaca mulatta*). Brain Res *96* 51–55

Benevento L & Rezak M (1976) The cortical projections of the inferior pulvinar and adjacent lateral pulvinar in the Rhesus monkey (*Macaca mulatta*). An autoradiographic study. Brain Res *108* 1–24

Benevento L & Standage G (1983) The organisation of projections of the retino-recipient and nonretinorecipient nuclei of the pretectal complex and layers of the superior colliculus to the lateral pulvinar and medial pulvinar in the macaque monkey. J Comp Neurol *217* 307–336

Benevento J & Yoshida K (1981) The afferent and efferent organisation of the lateral geniculo-prestriate pathways in the macaque monkey. J Comp Neurol *203* 455–474

Berardi N, Bisti S, Cattaneo A, Fiorentini A & Maffei L (1982) Correlation between the preferred orientation and spatial frequency of neurons in visual areas 17 and 18 of the cat. J Physiol *323* 603–618

Berkley M & Sprague J (1979) Striate cortex and visual acuity functions in the cat. J Comp Neurol *187* 679–703

Berman N & Cynader M (1972) Comparison of receptive field organisation of the superior colliculus in Siamese and normal cats. J Physiol *224* 363–389

Berman N & Cynader M (1975) Receptive fields in cat superior colliculus after visual cortex lesions. J Physiol *245* 261–270

Berman N, Blakemore C & Cynader M (1975) Binocular interaction in the cat's superior colliculis. J Physiol *246* 595–615

Berson D (1988) Retinal and cortical inputs to cat superior colliculus: Composition, convergence and laminar specificity (pp 17–26). In Hicks T & Benedek G (Eds), Vision within Extrageniculo-Striate Systems (Progress in Brain Research Series Vol 75). Elsevier, New York

Berson D & Graybiel A (1978) Parallel thalamic zones in the LP-pulvinar complex of the cat identified by their afferent and efferent connections. Brain Res *147* 139–148

Biernbaum M & Bownds D (1979) Influence of light and calcium on guanosine 5′ triphosphate in isolated frog rod outer segments. J Gen Physiol 74 649–669

Bishop P (1973) Neurophysiology of binocular single vision and stereopsis. In Jung R (Ed), Handbook of Sensory Physiology VII Vol. 3 Central Visual Information. Springer-Verlag, Berlin

Bishop P, Kozak W & Vakkur G (1962a) Some quantitative aspects of the cat's eye: axis and plane of reference, visual field coordinates and optics. J Physiol 163 466–502

Bishop P, Kozak W, Levick W & Vakkur G (1962b) The determination of the projection of the visual field on the lateral geniculate nucleus of the cat. J Physiol 163 503–539

Bishop P, Coombs J & Henry G (1971a) Responses to visual contours: spatio-temporal aspects of excitation in the receptive fields of simple striate neurons. J Physiol 219 625–657

Bishop P, Coombs J & Henry G (1971b) Interaction effects of visual contours on the discharge frequency of simple striate neurons. J Physiol 219 659–687

Bishop P, Coombs J & Henry G (1973) Receptive fields of simple cells in the cat striate cortex. J Physiol 231 31–60

Blakemore C & Campbell F (1969) On the existence of neurons in the human visual system selectively sensitive to orientation and size of retinal images. J Physiol 203 237–260

Blakemore C & Rushton W (1965) Dark adaptation and incremental threshold in a rod monochromat. J Physiol 181 612–628

Blakemore C & Vital-Durand F (1986) Organisation and postnatal development of the monkey's lateral geniculate. J Physiol 380 453–491

Blakemore C, Fiorenti A & Maffei L (1972) A second neural mechanism of binocular depth discrimination. J Physiol 226 725–749

Blasdel G & Lund J (1983) Termination of afferent axons in macaque striate cortex. J Physiol 3 1389–1413

Bodia R & Detwiler P (1985) Patch-clamp recordings of the light-sensitive dark noise in retinal rods from the lizard and frog. J Physiol 367 183–216

Bonnet C (1984) Two systems in the detection of visual motion. Ophthal Physiol Optics 4 61–65

Bons N & Petter A (1986) Afférences rétiniennes d'origine hypothalamique chez un primate prosimien: microcebus murinus. Etude à l'aide de traceurs fluorescents rétrograde. Comptes rendus de l'Académie des Sciences de Paris. 303 719–722

Boothe R, Dobson V & Teller D (1985) Postnatal development of vision in human and nonhuman primates. Annu Rev Neurosci 8 495–545

Bouman M (1955) Absolute thresholds for visual perception. J Opt Soc Am 45 36–43

Bowmaker J (1980) Colour vision in birds and the role of oil droplets. Trends Neurosci 3 196–199

Bowmaker J (1983) Trichromatic vision: why only three receptor channels? Trends Neurosci 6 41–43

Bowmaker J & Dartnall H (1980) Visual pigments of rods and cones in a human retina. J Physiol 298 501–511

Bowmaker J, Dartnall H & Mollon J (1980) Microspectrophotometric demonstration of four classes of receptor in an Old World Primate (*Macaca fascicularis*) J Physiol 289 131–143

Bownds D (1980) Biochemical steps in visual transduction. Roles for nucleotides and calcium ions. Photochem Photobiol 32 487

Boycott B & Wässle H (1974) The morphological types of ganglion cells of the domestic cat's retina. J Physiol 240 397–419

Boynton R (1979) Human Color Vision. Holt-Rinehart-Winston, New York.

Braddick O (1974) A short range process in apparent motion. Vision Res 14 519–527

Breitmeyer B (1973) A relationship between the size, rate, orientation, and direction in the human visual system. Vision Res 13 41–58

Brooks B & Jung R (1973) Neuronal physiology of the visual cortex (pp 325–440). In Jung R (Ed), Handbook of Sensory Physiology VII Vol. 3 Central Visual Information. Springer-Verlag, Berlin.

Brown J (1965) Afterimages (pp 479–503). In Graham C (Ed), Vision and Visual Perception. Wiley, New York.

Brown J, Coles J & Pinto L (1977) Effects of injections of calcium and EGTA into the outer segments of retinal rods of *Bufo marinus*. J Physiol 269 707–722

Brown K (1968) The electroretinogram: its components and their origin. Vision Res 8 633–677

Brown K & Murakami M (1964a) A new receptor potential of the monkey retina with no detectable latency. Nature 201 626–628

Brown K & Murakami M (1964b) Biphasic form of the early receptor potential of the monkey retina. Nature 204 739–740

Brown K & Wiesel T (1961) Localisation of the origins of electroretinogram components by intraretinal recording in the intact cat eye. J Physiol *158* 257–280

Brown P & Wald G (1963) Visual pigments in human and monkey retinas. Nature *200* 37–43

Brown R (1955) Velocity discrimination and the intensity-time relation. J Opt Soc Am *45* 189–192

Bullier J & Henry G (1979a) Ordinal position of neurons in cat striate cortex. J Neurophysiol *42* 1251–1263

Bullier J & Henry G (1979b) Neural path taken by afferent streams in striate cortex of the cat. J Neurophysiol *42* 1264–1270

Bullier J & Henry G (1979c) Laminar distribution of first order neurons and afferent terminals in cat striate cortex. J Neurophysiol *42* 1271–1281

Bullier J & Norton T (1977) Receptive field properties of X-, Y- and intermediate cells in the cat lateral geniculate nucleus. Brain Res *121* 151–156

Bullier J & Norton T (1978) X and Y relay cells in the cat lateral geniculate nucleus: quantitative analysis of receptive field properties and classification. J Neurophysiol *42* 244–273

Bullier J & Norton T (1979) Comparison of receptive field properties of X and Y ganglion cells with X and Y lateral geniculate cells in the cat. J Neurophysiol *42* 274–290

Bunt A, Hendrickson A, Lund J, Lund R, & Fuchs A (1975) Monkey retinal ganglion cells: morphometric analysis and tracing of axonal projections with a consideration of the peroxidase technique. J Comp Neurol *164* 265–286

Bunt A, Minckler D, Johanson G (1977) Demonstration of bilateral projection of the central retina of the monkey with horseradish peroxidase neuronography. J Comp Neurol *171* 619–630

Burr D & Ross J (1986) Visual processing of motion. Trends Neurosci *9* 304–307

Buser P & Imbert M (1992) Audition. MIT Press, Cambridge, Massachusetts

Camarda R & Rizzolatti G (1976) Receptive field of cells in the superficial layers of the cat's area 17. Exp Brain Res *24* 423–427

Campbell F & Gubisch R (1966) Optical quality of the human eye. J Physiol *186* 558–578

Campbell F & Maffei L (1970) Electrophysiological evidence for the existence of orientation and size detectors in the human visual system. J Physiol *207* 635–652

Campbell F & Robson J (1968) Application of Fourier analysis to the visibility of gratings. J Physiol *197* 551–566

Campbell F & Rushton W (1955) Measurement of the scotopic pigment in the living human eye. J Physiol *130* 131–147

Campbell F, Cooper G & Enroth-Cugell C (1969a) The spatial selectivity of the visual cells of the cat. J Physiol *203* 223–235

Campbell F, Cooper G, Robson J & Sachs M (1969b) The spatial selectivity of visual cells of the cat and the squirrel monkey. J Physiol *204* 120P

Campbell F, Maffei L & Piccolino M (1973) The contrast sensitivity of the cat. J Physiol *229* 719–731

Campion J, Latto R & Smith Y (1983) Is blindsight an effect of scattered light, spared cortex and near threshold vision? Behav Brain Res *6* 423–486

Caviness V Jr (1975) Architectonic map of neocortex of the normal mouse. J Comp Neurol *164* 247–263

Chabre M (1985a) Trigger and amplification phenomena in visual phototransduction. Annu Rev Biophys Chem *14* 331–360

Chabre M (1985b) From the photon to the neuronal signal. Europhysics News *16* 1–4

Chalupa L & Abramson B (1988) Receptive field properties in the tecto- and striate-recipient zones of the cat's lateral posterior nucleus (pp 85–94). In Hicks T & Benedek G (Eds), Vision within Extrageniculo-Striate Systems (Progress in Brain Research Series Vol 75). Elsevier, New York

Chevalier G & Deniau J (1984) Spatio-temporal organisation of a branched tecto-spinal/tecto-diencephalic neuronal system. Neuroscience *12* 427–439

Chevalier G, Deniau J, Thierry A & Féger J (1981) The nigro-tectal pathway: an electrophysiological reinvestigation in the rat. Brain Res *213* 253–263

Chow K, Mathers L & Spear P (1973) Spreading of uncrossed retinal projection in superior colliculus of neonatally enucleated rabbits. J Comp Neurol *151* 307–322

Cleland B, Dubin M & Levick W (1971) Sustained and transient neurones in the cat's retina and lateral geniculate nucleus. J Physiol *217* 473–496

Cleland B, Levick W & Sanderson K (1973) Properties of sustained and transient cells in the cat's retina. J Physiol *228* 649–680

Cohen A (1963) Vertebrate retinal cells and their organisation. Biol Rev *38* 427–449

Cohen A (1972) Rods and cones (pp 63–111). In Fuortes (Ed), Handbook of Sensory Physiology VII Vol. 2 Physiology of Photoreceptor organs. Springer-Verlag, Berlin

Cone R (1967) Early receptor potential: photoreversible charge displacement in rhodopsin. Science *155* 1128–1131

Cooper M, Lee G & Pettigrew J (1979) The decussation of the retinothalamic pathway in the cat with a note on the major meridians of the cat's eye. J Comp Neurol *187* 285–312.

Copenhagen D & Owen D (1980) Current voltage relations in the rod photoreceptor network of the turtle retina. J Physiol *308* 159–184

Cornsweet T (1970) Visual Perception. Academic Press, New York

Cowey A (1964) Projection of the retina on to striate and prestriate cortex in the squirrel monkey *Saimiri sciureus*. J Neurophysiol *27* 366–393

Cowey A (1967) Perimetric study of field defects in monkeys after cortical and retinal ablations. Q J Exp Psychol *19* 232–245

Craik K (1966) The native of psychology. A selection of papers, essays and other writings by the late KJW Craik. Sherwood. Cambridge University Press, Cambridge

Crawford B (1947) Visual adaptation in relation to brief conditioning stimuli. Proc R Soc [B] *134* 283–302

Crescitelli F (1972) The visual cells and visual pigments of the vertebrate eye (pp 245–363). In Dartnall H (Ed), Handbook of Sensory Physiology VII Vol 1 Photochemistry of Vision. Springer-Verlag, Berlin

Crescitelli F (1977) The visual pigment of geckos and other vertebrates (pp 392–449). Crescitelli (Ed), Handbook of Sensory Physiology VII Vol. V. The Visual System in Vertebrates. Springer-Verlag, Berlin

Creutzfeldt O, Innocenti G & Brooks D (1974) Vertical organisation in the visual cortex (area 17) in the cat. Exp Brain Res *21* 315–336

Creutzfeldt O, Lee B & Elepfandt A (1979) A quantitative study of chromatic organisation and receptive fields of cells in the lateral geniculate body of the rhesus monkey. Exp Brain Res *35* 527–545

Cynader M & Berman N (1972) Receptive field organisation of monkey superior colliculus. J Neurophysiol *35* 187–201

Cynader M & Regan D (1978) Neurones in cat parastriate cortex sensitive to the direction of motion in three dimensional space. J Physiol *274* 549–569

Daniel P & Whitteridge D (1961) The representation of the visual field on the cerebral cortex in monkeys. J Physiol *159* 203–221

Dartnall H (1962) Photobiology of visual processes (pp 323–533). In Davson H (Ed), The Eye. Academic Press, New York

Dartnall H (Ed) (1972) Handbook of Sensory Physiology VII Vol. 1 Photochemistry of Vision. Springer-Verlag, Berlin

Davson H (1976) The Physiology of the Eye (3rd Edition). Churchill, London.

de Monasterio F & Gouras P (1975) Functional properties of ganglion cells of the rhesus monkey retina. J Physiol *251* 167–195

de Monasterio F, Gouras P & Tolhurst D (1975) Trichromatic colour opponency in ganglion cells of the rhesus monkey retina. J Physiol *251* 197–216

Detwiler P & Hodgkin A (1979) Electrical coupling between cones in turtle retina. J Physiol *291* 75–100

De Valois R (1971) Contributions of different lateral geniculate cell types to visual behaviour. Vision Res *Suppl 2* 344–59

De Valois R (1973) Central mechanisms of color vision. In Jung R (Ed) Handbook of Sensory Physiology VII Vol. 3 Central Visual Information. Springer-Verlag, Berlin

De Valois R & De Valois K (1980) Spatial vision. Annu Rev Psychol *31* 309–341

De Valois R, Morgan H, Poloon M, Mead W & Hull E (1974) Psychological studies of monkey vision. I. Macaque luminosity and color vision test. Vision Res *14* 53–67

De Valois K, De Valois R & Yund W (1979) Responses of striate cortex cells to grating and checkerboard patterns. J Physiol *291* 483–496

De Valois R, Yund E & Hepler N (1982) The orientation and direction selectivity of cells in macaque visual cortex. Vision Res *22* 531–544

Derrington A & Lennie P (1984) Spatial and temporal contrast sensitivities of neurones in lateral geniculate nucleus of macaque. J Physiol *357* 219–240

Dick E & Miller R (1978) Light evoked potassium activity in mudpuppy retina: its relationship to the b-wave of the retinogram. Brain Res *154* 388–394

Dineen J & Keating E (1981) The primate visual system after bilateral removal of striate cortex. Exp Brain Res *41* 338–345

Dowling J (1960) Chemistry of visual adaptation in the rat. Nature *188* 114–118

Dowling J (1968) Synaptic organisation of the frog retina: an electron microscopic analysis comparing the retinas of frog and primates. Proc R Soc [B] *170* 205–228.

Dowling J (1979a) Information processing by local circuits: the vertebrate retina as a model system. In Schmitt F & Worden F (Eds), The Neurosciences: 4th Study Program. MIT Press, Cambridge, Massachusetts

Dowling J (1979b) A new retinal neuron—the interplexiform cell. Trends Neurosci *2* 189–191

Dowling J (1986) Dopamine: a retinal neuromodulator? Trends Neurosci *9* 236–240

Dowling J & Boycott B (1966) Organisation of the primate retina: electron microscopy. Proc R Soc [B] *166* 80–111

Dowling J & Werblin F (1969) Organisation of the retina of the Mudpuppy *Necturus maculosus*. I. Synaptic structure. J Neurophysiol *32* 315–338

Dräger U & Olsen J (1980) Origins of crossed and uncrossed retinal projections in pigmented and albino mice. J Comp Neurol *191* 383–412

Dratz E & Hargrave P (1983) The structure of rhodopsin and the rod outer segment disk membrane. Trends Biochem Sci *6* 128–131

Dreher B & Hoffman K (1973) Properties of excitatory and inhibitory regions in the receptive fields of single units in the cat's superior colliculus. Exp Brain Res *16* 333–353

Dreher B & Sanderson K (1973) Receptive field analysis: responses to moving visual contours by single lateral geniculate neurones in the cat. J Physiol *234* 95–118

Dreher B & Sefton A (1978) Properties of neurones in cat's dorsal lateral geniculate nucleus: a comparison between medial interlaminar and laminated parts of the nucleus. J Comp Neurol *183* 47–64

Dreher B, Fukada Y & Rodieck R (1976) Identification, classification and anatomical segregation of cells with X-like and Y-like properties in the lateral geniculate of old world monkeys. J Physiol *258* 433–452

Duke-Elder W (1958) The Eye in Evolution. Vol I. Mosby, St Louis

Eggers H & Blakemore C (1978) Physiological basis of anisometropic amblyopia. Science *201* 264–266

Enroth-Cugell C & Robson J (1966) The contrast sensitivity of the retinal ganglion cell of the cat. J Physiol *187* 517–552

Enroth-Cugell C & Shapley R (1973a) Flux, not retinal illumination is what cat retinal ganglion cells really care about. J Physiol *233* 311–326

Enroth-Cugell C & Shapley R (1973b) Adaptation and dynamics of cat retinal ganglion cells. J Physiol *233* 271–309

Fain G (1975) Quantum sensitivity of rods in the toad retina. Science *187* 838–841

Fain G, Gerschenfeld H & Quandt F (1980) Calcium spikes in toad rods. J Physiol *303* 495–513

Famiglietti E & Kolb H (1975) A bistratified amacrine cell and synaptic circuitry in the inner plexiform layer of the retina. Brain Res *84* 293–300

Feldon S, Feldon P & Kruger L (1970) Topography of the retinal projection upon the superior colliculus of the cat. Vision Res *10* 135–143

Ferster D (1981) A comparison of binocular depth mechanisms in area 17 and 18 of the cat visual cortex. J Physiol *311* 623–655

Fesenko E, Kolesnikov S & Lyubarsky A (1985) Induction by cyclic GMP of cationic conductance in plasma membrane retinal rod outer segment. Nature *313* 310–313

Finlay B, Schneps S, Wilson K & Schneider G (1978) Topography of visual and somatosensory projections to the superior colliculus of the golden hamster. Brain Res *142* 223–235

Fiorentini A (1972) Mach band phenomena (pp 188–201). In Jameson & Hurvitch (Eds), Handbook of Sensory Physiology VII Vol. 4 Visual Psychophysics. Springer-Verlag, Berlin

Foster K, Gaska J, Nagler M & Pollen D (1985) Spatial and temporal frequency selectivity of neurones in visual cortical areas V1 and V2 of the macaque monkey. J Physiol *365* 331–363

Freund H (1973) Neuronal mechanisms of the lateral geniculate body (pp 177–246). In Jung R (Ed), Handbook of Sensory Physiology VII Vol. 3 Central Visual Information. Springer-Verlag, Berlin

Friedländer M & Sherman M (1981) Morphology of physiologically identified neurons. Trends Neurosci *4* 211–214

Frumkes T, Miller R, Slaughter M & Dacheux R (1981) Physiological and pharmacological basis of GABA and Glycine action on neurons of mudpuppy retina III. Amacrine-mediated inhibitory influences on ganglion cell receptive field organisation: a model. J Neurophysiol *45* 783–804

Fukuda Y & Stone J (1974) Retinal distribution and central projections of X-, Y- and W-cells of the cat's retina. J Neurophysiol *37* 749–772

Fukuda Y & Stone J (1975) Direct identification of the cell bodies of Y-, X- and W-cells of the cat retina. Vision Res *15* 1034–1036

Fukuda Y & Stone J (1976) Evidence of differential inhibitory influences on X- and Y-type relay cells in the cat's lateral geniculate nucleus. Brain Res *113* 188–196

Fung B, Hurley J & Stryer L (1981) Flow of information in the light triggered cyclic nucleotide cascade of vision. Proc Natl Acad Sci USA *78* 152–156

Furukawa T & Hanawa I (1955) Effects of some common cations on electroretinogram of the toad. Jap J Physiol *5* 289–300

Galifret Y (1968) Les diverses aires fonctionelles de la rétine du pigeon. Z Zellforschungen *86* 535–545

Galifret Y & Piéron H (1948) Etude des fréquences critiques de fusion pour les stimulations chromatiques intermittentes à brillance constante. Ann Psychol *45, 46* 1–15

Garey L, Jones E & Powell T (1968) Interrelationships of striate and extrastriate cortex with the primary relay sites of the visual pathway. J Neurol Neurosurg Psychiatry *31* 135–157

Gattass R & Gross C (1981) Visual topography of the striate projection zone (MT) in the posterior superior temporal sulcus of the macaque. J Neurophysiol *46* 621–638

Gattass R, Gross C & Sandell J (1981) Visual topography of V2 in the macaque. J Comp Neurol *201* 519–539

Geisert E (1980) Cortical projections of the lateral geniculate nucleus in the cat. J Comp Neurol *190* 793–812

Gerschenfeld H, Neyton J, Piccolino M & Witkovsky P (1982) L-Horizontal cells of the turtle: network organisation and coupling modulation (pp 21–34). In Kaneko A et al (Eds), Neurotransmitters in the Retina and Visual Centres. Biomedical Research Foundation, Tokyo

Giaume C & Horn K (1983) Bidirectional transmission at the rectifying electronic synapse. Science *220* 84–87

Gilbert C (1977) Laminar differences in receptive field properties of cells in primary visual cortex. J Physiol *268* 391–421

Gilbert C (1983) Microcircuitry of the visual cortex. Annu Rev Neurosci *6* 217–247

Gilbert C & Kelly J (1975) The projections of cells in different layers of the cat's visual cortex. J Comp Neurol *163* 81–106

Gilbert C & Wiesel T (1981) Laminal specialization and intracortical connections in cat primary visual cortex (pp 163–194). In Schmitt FO et al (Eds), The organization of the cerebral cortex. MIT Press, Cambridge, Massachusetts

Gioanni H, Villalobos J, Rey J & Dalbera A (1983) Optokinetic nystagmus in the pigeon (*Columbia livia*). III. Role of nucleus ectomamillaris (nEM). Interactions in the accessory optic system. Exp Brain Res *50* 248–258

Giolli R & Guthrie M (1969) The primary optic projections in the rabbit. An experimental degeneration study. J Comp Neurol *136* 99–125

Glendenning K, Hall J, Diamond I & Hall W (1975) The pulvinar nucleus of *Galago*. J Neurophysiol *161* 419–458

Goldberg M & Robinson D (1978) Visual system: superior colliculus (pp 119–164). In Bruce & Masterton (Eds), Handbook of Behavioural Neurobiology. Plenum Press, New York

Goldberg M & Wurtz R (1972a) Activity of the superior colliculus in behaving monkey I. Visual receptive fields of single neurons. J Neurophysiol 35 542–549

Goldberg M & Wurtz R (1972b) Activity of superior colliculus in behaving monkey II. Effects of attention on neuronal responses. J Neurophysiol 35 560–574

Goodwin A & Henry G (1975) Direction sensitivity of complex cells in comparison with simple cells. J Neurophysiol 38 1524–1540

Goodwin A & Henry G (1978) The influences of stimulus velocity on the responses of single neurones in the striate cortex. J Physiol 277 467–482

Goodwin A, Henry G & Bishop P (1975) Direction sensitivity of simple striate cells: properties and mechanism. J Neurophysiol 38 1500–1523

Gouras P (1968) Identification of cone mechanisms in monkey ganglion cells. J Physiol 199 533–547

Gouras P (1969) Antidromic responses of orthodromically identified ganglion cells in monkey retina. J Physiol 204 407–419

Gouras P & Kruger J (1979) Responses of cells in foveal visual cortex of the monkey to pure color contrast. J Neurophysiol 42 850–860

Graham C (Ed) (1965) Vision and Visual Perception. Wiley, New York

Graham N (1977) Visual detection of aperiodic stimuli by probability summation among narrow band channels. Vision Res 17 637–652

Granit R (1947) Sensory Mechanisms of the Retina. Oxford University Press, Oxford

Grantyn A & Grantyn R (1980) Reticular substrates for coordination of horizontal eye movements and their relation to rectal efferent pathways (pp 211–225). In Hobson J & Brazier M (Eds), The Reticular Formation Revisited. Raven Press, New York.

Graybiel A & Berson D (1980) Histochemical identification and afferent connections of subdivisions in the lateralis posterior pulvinar complex and related thalamic nuclei in the cat. Neuroscience 5 1175–1238

Green D & Swets J (1966) Signal detection theory and psychophysics. Wiley, New York

Guillery R (1969) The organisation of synaptic interconnections in the laminae of the dorsal lateral geniculate nucleus of the cat. Z Zellforschung Mikroskopische Anatomie 96 1–38

Guillery R, Geisert E, Polley E & Mason C (1980) An analysis of the retinal afferents to the cat's medial interlaminar nucleus and to its rostral thalamic extension, "the geniculate wing." J Comp Neurol 194 117–147

Guitton D, Crommelinck & Roucoux (1980) Stimulation of the superior colliculus in the alert cat. Exp Brain Res *39* 63

Haimovic I & Pedley T (1982) Hemi-field pattern reversal of visual evoked potential I. Normal subjects. Electroencephalo Clin Neurophysiol *54* 111–120

Hammond P (1973) Contrasts in spatial organisation of receptive fields at geniculate and retinal levels: centre, surround and outer surround. J Physiol *228* 115–137

Hammond P & MacKay D (1975) Differential responses of cat visual cortical cells to textured stimuli. Exp Brain Res *22* 427–430

Hammond P & MacKay D (1977) Differential responsiveness of simple and complex cells in cat striate cortex to visual texture. Exp Brain Res *30* 275–296

Harting J & Guillery R (1976) Organisation of retinocollicular pathways in the cat. J Comp Neurol *166* 133–144

Harting J, Hall W & Diamond I (1972) Evolution of the pulvinar. Brain Behav Evol *6* 424–452

Harting J, Diamond I & Hall W (1973) Anterograde degeneration study of the cortical projections of the lateral geniculate and pulvinar nuclei in the tree shrew. J Comp Neurol *150* 393–439

Hartline H (1938) The response of single optic nerve fibers of the vertebrate eye to illumination of the retina. Am J Physiol *121* 400–415

Hashimoto Y & Ueki K (1982) The connectivity of cones and cone horizontal cells in Japanese Dace retina (pp 9–13). In Kaneko et al (Eds), Neurotransmitters in the Retina and the Visual Centres. Biomedical Research Foundation, Tokyo

Hawken M & Parker A (1984) Contrast sensitivity and orientation selectivity in lamina IV of the striate cortex of Old World monkeys. Exp Brain Res *54* 367–372

Hayhow W (1959) An experimental study of the accessory optic fibre system in the cat. J Comp Neurol *113* 282–315

Hayhow W, Sefton A & Webb C (1962) Primary optic centres in the rat in relation to the terminal distribution of the crossed and uncrossed nerve fibres. J Comp Neurol *118* 295–321

Haynes L & Yau K (1990) Single channel measurement from the cyclic GMP activated conductance of catfish retinal cones. J Physiol *429* 451–481

Heath C & Jones E (1971) The anatomical organisation of the supra sylvian cortex in the cat. Ergebnisse der Anatomie und Entwicklungsgeschichte *45* 1–64

Hecht S (1937) Rods, cones and the chemical basis of vision. Physiol Rev *17* 239–290

Hecht S & Mintz E (1939) The visibility of single lines at various illuminations. J Gen Physiol *22* 593–612

Hecht S, Haig C & Wald G (1935) The dark adaptation of retinal fields of different size and location. J Gen Physiol *19* 321–327

Hecht S & Shlaer S (1936) Intermittent stimulation by light. V. The relation between intensity and critical frequency for different parts of the spectrum. J Gen Physiol *19* 965–979

Hecht S & Shlaer S (1938) An adaptometer for measuring human dark adaptation. J Opt Soc Am *28* 269–275

Hecht S & Smith E (1936) Intermittent stimulation by light. VI. Area and the relation between critical frequency and intensity. J Gen Physiol *19* 979–991

Hecht S, Shlaer S & Pirenne M (1942) Energy, quanta and vision. J Gen Physiol *25* 819–840

Hecht S, Shlaer S, Smith E, Haig C & Peskin J (1948) The visual functions of the complete colorblind. J Gen Physiol *31* 459–472

Heinemann E (1955) Simultaneous brightness induction as a function of inducing and test field luminances. J Exp Psychol *50* 89–96

Hendrickson A, Wilson J & Ogren M (1978) The neuroanatomical organisation of pathways between the dorsal lateral geniculate nucleus and visual cortex in Old World and New World primates. J Comp Neurol *182* 123–136

Henry G (1977) Receptive field classes of cells in the striate cortex of the cat. Brain Res *133* 1–28

Henry G, Bishop P, Tupper R & Dreher B (1973) Orientation specificity and response variability of cells in the striate cortex. Vision Res *13* 1771–1779

Henry G, Dreher D & Bishop P (1974) Orientation specificity of cells in cat striate cortex. J Neurophysiol *37* 1394–1409

Henry G, Lund J & Harvey A (1978) Cells of the striate cortex projecting to the Clarke-Bishop area of the cat. Brain Res *151* 154–159

Herz A, Creutzfeldt O & Fuster J (1964) Statistische Eigenschaften der Neuronenaktivität in ascendierenden visuellen System. Kybernetik *2* 61–71

Hick W (1950) The threshold for sudden changes in velocity of a seen object. Q J Exp Psychol *2* 23–41

Hitchcock P & Hickey T (1983) Morphology of C-laminae neurons in the dorsal lateral geniculate nucleus of the cat: a Golgi impregnation study. J Comp Neurol *220* 137–146

Hochstein S & Shapley R (1976) Linear and nonlinear spatial subunits in Y cat retinal ganglion cells. J Physiol *262* 265–284

Hochstein S & Shapley R (1976) Quantitative analysis of retinal ganglion cell classification. J Physiol *262* 237–264

Hodgkin A, McNaughton P, Nunn B & Yau K (1984) Effects of ions on retinal rods from *Buffo marinus*. J Physiol *350* 649–680

Hoffman K & Stone J (1973a) Conduction velocity of afferents to cat visual cortex: a correlation with cortical receptive field properties. Brain Res *32* 640–646

Hoffman K & Stone J (1973b) Central termination of W, X and Y ganglion cells from cat retina. Brain Res *49* 500–501

Hoffman K, Stone J & Sherman M (1972) Relay of receptive field properties in dorsal lateral geniculate nucleus of the cat. J Neurophysiol *35* 518–531

Holländer H & Martinez-Millan L (1975) Autoradiographic evidence for a topographically organised projection from the striate cortex to the lateral geniculate nucleus in the rhesus monkey. Brain Res *100* 407–411

Holländer H & Vanegas H (1977) The projection from the lateral geniculate nucleus on to the visual cortex in the cat. A quantitative study with horseradish peroxidase. J Comp Neurol *173* 519–536

Holmes, G (1945) The organisation of the visual cortex in man. Proc R Soc *132B* 348–361

Hubel D & Freeman D (1977) Projection into the visual field of ocular dominance columns in macaque monkey. Brain Res *122* 336–343

Hubel D & Wiesel T (1959) Receptive fields of single neurons in the cat's striate cortex. J Physiol *148* 574–591

Hubel D & Wiesel T (1962) Receptive fields, binocular interaction and functional architecture in the cat's visual cortex. J Physiol *160* 106–154

Hubel D & Wiesel T (1965) Receptive fields and functional architecture in two non striate visual areas (18 and 19) of the cat. J Neurophysiol *28* 1041–1059

Hubel D & Wiesel D (1968) Receptive fields and functional architecture of monkey striate cortex. J Physiol *195* 215–243

Hubel D & Wiesel T (1972) Laminar and columnar distribution of geniculo-cortical fibres in the macaque monkey. J Comp Neurol *146* 421–450

Hubel D, Wiesel T & LeVay S (1976) Functional architecture of area 17 in normal and monocularly deprived macaque monkeys. Cold Spring Harbor Symposium in Quantitative Biology *40* 581–589

Hubel D, Wiesel T & Stryker M (1978) Anatomical demonstration of orientation selectivity. J Comp Neurol *177* 361–380

Hughes A (1972) A schematic eye for the rabbit. Vision Res *12* 123–138

Hughes A (1976) A supplement to the cat schematic eye. Vision Res *16* 149–154

Hughes A (1977) The topography of vision in mammals of contrasting life style:

comparative optics and retinal organisation. In Crescitelli F (Ed), Handbook of Sensory Physiology VII Vol V. The Visual System in Vertebrates. Springer-Verlag, Berlin

Hughes A (1979) A schematic eye for the rat. Vision Res 19 569–588

Hughes A & Vaney D (1982) The organisation of binocular cortex in the primary visual area of the rabbit. J Comp Neurol 204 151–164

Hughes A & Wilson M (1969) Callosal terminations along the boundary between visual areas I and II in the rabbit. Brain Res 12 19–25

Humphrey N (1970) What the frog's eye tells the monkey's brain. Brain Behav Evol 3 324–337

Humphrey N & Weiskrantz L (1967) Vision in monkeys after removal of the striate cortex. Nature 215 595–597

Humphrey A & Norton T (1980) Topographic organisation of the orientation column system in the striate cortex of the tree shrew. I. Microelectrode recording. J Comp Neurol 192 539–548

Humphrey A, Skeen L & Norton T (1980) Topographic organisation of the orientation column system in the striate cortex of the tree shrew II. Deoxyglucose mapping. J Comp Neurol 192 549–566

Hurvich L (1985) Opponent colours theory. In Ottoson D & Zeki S (Eds), Central and Peripheral Mechanisms in Colour Vision. Macmillan, London

Hutchins B & Weber J (1985) The pretectal complex of the monkey: a reinvestigation of the morphology and retinal termination. J Comp Neurol 232 425–442

Ikeda H (1979) Physiological basis of amblyopia. Trends Neurosci 2 209–213

Ikeda H & Wright M (1972) Receptive field organisation of "sustained" and "transient" retinal ganglion cells which subserve different functional roles. J Physiol 227 769–800

Ikeda H & Wright M (1975a) Spatial temporal properties of "sustained" and "transient" cortical neurones in area 17 of the cat's visual cortex. Exp Brain Res 22 363–383

Ikeda H & Wright M (1975b) Retinotopic distribution, visual latency and orientation tuning of "sustained" and "transient" cortical neurones in area 17 of the cat. Exp Brain Res 22 385–398

Illing R & Wässle H (1981) The retinal projection to the thalamus in the cat: a quantitative investigation and a comparison with the retinotectal pathway. J Comp Neurol 202 265–285

Ito K, Mizuno N & Kudo M (1983) Direct retinal projections to the lateroposterior and pulvinar nuclear complex (LP-PUL) in the cat as revealed by the anterograde HRP method. Brain Res 276 325–328

Jameson D (1985) Opponent colours in the light of physiological findings. In Ottoson D & Zeki S (Eds), Central and Peripheral Mechanisms in Colour Vision. Macmillan, London

Jeffreys D & Axford J (1972) Source locations of pattern specific components of human visual evoked potentials. I. Component of striate cortical origin. Exp Brain Res 16 1–21

Joshua D & Bishop G (1970) Binocular single vision and depth discrimination. Receptive field disparities for central and peripheral vision and binocular interaction on peripheral units in cat striate cortex. Exp Brain Res 10 389–416

Judd D (1951) Basic correlates of the visual stimulus (pp. 811–867). In Stevens S (Ed), Handbook of Experimental Psychology. Wiley, New York

Julesz B (1978) Global stereopsis: cooperative phenomena in stereoscopic depth perception (pp 215–252). In Held, Leibovitz & Teuber (Eds), Handbook of Sensory Physiology VIII. Perception. Springer-Verlag, Berlin

Jung R (Ed) (1973) Central Processing of Visual Information. Handbook of Sensory Physiology. VII 13 Springer-Verlag, Berlin

Jung R (1978) Einführung in die Physiologie des Sehens (pp 3–140). In Gauer, Kramer & Jung (Eds), Physiologie des Menschen. Vol. 13. Das Sehen. Urban & Schwartzenberg, München

Kaas J, Harting J & Guillery R (1974) Representation of the complete retina in the contralateral superior colliculus of some mammals. Brain Res 65 343–346

Kabrisky M, Tallman O, Day C & Radoy C (1970) A theory of pattern perception based on human physiology. Ergonomics 13 129–142

Kanaseki T & Sprague J (1974) Anatomical organisation of pretectal nuclei and tectal laminae in the cat. J Comp Neurol 158 319–337

Kaneko A (1983) Retinal bipolar cells: their function and morphology. Trends Neurosci 6 219–223

Kaneko A & Tachibana M (1981) Retinal bipolar cells with double colour-opponent receptive fields. Nature 293 220–222

Kaneko A, Yang X & Tauchi M (1982) Interaction between red-sensitive and green-sensitive cones in the goldfish retina: an observation made in L-type external horizontal cells (pp 15–20). In Kaneko et al (Eds), Neurotransmitters in the Retina. Tokyo.

Kaplan E & Shapley R (1982) X and Y cells in the lateral geniculate nucleus of macaque monkeys. J Physiol 330 125–143

Kappers C, Huber C & Crosby E (1960) The Comparative Anatomy of the Nervous System of Vertebrates Including Man. Hafner, New York

Kaupp U (1991) The cyclic nucleotide-gated channels of vertebrate photoreceptors and olfactory epithelium. Trends Neurosci 14 150–157

Kawamura S & Bownds D (1981) Light adaptation of the cyclic GMP phosphodiesterase of frog photoreceptor membranes mediated by ATP and calcium ions. J Gen Physiol 77 571–591

Keating E & Dineen J (1982) Visuomotor transformations of the primate tectum (pp 335–365). In Ingle D, Goodale M & Mansfield R (Eds), Analysis of Visual Behavior. MIT Press, Cambridge, Massachusetts

Kelly D (1961) Visual responses to time-dependent stimuli. I. Amplitude sensitivity measurements. J Opt Soc Am 51 422–429

Kelly J & Gilbert C (1975) The projections of different morphological types of ganglion cells in the cat retina. J Comp Neurol 163 65–80

Kennedy H & Bullier J (1985) A double investigation of the afferent connectivity to cortical areas V1 and V2 of the macaque monkey. J Neurosci 5 2815–2830

Kilbride P & Ebrey T (1979) Light initiated changes of cyclic guanosine monophosphate levels in the frog retina measured with quick-freezing techniques. J Gen Physiol 74 415–426

Kingston W, Vadas M & Bishop P (1969) Multiple projection of the visual field to the medial portion of the dorsal lateral geniculate nucleus and the adjacent nuclei of the thalamus of the cat. J Comp Neurol 136 295–315

Kline R, Ripps H & Dowling J (1978) Generation of b-wave currents in the skate retina. Proc Natl Acad Sci USA 75 5727–5731

Klüver H (1941) Visual functions after the removal of the occipital lobes in monkeys. J Physiol 11 23–45

Kolb H (1958) Organisation of the outer plexiform layer of the primate retina: electron microscopy of Golgi impregnated cells. Philos Trans R Soc [B] 258 261–283

Kolb H (1970) The inner plexiform layer in the retina of the cat: electron microscope observations. J Neurocytol 8 295–329

Kolb H & West R (1977) Synaptic connections of the interplexiform layer cells in the retina of the cat. J Neurocytol 6 155–170

Kolb H, Nelson R & Mariani A (1981) Amacrine cells, bipolar cells and ganglion cells of the cat retina: a Golgi study. Vision Res 21 1081–1114

Korte A (1915) Kinematosckopische Untersuchungen. Z Psychol 72 193–296

Kropf A (1972) The structure and reactions of visual pigments (pp 239–278). In Fuortes (Ed), Handbook of Sensory Physiology VII Vol 2 Physiology of Photoreceptor Organs. Springer-Verlag, Berlin

Kuffler S (1953) Discharge patterns and functional organisation of mammalian retina. J Neurophysiol 16 37–68

Kuffler S & Nicholls J (1966) The physiology of neuroglial cells. Ergebnisse der Physiologie 57 1–90

Kulikowski J & Tolhurst D (1973) Psychophysical evidence for sustained and transient detectors in human vision. J Physiol 232 149–162

Lamb T (1976) Spatial properties of horizontal cell responses in the turtle retina. J Physiol 263 239–255

Lamb T (1986) Transduction in vertebrate photoreceptors: the roles of cyclic GMP and calcium. Trends Neurosci 9 224–228

Lamb T & Simon E (1976) Analysis of electrical noise in turtle cones. J Physiol 273 435–468

Lamb T & Simon E (1977) The relation between intercellular coupling and electrical noise in turtle photoreceptors. J Physiol 263 257–286

Lamb T, McNaughton P & Yau K (1981) Spatial spread of activation and background desensitization in toad rod outer segments. J Physiol 319 463–496

Lamb T, Matthews H & Torre V (1986) Incorporation of calcium buffers into salamander retinal rods: a rejection of the calcium hypothesis of phototransduction. J Physiol 372 315–349

Land E (1974) The retinex theory of colour vision. Proc R Inst Great Britain 47 23–58

Land E (1983) Recent advances in retinex theory and some implications for cortical computations: color vision and the natural image. Proc Natl Acad Sci USA 80 5163–5169

Lane R, Kaas J & Allman J (1974) Visuotopic organisation of the superior colliculus in normal and siamese cats. Brain Res 70 413–430

Legge G (1978) Sustained and transient mechanisms in human vision: temporal and spatial properties. Vision Res 18 69–81

Le Grand Y (1964) Optique Physiologique. Editions de la Review d'Optique, Paris.

Lehmkühle S, Kratz K, Mangel S & Sherman M (1980) Spatial and temporal sensitivity of X and Y-cells in dorsal lateral geniculate nucleus of the cat. J Neurophysiol 43 520–541

Leibowitz H (1955) The relation between the rate threshold for the perception of movement and luminance for various durations of exposure. J Exp Psychol *49* 209–214

Lesèvre N & Joseph J (1979) Codification of the pattern-evoked potential (PEP) in relation to the stimulated part of the visual field. Electroencephalog Clin Neurophysiol *47* 183–203

LeVay S & Gilbert C (1976) Laminar patterns of geniculocortical projection in the cat. Brain Res *113* 1–19

LeVay S, Hubel D & Wiesel T (1975) The pattern of ocular dominance columns in macaque visual cortex revealed by reduced silver stain. J Comp Neurol *159* 559–576

LeVay S, Stryker M & Schatz C (1978) Ocular dominance columns and their development in layer IV of the cat's visual cortex: a quantitative study. J Comp Neurol *179* 223–244

Leventhal A (1979) Evidence that the different classes of relay cells of the cat's lateral geniculate nucleus terminate in different layers of the striate cortex. Exp Brain Res *37* 349–372

Leventhal A, Rodieck R & Dreher B (1981) Retinal ganglion cell classes in the old world monkey: morphology and central projections. Science *213* 1139–1142

Levick W (1972) Receptive fields of retinal ganglion cells (pp 535–566). In Fuortes M (Ed), Handbook of Sensory Physiology VII Vol 2 Physiology of Photoreceptor Organs. Springer-Verlag, Berlin

Levick W & Thibos L (1980) Orientational bias of cat retinal ganglion cells. Nature *286* 389–390

Levick W, Thibos L, Cohn T, Catanzaro D & Barlow H (1983) Performance of cat retinal ganglion cells at low light levels. J Gen Physiol *82* 405–426

Lin C, Wagor E & Kaas J (1974) Projections from the pulvinar to the middle temporal visual area (MT) in the owl monkey. Brain Res *76* 145–149

Linsenmeir R & Steinberg R (1984) Delayed basal hyperpolarisation of cat retinal pigment epithelium and its relationship to the fast oscillation of the DC electroretinogram. J Gen Physiol *83* 213–232

Livingstone M & Hubel D (1982) Thalamic inputs to cytochrome oxidase rich regions in monkey visual cortex. Proc Natl Acad Sci USA *79* 6098–6101

Livingstone M & Hubel D (1984a) Anatomy and physiology of color system in the primate visual cortex. J Neurosci *4* 309–356

Livingstone M & Hubel D (1984b) Specificity of intrinsic connections in primate primary visual cortex. Journal of Neuroscience *4* 2830–2835

Lochrie M, Hurley J & Simon M (1985) Sequence of the alpha subunit of photoreceptor G protein: homologies between tranducin, *ras* and elongation factor. Science *228* 96–99

Lund J (1981) Intrinsic organisation of the primate visual cortex, area 17, as seen in Golgi preparations (pp 325–345). In Schmitt F, Worden F, Adelman G & Gennis S (Eds), The Organization of the Cerebral Cortex. MIT Press, Cambridge, Massachusetts

Lund R, Lund J & Wise R (1974) The organisation of the retinal projection to the lateral geniculate nucleus in pigmented and albino rats. J Comp Neurol *158* 383–403

Lund J, Henry G, Macqueen C & Harvey A (1979) Anatomical organisation of the primary visual cortex (area 17) of the cat. A comparison with area 17 of the macaque monkey. J Comp Neurol *184* 599–618

MacLeish P, Schwartz E & Tachibana M (1984) Control of the generator current in solitary rods of the *amblistoma tigrinum* retina. J Physiol *348* 645–664

MacNichol E (1964) Three pigment color vision. Sci Am *211* 48–56

Maffei L (1978) Spatial frequency channels: neural mechanisms (pp 39–66). In Held, Leibovitz & Teuber (Eds), Handbook of Sensory Physiology. VIII Perception. Springer-Verlag, Berlin

Maffei L & Fiorentini (1973) The visual cortex as a spatial frequency analyser. Vision Res *36* 1255–1267

Maffei L & Fiorentini A (1976) Monocular deprivation in kittens impairs the spatial resolution of geniculate neurons. Nature *264* 754–755

Maffei L & Fiorentini A (1977) Spatial frequency rows in striate visual cortex. Vision Res *17* 257–264

Malpeli J & Baker F (1975) The representation of the visual field in the lateral geniculate nucleus of *macaca mulatta*. J Comp Neurol *161* 569–594

Mandelbaum J & Sloan L (1947) Peripheral visual acuity. Am J Ophthalmol *30* 581–588

Marg (1973) Neurophysiology of the accessory optical system (pp 103–111). In Jung R (Ed) Handbook of Sensory Physiology VII Vol 3 Central Visual Information. Springer-Verlag, Berlin

Marks W (1965) Visual pigments of single goldfish cones. J Physiol *178* 14–32

Marks W, Dobelle W & MacNichol E (1964) Visual pigments of single primate cones. Science *143* 1181–1183

Marr D & Hildreth E (1980) Theory of edge detection. Proc R Soc [B] *207* 187–217

Marr D & Poggio T (1976) Cooperative computation of stereo disparity. Science *194* 283–287

Marr D & Ullman S (1981) Directional sensitivity and its use in early visual processing. Proc R Soc [B] *211* 151–180

Marriott F (1959) Color naming experiments and the two quanta theory. J Opt Soc Am *49* 1022

Marriott F (1962) Colour Vision (Chs 12–16). In Davson H (Ed), The Eye. Vol II, The Visual Process, Academic Press, New York

Marrocco R (1976) Sustained and transient cells in monkey lateral geniculate nucleus: conduction velocities and response properties. J Neurophysiol *39* 340–353

Marrocco R (1982) Spatial summation and conduction latency classification of cells of the lateral geniculate nucleus of macaque. J Neurosci *2* 1275–1291

Martinoya C, Rey J & Bloch S (1981) Limits of the pigeon's binocular field and direction for best binocular viewing. Vision Res *21* 1197–1200

Masland R & Mills J (1979) Autoradiographic identification of acetylcholine in the rabbit retina. J Cell Biol *83* 159–178

Mason R (1975) Cell properties in the intermediate interlaminar nucleus of the cat's lateral geniculate complex in relation to the transient/sustained classification. Exp Brain Res *22* 327–329

Matsuura T (1984) Effects of barium on separately recorded fast and slow P III responses in bull-frog retina. Experientia *40* 811–819

Matsuura T, Miller W & Tomita T (1978) Cone-specific T wave in the turtle retina. Vision Res *18* 767–775

Matthews G (1983) Physiological characteristics of single green rod photoreceptors from toad retina. J Physiol *342* 347–359

Matthews G (1984) Dark noise in the outer segment membrane current of green rod photoreceptors in the toad retina. J Physiol *349* 607–618

Maturana H & Frenk S (1965) Synaptic connections of the centrifugal fibres in the pigeon retina. Science *150* 359–361

Maunsell J & Van Essen D (1983a) Functional properties of neurons in middle temporal visual area of the macaque monkey I. Selectivity for stimulus direction, speed and orientation. J Neurophysiol *49* 1127–1147

Maunsell J & Van Essen D (1983b) Functional properties of neurons in middle temporal visual area of the macaque monkey II. Binocular interactions and sensitivity to binocular disparity. J Neurophysiol *49* 1148–1167

Mayhew J & Longuet-Higgins C (1982) A computational model of binocular depth perception. Nature *297* 376–378

McAdam D (1942) Visual sensitivities to color differences in daylight. J Opt Soc Am *32* 247–274

McGuire B, Stevens J & Sterling P (1984) Microcircuitry of bipolar cells in the cat's retina. J Neurosci *4* 2920–2938

McIlwain J (1975) Visual receptive fields and their images in superior colliculus of the cat. J Neurophysiol *38* 219–230

McIlwain J (1976) Large receptive fields and spatial transformation in the visual system (pp 223–48). In Porter R (Ed), International Review of Physiology. Neurophysiology. Vol *10*. University Park Press, Baltimore

McIlwain J (1977) Topographic organisation and convergence in cortico-tectal projections from areas 17, 18 and 19 in the cat. J Neurophysiol *40* 189–198

McIlwain J & Buser P (1968) Receptive fields of single cells in the cat's superior colliculus. Exp Brain Res *5* 314–325

Meyer D (1977) The avian eye and its adaptations (pp 549–612). In Crescitelli F (Ed), Handbook of Sensory Physiology VII Vol V. The Visual System in Vertebrates. Springer-Verlag, Berlin

Meyer G & Albus K (1981) Topography and cortical projections of morphologically identified neurons in the visual thalamus of the cat. J Comp Neurol *201* 353–374

Michael C (1968a) Receptive fields of single optic nerve fibres in a mammal with an all-cone retina. I. Contrast sensitive units. J Neurophysiol *31* 249–256

Michael C (1968b) Receptive fields of single optic nerve fibres in a mammal with an all-cone retina. II. Directional sensitive units. J Neurophysiol *31* 257–267

Michael C (1968c) Receptive fields of single optic nerve fibres in an all-cone retina. J Neurophysiol *31* 268–282

Michael C (1973) Opponent color and opponent contrast cells in lateral geniculate nucleus of the ground squirrel. J Neurophysiol *36* 536–550

Michael C (1978a) Color vision mechanisms in monkey striate cortex: dual opponent cells with concentric receptive fields. J Neurophysiol *41* 572–588

Michael C (1978b) Color vision mechanisms in monkey striate cortex: simple cells with dual opponent color receptive fields. J Neurophysiol *41* 1233–1249

Michael C (1979a) Color-sensitive complex cells in monkey striate cortex. J Neurophysiol *41* 1250–1266

Michael C (1979b) Color sensitive hypercomplex cells in monkey striate cortex. J Neurophysiol *42* 7244

Michael C (1981) Columnar organisation of color cells in monkey's striate cortex. J Neurophysiol *46* 587–604

Mikami A, Newsome W & Wurtz R (1986a) Motion selectivity in macaque visual cortex. I. Mechanisms of direction and speed selectivity in extrastriate area MT. J Neurophysiol *55* 1308–1327

Mikami A, Newsome W & Wurtz R (1986b) Motion selectivity in macaque visual cortex. II. Spatiotemporal range of directional interactions in MT and V1. J Neurophysiol 55 1328–1339

Miller A & Schwartz E (1983) Evidence for the identification of synaptic transmitters released by photoreceptors of the toad retina. J Physiol 334 325–349

Miller R & Dacheux R (1976a) Synaptic organisation and ionic basis of on and off channels in mudpuppy retina. I. Intracellular analysis of chloride sensitive electrogenic properties of receptors, horizontal cells, bipolar cells and amacrine cells. J Gen Physiol 67 639–659

Miller R & Dacheux R (1976b) Synaptic organisation and ionic basis of on and off channels in mudpuppy. II. Chloride dependent ganglion cell mechanisms. J Gen Physiol 67 661–678

Miller R & Dacheux R (1976c) Synaptic organisation and ionic basis of on and off channels in mudpuppy retina. III. A model of ganglion cell receptive field organisation based on chloride-free experiments. J Gen Physiol 67 679–690

Miller R & Dowling J (1970) Intracellular responses of the Müller (glial) cells of the mudpuppy retina: their relation to the b-wave of the electroretinogram. J Neurophysiol 33 323–341

Miller R & Slaughter M (1986) Excitatory amio acid receptors of the retina: diversity of subtypes and conductance mechanisms. Trends Neurosci 9 211–218

Miller R, Frumkes T, Slaughter M & Dacheux R (1981a) Physiological and pharmacological basis of GABA and glycine action on neurons of mudpuppy retina. I. receptors, horizontal cells, bipolar and G-cells. J Neurophysiol 45 743–763

Miller R, Frumkes T, Slaughter M & Dacheux R (1981b) Physiological and pharmacological basis of GABA and glycine action on neurons of mudpuppy retina. II. Amacrine and ganglion cells. J Neurophysiol 45 764–782

Miller W (1982) Physiological evidence that light mediated decrease in cyclic GMP is an intermediary process in retinal rod transduction. J Gen Physiol 80 103–123

Mohler C & Wurtz R (1976) Organisation of monkey superior colliculus: intermediate layer cells discharging before eye movements. J Neurophysiol 39 722–744

Mollon J (1982) Color vision. Annu Rev Psychol 33 42–85

Mollon J (1982) Colour vision and colour blindness (pp 165–191). In Barlow H & Mollon J (Eds), The Senses. Cambridge University Press, Cambridge

Mollon J & Polden P (1977) An anomaly in the response of the eye to short wavelengths. Philos Trans R Soc London [B] 278 207–240

Montero V (1980) Patterns of connections from the striate cortex to cortical visual areas in superior temporal sulcus of macaque and middle temporal gyrus of owl monkey. J Comp Neurol 189 45–59

Montero V & Scott G (1981) Synaptic terminals in the dorsal lateral geniculate nucleus from neurons in the thalamic reticular nucleus: a light and electron microscope autoradiographic study. Neuroscience 6 2561–2577

Montero V, Brugge J & Beitel R (1968) Relation of the visual field to the lateral geniculate body of the albino rat. J Neurophysiol 31 221–236

Morton R (1972) The chemistry of visual pigments (pp 33–38). In Dartnall H (Ed), Handbook of Sensory Physiology VII Vol 1 Photochemistry of Vision. Springer-Verlag, Berlin

Mucke L, Norita M, Benedek G & Creutzfeldt O (1982) Physiologic and anatomic investigation of a visual cortical area situated in the ventral bank of the anterior ectosylvian sulcus of the cat. Exp Brain Res 46 1–11

Mullikin W, Jones J & Palmer L (1984a) Receptive field properties and laminar distribution of X-like and Y-like simple cells in cat area 17. J Neurophysiol 52 350–371

Mullikin W, Jones J & Palmer L (1984b) Periodic simple cells in cat area 17. J Neurophysiol 52 372–390

Murakami M & Shimoda Y (1977) Identification of amacrine and ganglion cells in the carp retina. J Physiol 264 801–818

Nagel A (1861) Das sehen mit zwei Augen. Winter, Leipzig

Naka K & Rushton W (1966a) S potentials from colour units in the retina of fish (*Cyprinidae*). J Physiol 185 536–555

Naka K & Rushton W (1966b) An attempt to analyse colour perception by electrophysiology. J Physiol 185 555–586

Nathans J, Thomas D & Hogness D (1986a) Molecular genetics of human color vision: the genes encoding blue, green and red pigments. Science 232 193–202

Nathans J, Piantanida T, Eddy R, Shows T & Hogness D (1986b) Molecular genetics of inherited variation in human color vision. Science 232 203–210

Nelson R & Kolb H (1983) Synaptic patterns and response properties of bipolar and ganglion cells in the cat retina. Vision Res 23 1183–1195

Nelson J, Kato H & Bishop P (1977) Discrimination of orientation and position disparities by binocularly activated neurons in cat striate cortex. J Neurophysiol 40 260–283

Nelson R, Famiglietti E & Kolb H (1978) Intracellular staining reveals different levels of stratification for on- and off-center ganglion cells in cat retina. J Neurophysiol 41 472–483

Neuhaus W (1930) Experimentelle Untersuchung der Scheinbewegung. Arch ges Physiol 75 315–458

Newmann E (1980) Current source density analysis of the b-wave of the frog retina. J Neurophysiol 43 1355–1366

Newmann E & Odette L (1984) Model of electroretinogram b-wave generation: a test of the K+ hypothesis. J Neurophysiol 51 164–182

Newsome W, Mikami A & Wurtz R (1986) Motion selectivity in macaque visual cortex. III. Psychophysics and physiology of apparent motion. J Neurophysiol 55 1340–1351

Neyton H & Trautmann A (1985) Single channel currents of an intercellular junction. Nature 317 331–335

Nicol G & Miller W (1981) Cyclic GMP injected into retinal rod outer segments increases latency and amplitude of response to illumination. Proc Natl Acad Sci USA 75 5217–5220

Nikara T, Bishop P & Pettigrew J (1968) Analysis of retinal correspondence by studying receptive fields of binocular single units in cat striate cortex. Exp Brain Res 6 353–372

Nishimura Y, Shimai K, Tauchi M & Kaneko A (1982) (pp 45–49). In Kaneko A et al. (Eds), Neurotransmitters in the Retina and Visual Centers. Biomedical Research Foundation, Tokyo

Niven J & Brown R (1944) Visual resolution as a function of intensity and exposure time in the human fovea. J Opt Soc Am 34 738–743

Norman R & Pearlman I (1979) Signal transmission from red cones to horizontal cells in the turtle retina. J Physiol 286 509–524

Notterman J & Page D (1957) Weber's law and the difference threshold for the velocity of a seen object. Science 126 652

Oakley B II (1979) Potassium and photoreceptor-dependent pigment epithelial hyperpolarisation. J Gen Physiol 70 405–425

Oakley B II & Green D (1976) Correlation of light induced changes in retinal extracellular potassium concentration with c-wave of the electroretinogram. J Neurophysiol 39 1117–1132

Oakley B II, Flaming D & Brown K (1979) Effect of the rod receptor potential upon retinal extracellular K concentration. J Gen Physiol 74 713–737

Ogle K (1962) The optical space sense (pp 211–432). In Davson H (Ed), The Eye. Vol 4. Academic Press, New York

Orban G & Callens M (1977) Receptive field types of area 18 neurones in the cat. Exp Brain Res 30 107–123

Orban G & Kennedy H (1981) The influence of eccentricity on receptive field types and orientation selectivity in areas 17 and 18 of the cat. Brain Res *208* 203–208

Orban G, Callens M & Colle J (1975) Unit responses to moving stimuli in area 18 of the cat. Brain Res *90* 205–219

Orban G, Kennedy H & Maes H (1981) Response to movement of neurons in areas 17 and 18 of the cat: velocity selectivity. J Neurophysiol *45* 1043–1073

Otsuka & Hassler R (1962) Ueber Aufbau und Gliederung der corticalen Sehsphäre bei der Katze. Archiv für Psychiatrie und Nervenkrankheiten *203* 212–234

Oyster C (1968) The analysis of image motion by the rabbit retina. J Physiol *199* 613–635

Palmer L, Rosenquist A & Tusa R (1978) The retinotopic organisation of the lateral suprasylvian visual areas in the cat. J Comp Neurol *177* 237–256

Pantle A (1970) Adaptation to spatial pattern frequency: effects on visual movement selectivity in humans. J Opt Soc Am *60* 1120–1124

Pantle A & Sekuler R (1969) Contrast response of human visual mechanisms sensitive to orientation and direction of motion. Vision Res *9* 397–406

Pasik T & Pasik P (1973) The visual world of monkeys deprived of striate cortex: effective stimulus parameters and the importance of the accessory optic system. Vision Res *Suppl 3* 419–435

Pasik T & Pasik P (1982) Visual functions in monkeys after total removal of visual cerebral cortex (pp 147–200). In Neff W (Ed), Contributions to Sensory Physiology *7*. Academic Press, New York

Payne B & Berman N (1983) Functional organisation of neurons in cat striate cortex: variations in preferred orientation and orientation selectivity with receptive field type, ocular dominance and location in visual field map. J Neurophysiol *49* 1051–1072

Peck C, Schlag-Rey M & Schlag J (1980) Visuo-oculomotor properties of cells in the superior colliculus of the alert cat. J Comp Neurol *194* 97–116

Perenin M & Jeannerod M (1975) Residual vision in cortically blind hemifield. Neuropsychologia *13* 1–7

Perenin M & Jeannerod M (1978a) Visual function within the hemianopic field following early cerebral hemidecortication in man. I. Spatial localisation. Neuropsychologia *16* 1–13

Perenin M & Jeannerod M (1978b) Visual function within the hemianopic field following early cerebral hemidecortication in man. II. Pattern discrimination. Neuropsychologia *16* 697–708

Perry V & Cowey A (1981) The morphological correlates of X- and Y-like characteristics. Exp Brain Res *43* 226–228

Perry V & Cowey A (1984) Retinal ganglion cells that project to the superior colliculus and pretectum in the macaque monkey. Neuroscience *12* 1125–1135

Perry V, Oehler R & Cowey A (1984) Retinal ganglion cells that project to the dorsal lateral geniculate nucleus in the macaque monkey. Neuroscience *12* 1101–1123

Peters A & Palay S (1966) The morphology of laminae A and A1 of the dorsal nucleus of the lateral geniculate body of the cat. J Anat *100* 451–486

Pettigrew J, Nikara T & Bishop P (1968a) Responses to moving slits by single units in cat striate cortex. Exp Brain Res *6* 373–390

Pettigrew J, Nikara T & Bishop P (1968b) Binocular interaction on single units in cat striate cortex: simultaneous stimulation by single moving slits with receptive field in correspondence. Exp Brain Res *6* 391–410

Piccolino M, Witkovsky P, Neyton H, Gerschenfeld H & Trimarchi C (1985) Modulation of gap junction permeability by dopamine and GABA in the network of horizontal cells of the turtle retina (pp 66–76). In Gallego A & Gouras P (Eds), Neurocircuitry of the Retina. A Cajal Memorial. Elsevier, New York.

Piccolino M, Neyton J, Witkovsky P & Gerschenfeld (1982) Gamma-aminobutyric acid antagonists decrease junctional communication between L-horizontal cells of the retina. Proc Natl Acad Sci USA *79* 3671–3675

Piéron H (1945) La Sensation: Guide de Vie. Gallimard, Paris

Pinegin N (1958) Independence of wavelength of the threshold number of quanta for peripheral rod and foveal cone vision (pp 727–729). In Visual Problems of Colour. Symposium *8*. National Physical Laboratory, London

Pirenne M & Marriott F (1962) Visual functions in man (pp 3–217). In Davson H (Ed), The Eye. Vol II. The visual process. Academic Press, New York

Pirenne M & Marriott F (1959) The quantum theory of light and the psychophysiology of vision (pp 288–361). In Psychology: A Study of Science. I. McGraw-Hill, New York

Pitt F (1935) Characteristics of dichromatic vision. Medical Research Council Special Report Series (London) *200* 1–58.

Pitt F (1944) The nature of normal trichromatic and dichromatic vision. Proc R Soc [B] *132* 101–117

Plateau M (1872) Sur la mesure des sensations physiques et sur la loi qui lie l'intensité de ces sensations à l'intensité de la cause excitante. Bull Acad Roy Belg *3* 376–388.

Poggio G (1979) Mechanisms of stereopsis in monkey visual cortex. Trends Neurosci 2 199–201

Poggio G & Fisher B (1977) Binocular interaction and depth sensitivity of striate and prestriate cortical neurons of the behaving rhesus monkey. J Neurophysiol 40 1392–1405

Poggio G & Poggio T (1984) The analysis of stereopsis. Annu Rev Neurosci 7 379–412

Poggio G & Talbot W (1981) Mechanisms of static and dynamic stereopsis in foveal cortex of rhesus monkey. J Physiol 315 469–492

Pokorny J & Smith V (1986) Colorimetry and color discrimination (pp 8–1 to 8–51). In Boff K, et al. (Eds), Handbook of Perception and Human Performance. Vol 1. Sensory Processes and Perception. Wiley, New York

Pokorny J, Smith V, Verriest G & Pinckers A (1979) Congenital and Acquired Color Vision Defects. Grune & Stratton, New York

Polans A, Hermolin J & Bownds D (1979) Light induced dephosphorylation of two proteins in frog outer segment. J Gen Physiol 74 595–613

Polyak S (1941) The Vertebrate Visual System. Chicago University Press, Chicago

Pöppel E, Held R & Frost D (1973) Residual visual functions after brain wounds involving the central visual pathways in man. Nature 243 295–296

Powell T (1976) Bilateral cortico-tectal projection from the visual cortex in the cat. Nature 260 526–527

Provis I (1979) The distribution and size of ganglion cells in the retina of the pigmented rabbit. J Comp Neurol 185 121–138

Provis J & Watson C (1981) The distribution of ipsilaterally and contralaterally projecting ganglion cells in the retina of the pigmented rabbit. Exp Brain Res 44 82–92

Raczkowski D & Rosenquist A (1983) Connections of the multiple visual cortical areas with the lateral posterior-pulvinar complex and adjacent thalamic nuclei in the cat. J Neurosci 3 1912–1942

Raisanen J & Dawis S (1983) A reweighting of receptor mechanisms in the ground squirrel retina: PIII and B-wave spectral sensitivity functions. Brain Res 270 311–318

Rapaport D & Stone J (1984) The area centralis of the retina in the cat and other mammals: focal point for function and development of the visual system. Neuroscience 11 289–301

Reese B & Jeffrey G (1983) Crossed and uncrossed visual topography in dorsal lateral geniculate nucleus of the pigmented rat. J Neurophysiol 43 877–890

Réperant J, Vesselkin N, Rio J, Ermakova T, Miceli D, Peyrichoux J & Weidner C (1981) La voie centrifuge n'existe-t-elle que chez les oiseaux? Rev Can Biol 40 29–46

Rezak M & Benevento L (1977) A redefinition of pulvinar subdivisions in the macaque monkey: evidence for three distinct subregions within classically defined lateral pulvinar. Soc Neurosci Abstr 3 574

Ribak C (1978) Aspinous and sparsely spinous stellate neurons in the visual cortex of rats contain glutamic acid decarboxylase. J Neurocytol 7 461–478

Richards W (1970) Stereopsis and stereoblindness. Exp Brain Res 10 380–388

Richards W & Kaye M (1974) Local vs global stereopsis. Vision Res 14 1345–1347

Riggs L, Armington J & Ratliff F (1954) Motions of the retinal image during fixation. J Opt Soc Am 44 315–321

Rioch D (1929) Studies on the diencephalon of carnivora. I. The nucleus configuration of the thalamus, epithalamus, and hypothalamus of the dog and cat. J Comp Neurol 49 1–119

Robinson D (1972) Eye movements evoked by collicular stimulation in the alert monkey. Vision Res 12 1795–1808

Robinson P, Kawamura S, Abramson B & Bownds D (1980) Control of the cyclic GMP phosphodiesterase of frog photoreceptor membranes. J Gen Physiol 76 631–645

Rock I (1975) An Introduction to Perception. Macmillan, New York.

Rockland K & Pandya D (1979) Laminar origins and terminations of cortical connections of the occipital lobe in the rhesus monkey. Brain Res 179 3–20

Rockland K & Pandya D (1981) Cortical connections of the occipital lobe in the rhesus monkey: interconnections between areas 17, 18, 19 and the superior temporal sulcus. Brain Res 212 249–270

Rodieck R (1972) Components of the electroretinogram: a reappraisal. Vision Res 12 773–780

Rodieck R (1973) The Vertebrate Retina: Principles of Structure and Function. Freeman, San Francisco.

Rodieck R & Stone J (1975a) Response of cat retinal ganglion cells to moving visual patterns. J Neurophysiol 38 819–833

Rodieck R & Stone J (1975b) Analysis of receptive fields of cat retinal ganglion cells. J Neurophysiol 38 833–849

Rodrigo-Angulo M & Reinoso-Suarez F (1982) Topographical organisation of the brainstem cells to the lateral posterior-pulvinar thalamic complex in the cat. Neuroscience 7 1495–1508

Rolls E & Cowey A (1970) Topography of the retina and striate cortex and its relationship to visual acuity in rhesus monkeys and squirrel monkeys. Exp Brain Res 10 298–310

Rose D (1977) Responses of single units in cat visual cortex to moving bars of light as a function of bar length. J Physiol 271 1–23

Rose D & Blakemore C (1974a) An analysis of orientation selectivity in the cat's visual cortex. Exp Brain Res 20 1–17

Rose D & Blakemore C (1974b) Effects of bicuculline on function of inhibition in visual cortex. Nature 249 375–377

Roucoux A, Guitton D & Crommelinck M (1980) Stimulation of the superior colliculus in the alert cat. II. Eye and head movements evoked when the head is unrestrained. Exp Brain Res 39 75–85

Rowe M & Dreher B (1982) Retinal W-cell projections to the medial interlaminar nucleus in the cat: implications for ganglion cell classification. J Comp Neurol 204 117–133

Rushton W (1956) The rhodopsin density in human rods. J Physiol 134 30–46

Rushton W (1961) Rhodopsin measurement and dark adaptation in a subject deficient in cone vision. J Physiol 156 193–205

Rushton W (1963) A cone pigment in the protanope. J Physiol 168 345–359

Rushton W (1965a) A foveal pigment in the deuteranope. J Physiol 176 24–37

Rushton W (1965b) Bleached rhodopsin and visual adaptation. J Physiol 181 645–655

Rushton W (1965c) Stray light and the measurement of mixed pigments in the retina. J Physiol 176 46–55

Rushton W (1972) Pigments and signals in colour vision. J Physiol 220 1–31P.

Rushton W & Campbell F (1954) Measurement of rhodopsin in the living eye. Nature 174 1096–1097

Rushton W & Westheimer G (1962) The effect upon the rod threshold of bleaching neighbouring rods. J Physiol 164 318–329

Saito H, Yukie M, Tanaka K, Hikosaka K, Fukada Y & Iwai E (1986) Integration of direction signals of image motion in the superior temporal sulcus of the macaque monkey. J Neurosci 6 145–157

Sakai H & Naka K (1982) Structural differences between dendrites of on- and off-center bipolar cells in catfish retina (pp 61–66). In Kaneko A et al. (Eds), Neurotransmitters in the Retina and the Visual Centers. Biomedical Research Foundation, Tokyo

Sanderson K (1971) The projection of the visual field to the lateral geniculate and medial intralaminar nuclei in the cat. J Comp Neurol *143* 101–118

Sanderson K (1971) Visual field projection columns and magnification factors in the lateral geniculate nucleus of the cat. Exp Brain Res *13* 159–177

Sanderson K, Bishop G & Darian-Smith I (1971) The properties of the binocular receptive fields of lateral geniculate neurons. Exp Brain Res *13* 178–207

Sanderson K & Sherman M (1971) Nasotemporal overlap in visual field projected to the lateral geniculate nucleus in the cat. J Neurophysiol *34* 453–466

Scalia F & Arango V (1979) Topographic organisation of the projections of the retina to the pretectal region in the rat. J Comp Neurol *186* 271–292

Schiller P & Malpeli J (1978) Properties of tectal projections of monkey retinal ganglion cells. J Neurophysiol *41* 428–447

Schiller P, Pasik P & Pasik T (1972) Extrageniculostriate vision in the monkey. Exp Brain Res *14* 436–448

Schiller P, Finlay B & Volman S (1976a) Quantitative studies of single-cell properties in monkey striate cortex. I. Spatiotemporal organisation of receptive fields. J Neurophysiol *39* 1288–1319

Schiller P, Finlay B & Volman S (1976b) Quantitative studies of single cell properties in monkey striate cortex. II. Orientation specificity and ocular dominance. J Neurophysiol *39* 1320–1333

Schiller P, Finlay B & Volman S (1976c) Quantitative studies of single cell properties in monkey striate cortex. III. Spatial frequency. J Neurophysiol *39* 1334–1351

Schnapf J (1983) Dependence of the single photon response on longitudinal position of absorption in toad rod outer segments. J Physiol *343* 147–159

Schneider G (1967) Contrasting visuomotor functions of tectum and cortex in the golden hamster. Psychologische Forschungen *31* 52–62

Schneider G (1969) Two visual systems: brain mechanisms for localisation and discrimination are dissociated by tectal and cortical lesions. Science *163* 895–902

Schwartz E (1977) Voltage noise observed in rods of the turtle retina. J Physiol *272* 217–246

Schwartz E (1975) Rod-rod interaction in the retina of the turtle. J Physiol *246* 617–663

Sekuler R, Pantle A & Levinson L (1978) Physiological basis of motion perception (pp 67–110). In Teuber H (Ed), Handbook of Sensory Physiology VIII. Perception. Springer-Verlag, Berlin

Seltzer B & Pandya D (1978) Afferent cortical connections and architectonics of the superior temporal sulcus and surrounding cortex in the rhesus monkey. Brain Res *149* 1–24

Shapley R & Lennie P (1985) Spatial frequency analysis in the visual system. Annu Rev Neurosci *8* 577–583

Shapley R & Perry V (1986) Cat and monkey retinal ganglion cells and their visual functional roles. Trends Neurosci *9* 229–235

Shapley R, Kaplan E & Soodak R (1981) Spatial summation and contrast sensitivity of the X and Y cells in the lateral geniculate nucleus of the macaque monkey. Nature *202* 543–545

Sherman S (1985) Functional organisation of the W-, X-, and Y-pathways in the cat: a review and hypothesis (pp 233–314). In Sherman S, Sprague J & Epstein A (Eds), Progress in Psychobiology and Physiological Psychology. Academic Press, New York

Sherman S (1979) The functional significance of X and Y cells in normal and visually deprived cats. Trends Neurosci *2* 192–196

Sherman S, Watkins D & Wilson J (1976a) Further differences in receptive field properties of simple and complex cells in cat striate cortex. Vision Res *16* 919–927

Sherman S, Wilson J, Kaas J & Webb S (1976b) X and Y cells in the dorsal lateral geniculate nucleus of the owl monkey. Science *192* 475–477

Shlaer S (1937) The relation between visual acuity and illumination. J Gen Physiol *21* 165–168

Shlaer S, Smith E & Chase A (1942) Visual acuity and illumination in different spectral regions. J Gen Physiol *25* 553–569

Sillito A (1975a) The effectiveness of bicuculline as an antagonist of GABA and visually evoked inhibition in the cat's striate cortex. J Physiol *250* 287–304

Sillito A (1975b) The contribution of inhibitory mechanisms to the receptive field properties of neurones in the striate cortex of the cat. J Physiol *250* 305–329

Sillito A (1977) Inhibitory processes underlying the directional specificity of simple, complex and hypercomplex cells in the cat's visual cortex. J Physiol *271* 699–720

Sillito A, Kemp J, Milson J & Bernardi N (1980) A re-evaluation of the mechanism underlying simple cell orientation selectivity. Brain Res *194* 517–520

Simon E, Lamb T & Hodgkin A (1975) Spontaneous voltage fluctuations in retinal cones and bipolar cells. Nature *256* 661–662

Simpson J (1984) The accessory optic system. Annu Rev Neurosci *7* 13–41

Simpson J, Soodak R & Hess R (1979) The accessory optic system and its relation to the vestibulocerebellum. Prog Brain Res *50* 715–724

Singer W (1977) Control of thalamic transmission by corticofugal and ascending reticular pathways in the visual system. Physiol Rev 57 386–425

Singer W (1981) Topographic organisation of orientation columns in the cat visual cortex. A deoxyglucose study. Exp Brain Res 44 431–436

Singer W & Bedworth N (1973) Inhibitory interaction between X and Y units in the cat's lateral geniculate nucleus. Brain Res 49 291–307

Singer W & Creutzfeldt O (1970) Reciprocal lateral inhibition of on- and off-center neurones in the lateral geniculate body. Exp Brain Res 10 311–330

Singer W, Tretter F & Cynader M (1975) Organisation of cat striate cortex: a correlation of receptive field properties with afferent and efferent connections. J Neurophysiol 38 1080–1098

Sparks D & Mays L (1980) Movement fields of saccade-related burst neurons in the monkey superior colliculus. Brain Res 190 39–50

Sparks D & Mays L (1986) Translation of sensory signals into commands for control of saccadic eye movements: role of the superior colliculus. Annu Rev Neurosci 9 118–171

Sprague J, Berlucchi G & Rizzolatti G (1973) The role of the superior colliculus and pretectum in vision and visually guided behaviour (pp 27–101). In Jung R (Ed), Handbook of Sensory Physiology VII Vol 3 Central Visual Information. Springer-Verlag, Berlin

Standage G & Benevento L (1983) The organisation of connections between the pulvinar and visual area MT in the macaque. Brain Res 262 288–294

Stein B (1988) Superior colliculus-mediated visual behaviors in cat and the concept of two corticotectal systems (pp 37–53). In Hicks T & Benedek G (Eds), Vision within Extrageniculo-Striate Systems (Progress in Brain Research Series Vol 75). Elsevier, New York

Stein A, Mullkin W & Stevens J (1983) The spatiotemporal building blocks of X-, Y- and W-ganglion cell receptive fields of the cat's retina. Exp Brain Res 49 341–352

Stein B, Magalhaes-Castro B & Kruger L (1976) Relationship between visual and tactile representation in cat superior colliculus. J Neurophysiol 39 401–419

Steinberg R, Reid M & Lacy P (1973) The distributon of rods and cones in the retina of the cat (Felis domesticus). J Comp Neurol 148 229–248

Steinberg R, Fisher S & Anderson D (1980) Disc morphogenesis in vertebrate photoreceptors. J Comp Neurol 190 501–518

Steinberg R, Linsenmeier R & Griff E (1983) Three light-evoked responses of the retinal pigment epithelium. Vision Res 23 1315–1323

Stell W (1972) The morphological organisation of the retina (pp 111–213). In Fuortes (Ed), Handbook of Sensory Physiology VII Vol 2 Physiology of Photoreceptor Organs. Springer-Verlag, Berlin

Sterling P, Freed M & Smith R (1986) Microcircuitry and functional architecture of the cat retina. Trends Neurosci 9 186–192

Stevens J & Gerstein G (1976) Spatiotemporal organisation of cat lateral geniculate receptive fields. J Neurophysiol 39 213–238

Stevens J & Gerstein G (1976) Interactions between cat lateral geniculate neurons. J Neurophysiol 39 236–256

Stewart D, Chow K & Masland R (1971) Receptive field characteristics of lateral geniculate neurons in the rabbit. J Neurophysiol 34 139–147

Stiles W (1939) The directional selectivity of the retina and the spectral selectivity of the rods and cones. Proc R Soc [B] 127 64–105

Stiles W & Crawford B (1933) The luminous efficiency of rays entering the pupil at different points. Proc Roy Soc [B] 112 428–450

Stiles W & Crawford B (1934) The liminal brightness increment for white light for different conditions of the foveal and parafoveal retina. Proc R Soc [B] 116 55–102

Stiles W & Crawford B (1937) The effect of a glaring light source on extra-foveal vision. Proc R Soc [B] 122 255–280

Stone J (1966) The naso-temporal division of the cat's retina. J Comp Neurol 126 585–600

Stone J (1978) The number and distribution of ganglion cells in the cat retina. J Comp Neurol 180 753

Stone J & Campion C (1978) Estimates of the number of myelinated axons in the cat's optic nerve. J Comp Neurol 180 799–806

Stone J & Dreher B (1973) Projection of X- and Y-cells of the cats lateral geniculate nucleus to areas 17 and 18 of visual cortex. J Neurophysiol 36 551–567

Stone J & Fukada Y (1974) The nasotemporal division of the cat's retina reexamined in terms of W-, X-, and Y-cells. J Comp Neurol 155 377–394

Stone J, Leicester J & Sherman S (1973) The naso-temporal division of the monkey's retina. J Comp Neurol 150 333–348

Stone J, Dreher B & Leventhal A (1979) Hierarchical and parallel mechanisms in the organisation of the visual cortex. Brain Res Rev 1 345–394

Straschill M & Taghavy A (1967) Neuronale Reactionen im Tectum opticum der Katze auf bewegte und stationäre Lichtreize. Exp Brain Res 3 353–367

Stryer L (1986) Cyclic GMP cascade in vision. Annu Rev Neurosci 9 87–119

Stryer L, Hurley J & Fung B (1981) Transducin: an amplifier protein in vision. Trends Biochem Sci 6 245–247

Stryker M & Schiller P (1975) Eye and head movements evoked by electrical stimulation of monkey superior colliculus. Exp Brain Res 23 103–112

Susuki H & Takahashi M (1970) Organisation of the lateral geniculate neurons in binocular inhibition. Brain Res 23 261–264

Szentagothai J (1973) Neuronal and synaptic architecture of the lateral geniculate nucleus (pp 141–176). In Jung (Ed), Handbook of Sensory Physiology, VII Vol 3 Central Visual Information. Springer-Verlag, Berlin

Szentagothai J (1973) Synaptology of the visual cortex (pp 269–324). In Jung R (Ed), Handbook of Sensory Physiology VII Vol 3 Central Visual Information. Springer-Verlag, Berlin

Tiao Y & Blakemore C (1976) Functional organisation in the visual cortex of the golden hamster. J Comp Neurol 168 439–482

Tolhurst D (1973) Separate channels for the analysis of the shape and the movements of a moving visual stimulus. J Physiol 231 385–402

Tomita T (1963) Electrical activity in the vertebrate retina. J Opt Soc Am 53 49–57

Tomita T (1972) Light induced potential and resistance changes in vertebrate photoreceptors (pp 483–511). In Fuortes M (Ed), Handbook of Sensory Physiology VII Vol 2 Physiology of Photoreceptor Organs. Springer-Verlag, Berlin

Tomita T, Murakami M & Pautler E (1967) Spectral response curves of single cones in the carp. Vision Res 7 519–531

Tretter F, Cynader M & Singer W (1975) Cat parastriate cortex: a primary or secondary visual area. J Neurophysiol 38 1099–1113

Tsumoto T, Eckart W & Creutzfeldt O (1982) A role of Gabaergic inhibition in feature detecting properties of neurons in the cat visual cortex (pp 95–100). In Kaneko et al. (Eds), Neurotransmitters in the Retina and the Visual Centers. Tokyo.

Tusa R & Palmer J (1980) Retinotopic organisation of areas 20 and 21 in the cat. J Comp Neurol 193 147–164

Tusa R, Palmer L & Rosenquist A (1978) The retinotopic organisation of area 17 (striate cortex) in the cat. J Comp Neurol 177 213–236

Tusa R, Rosenquist A & Palmer L (1979) Retinotopic organisation of areas 18 and 19 in the cat. J Comp Neurol 185 657–678

Ungerleider L & Mishkin M (1983) Two cortical visual systems (pp 307–586). In Ingle, Goodale & Mansfield (Eds), Analysis of Visual Behaviour. J Comp Neurol vol 217.

Ungerleider L, Glakin T & Mishkin M (1983) Visuotopic organisation of projections from striate cortex to inferior and lateral pulvinar in rhesus monkey. J Comp Neurol 39 239–256

Updyke B (1976) Retinotopic organisation of the pulvinar and lateral posterior nucleus of the cat. Anat Rec 184 552

Updyke B (1981a) Projections from visual areas of the middle suprasylvian sulcus onto the lateral posterior complex and adjacent thalamic nuclei in the cat. J Comp Neurol 201 477–506

Updyke B (1981b) Multiple representations of the visual field: corticothalamic and thalamic organisation in the cat (pp 83–101). In Woolsey C (Ed), Cortical Sensory Organisation. Vol 2. Multiple Visual Areas. Humana Press, Clifton, NJ

Updyke V (1983) A re-evaluation of the functional organisation and cytoarchitecture of the feline lateral posterior complex, with observations on adjoining cell groups. J Comp Neurol 219 143–181

Vakkur G & Bishop P (1963) The schematic eye in the cat. Vision Res 3 357–381

Van Essen D (1985) Functional organisation of primate visual cortex (pp 259–329). In Peters & Jones (Eds), Cerebral Cortex. Vol 3. Plenum, New York

Van Essen D & Zeki S (1978) The topographic organisation of rhesus monkey prestriate cortex. J Physiol 277 193–226

Van Essen D, Maunsell J & Bixby J (1981) The middle temporal visual area in the macaque: myeloarchitecture, connections, functional properties and topographic organisation. J Comp Neurol 199 293–326

Van Nes F & Bouman M (1967) Spatial modulation transfer in the human eye. J Opt Soc Am 57 401–406

Wagor E, Lin C & Kaas J (1975) Some cortical projections of the dorsomedial visual area (DM) of association cortex in the owl monkey Aotus trivirgatus. J Comp Neurol 163 227–250

Wagor E, Mangini N & Pearlman A (1980) Retinotopic organisation of striate and extrastriate visual cortex in the mouse. J Comp Neurol 193 187–202

Wald G & Brown P (1965) Human color vision and color blindness. Cold Spring Harbor Symposium in Quantitative Biology 30 345–361

Wald G, Brown P & Smith P (1955) Iodopsin. J Gen Physiol 38 703–713.

Waloga G & Park W (1978) Ionic mechanism for the generation of horizontal cell potentials in isolated axolotl retina. J Gen Physiol 71 69–92

Walraven P (1961) On the Bezold-Brücke phenomenon. J Opt Soc Am 51 1113–1116

Wässle H, Peichl L & Boycott B (1983) Mosaic and territories of cat retinal ganglion cells. (pp 183–190). In Changeux P, et al (Eds), Progress in Brain Research. *Vol 58*. Elsevier, Holland.

Wässle H, Levick W & Cleland B (1975) The distribution of the alpha type of ganglion cells in the cat's retina. J Comp Neurol *159* 419–438

Watanabe A, Mori T, Nagata S & Hiwatashi K (1968) Spatial sinewave response of the human visual system. Vision Res *8* 1245–1263

Weale R (1959) Photosensitive reactions in foveae of normal and cone monochromatic onservers. Optica Acta *6* 158–174

Weidner C (1976) The c-wave in the ERG of albino rat. Vision Res *16* 753–763

Weiskrantz L (1972) Behavioural analysis of the monkey's visual nervous system. Proc R Soc [B] *182* 427–455

Weiskrantz L & Cowey A (1967) A comparison of the effects of striate cortex and retinal lesions on visual acuity in the monkey. Science *155* 104–106

Weiskrantz L, Warrington E, Sanders M & Marshall J (1974) Visual capacity of the hemianopic field following a restricted cortical ablation. Brain *97* 709–728

Weiskrantz L, Cowey A & Passingham C (1977) Spatial responses to brief stimuli by monkeys with striate cortex ablations. Brain *100* 655–670

Weller R & Kaas J (1983) Retinotopic patterns of connections of area 17 with visual areas V-II and MT in macaque monkeys. J Comp Neurol *220* 253–279

Werblin F (1977) Regenerative amacine cell depolarisation and formation of on-off ganglion cell response. J Physiol *264* 767–785

Werblin F & Copenhagen D (1974) Control of retinal sensitivity. III Lateral interactions at the inner plexiform layer. J Gen Physiol *63* 472–478

Werblin F & Dowling J (1969) Organisation of the retina of the mudpuppy *Necturus maculosus*. J Neurophysiol *32* 339–355

Wertheimer M (1912) Experimentelle Studien über das Sehen von Bewegung. Z Psycholog *61* 161–265

Westheimer G (1972) Visual acuity and spatial modulation thresholds (pp 188–201). In Jung (Ed), Handbook of Sensory Physiology VII Vol 3 Central Visual Information. Springer-Verlag, Berlin

Whitteridge D (1973) Projection of Optic Pathways to the Visual Cortex (pp 247–268). In Jung (Ed), Handbook of Sensory Physiology VII Vol 3 Central Visual Information. Springer-Verlag, Berlin

Wiesel T & Gilbert C (1983) Morphological basis of visual cortical function. The Sharpey-Schafer Lecture. Q J Exp Physiol *68* 525–543

Wiesel T & Hubel D (1966) Spatial and chromatic interactions in the lateral geniculate body of the rhesus monkey. J Neurophysiol 29 1115–1156

Wiesel T, Hubel D & Lam D (1974) Autoradiographic demonstration of ocular dominance columns in the monkey striate cortex by means of transneuronal transport. Brain Res 79 273–279

Wilson J (1978) Visual system: pulvinar-extrastriate cortex (pp 209–247). In Bruce & Masterton (Eds), Handbook of Behavioral Neurobiology. Plenum Press, New York

Wilson J (1982) An electron microscopic comparison of the medial interlaminar nucleus and the A laminae in the dorsal lateral geniculate nucleus of the cat. J Comp Neurol 212 89–101

Wilson P & Stone J (1975) Evidence of W-cell input to the cat's visual cortex via the C laminae of the lateral geniculate nucleus. Brain Res 92 472–478

Witkovsky P, Dudek F & Ripps H (1975) Slow PIII component of the carp electroretinogram. J Gen Physiol 63 119–134

Woodhouse J & Barlow H (1982) Spatial and temporal resolution and analysis (pp 133–164). In Barlow H & Mollon J (Eds), The Senses. Cambridge University Press, Cambridge

Woodruff M & Fain G (1982) Ca^{2+} dependent changes in cyclic GMP levels are not correlated with opening and closing of the light-dependent permeability of toad photoreceptors. J Gen Physiol 80 537–555

Woodruff M & Bownds D (1979) Amplitude, kinetics and reversibility of a light-induced decrease in guanosine 3'5' cyclic monophosphate in frog photoreceptor membranes. J Gen Physiol 73 629–653

Woodruff M, Fain G & Bastian B (1982) Light-dependent ion influx into toad photoreceptors. J Gen Physiol 80 517—536

Woolsey C (Ed) (1981) Cortical Sensory Organization Vol 2. Multiple Visual Areas. Humana Press, Clifton, NJ

Wright W (1946) Researches on Normal and Defective Colour Vision. Kimpton, London

Wu S & Dowling J (1980) Effects of GABA and Glycine on the distal cells of the cyprinid retina. Brain Res 19 401–414

Wunk D & Werblin F (1979) Synaptic inputs to the ganglion cells in the Tiger salamander. J Gen Physiol 73 265–286

Wurtz R & Goldberg M (1972) Activity of superior colliculus in behaving monkey. III. Cells discharging before eye movements. J Neurophysiol 35 575–587

Wurtz R & Goldberg M (1972) Activity of superior colliculus in behaving monkey. IV. Effects of lesions on eye movements. J Neurophysiol 35 587–596

Wurtz R & Mohler C (1976) Organisation of monkey superior colliculus: enhanced visual response of superficial layers. J Neurophysiol *39* 745–765

Yazulla S (1974) Intraretinal differentiation in the synaptic organisation of the inner plexiform layer of the pigeon retina. J Comp Neurol *153* 309–324

Yoshikama S & Hagins W (1973) Control of the dark current in vertebrate rods and cones (pp 245–255). In Langer H (Ed), Biochemistry and Physiology of the Visual Pigments. Springer-Verlag, Berlin

Zeki S (1974) Functional organisation of a visual area in the posterior bank of the superior temporal sulcus of the rhesus monkey. J Physiol *236* 549–573

Zeki S (1978a) The cortical projections of foveal striate cortex in the rhesus monkey. J Physiol *277* 227–244

Zeki S (1978b) The third visual complex of rhesus monkey prestriate cortex. J Physiol *277* 245–272

Zeki S (1978c) Functional specialisation in the visual cortex of the rhesus monkey. Nature *274* 423–428

Zeki S (1980a) A direct projection from area VI to area V3A of rhesus monkey visual cortex. Proc R Soc [B] *207* 499–506

Zeki S (1980b) The representation of colours in the cerebral cortex. Nature *284* 412–418

Zeki S (1983) Colour coding in the cerebral cortex: the reaction of cells in monkey visual cortex to wavelengths and colours. Neuroscience *9* 741–765

Zeki S (1990) Colour vision and functional specialisation in the visual cortex. Discussion Neurosci *6* (2)

Zeki S & Shipp S (1988) The functional logic of cortical connections. Nature *335* 311–317

Zihl J (1980) Blindsight: improvement of visually guided eye movements by systematic practice in patients with cerebral blindness. Neuropsychologia *18* 71–77

Zihl J (1981) Recovery of visual functions in patients with cerebral lesions. Neuropsychologia *44* 159–169

Zihl J & von Cramon D (1982) Restitution of visual field in patients with damage to the geniculostriate visual pathway. Hum Neurobiol *1* 5–8

Zihl J, von Cramon D & Mai N (1983) Selective disturbances of movement vision after bilateral brain damage. Brain *106* 313–340

Zuidam I & Collewijn H (1979) Vergence eye movements of the rabbit in visuomotor behaviour. Vision Res *19* 185–194

Index